Imaging of the Post Treatment Head and Neck

Editors

PRASHANT RAGHAVAN
ROBERT E. MORALES
SUGOTO MUKHERJEE

NEUROIMAGING CLINICS OF NORTH AMERICA

www.neuroimaging.theclinics.com

Consulting Editor
SURESH K. MUKHERJI

February 2022 • Volume 32 • Number 1

ELSEVIER

1600 John F. Kennedy Boulevard • Suite 1800 • Philadelphia, Pennsylvania, 19103-2899

http://www.neuroimaging.theclinics.com

NEUROIMAGING CLINICS OF NORTH AMERICA Volume 32, Number 1
February 2022 ISSN 1052-5149, ISBN 13: 978-0-323-79843-3

Editor: John Vassallo (j.vassallo@elsevier.com)
Developmental Editor: Karen Solomon

Neuroimaging Clinics of North America (ISSN 1052-5149) is published quarterly by Elsevier Inc., 360 Park Avenue South, New York, NY 10010-1710. Months of issue are February, May, August, and November. Business and editorial offices: 1600 John F. Kennedy Blvd., Suite 1800, Philadelphia, PA 19103-2899. Business and editorial offices: 6277 Sea Harbor Drive, Orlando, FL 32887-4800. Periodicals postage paid at New York, NY, and additional mailing offices. Subscription prices are USD 401 per year for US individuals, USD 932 per year for US institutions, USD 100 per year for US students and residents, USD 469 per year for Canadian individuals, USD 946 per year for Canadian institutions, USD 546 per year for international individuals, USD 946 per year for international institutions, USD 100 per year for Canadian students and residents and USD 260 per year for foreign students and residents. To receive student/resident rate, orders must be accompanied by name of affiliated institution, date of term, and the *signature* of program/residency coordinator on institution letterhead. Orders will be billed at individual rate until proof of status is received. Foreign air speed delivery is included in all *Clinics* subscription prices. All prices are subject to change without notice. POSTMASTER: Send address changes to *Neuroimaging Clinics of North America*, Elsevier Health Sciences Division, Subscription **Customer Service, 3251 Riverport Lane, Maryland Heights, MO 63043. Telephone: 1-800-654-2452 (U.S. and Canada); 314-447-8871 (outside U.S. and Canada). Fax: 314-447-8029. E-mail: journalscustomerservice-usa@elsevier.com (for print support); journalsonlinesupport-usa@elsevier.com (for online support).**

Reprints. For copies of 100 or more of articles in this publication, please contact the Commercial Reprints Department, Elsevier Inc., 360 Park Avenue South, New York, NY 10010-1710. Tel.: 212-633-3874; Fax: 212-633-3820; E-mail: reprints@elsevier.com.

Neuroimaging Clinics of North America is covered by *Excerpta Medical/EMBASE,* the RSNA Index of Imaging Literature, *MEDLINE/PubMed (Index Medicus),* MEDLINE/MEDLARS, SciSearch, Research Alert, and Neuroscience Citation Index.

PROGRAM OBJECTIVE

The goal of Neuroimaging Clinics of North America is to keep practicing radiologists and radiology residents up to date with current clinical practice in radiology by providing timely articles reviewing the state of the art in patient care.

TARGET AUDIENCE

Practicing radiologists, radiology residents, and other healthcare professionals who utilize neuroimaging findings to provide patient care.

LEARNING OBJECTIVES

Upon completion of this activity, participants will be able to:

1. Review use of NI-RADS to assess residual or recurrent head and neck squamous cell carcinoma.
2. Discuss use of advanced CT, MRI, and metabolic imaging in detecting recurrent head and neck cancer.
3. Recognize the complexity and range of imaging after varying surgeries.

ACCREDITATION

The Elsevier Office of Continuing Medical Education (EOCME) is accredited by the Accreditation Council for Continuing Medical Education (ACCME) to provide continuing medical education for physicians.

The EOCME designates this journal-based CME activity for a maximum of 15 *AMA PRA Category 1 Credit*(s)™. Physicians should claim only the credit commensurate with the extent of their participation in the activity.

All other healthcare professionals requesting continuing education credit for this enduring material will be issued a certificate of participation.

DISCLOSURE OF CONFLICTS OF INTEREST

The EOCME assesses conflict of interest with its instructors, faculty, planners, and other individuals who are in a position to control the content of CME activities. All relevant conflicts of interest that are identified are thoroughly vetted by EOCME for fair balance, scientific objectivity, and patient care recommendations. EOCME is committed to providing its learners with CME activities that promote improvements or quality in healthcare and not a specific proprietary business or a commercial interest.

The planning committee, staff, authors, and editors listed below have identified no financial relationships or relationships to products or devices they or their spouse/life partner have with commercial interest related to the content of this CME activity:

Jennifer C. Alyono, MD; Yoshimi Anzai, MD, MPH; Nafi Aygun, MD; J. Rajiv Bapuraj, MD; Kristen L. Baugnon, MD; Zoe P. Berman, MD; Paraag R. Bhatt, MD; Regina Chavous-Gibson, MSN, RN; David Dreizin, MD; Nancy J. Fischbein, MD; Daniel T. Ginat, MD, MS; Michael Gunson, DDS, MD; Mari Hagiwara, MD; Jeffrey D. Hooker, MD; Jason Hostetter, MD; Mark J. Jameson, MD; David Joyner, MD; Tuba Kalelioglu, MD; Pradeep Kuttysankaran; Remy Lobo, MD; Jose Mattos, MD, PhD; Robert E. Morales, MD; Sugoto Mukherjee, MD; Rohini Narahari Nadgir, MD; Gopi K. Nayak, MD; Lakir D. Patel, MD; Sohil H. Patel, MD; Mrudula Penta, MD; Prashant Raghavan, MBBS; Kalen Riley, MD, MBA; Tanvir Rizvi, MD; Eduardo D. Rodriguez, MD, DDS; Elana B. Smith, MD; Ashok Srinivasan, MD, FACR; Dania Tamimi, BDS, DMSc; Sevcan Turk, MD; Kalpesh Vakharia, MD, MS; Matthew E. Witek, MD, MS; Jeffrey Xi Yang, MD; Sandrine Yazbek, MD

The planning committee, staff, authors and editors listed below have identified financial relationships or relationships to products or devices they or their spouse/life partner have with commercial interest related to the content of this CME activity:

Gloria J. Guzmán Pérez-Carrillo, MD, MSc, MPH: Consultant: Medtronic

Jana Ivanidze, MD, PhD: Researcher: Novartis Pharmaceuticals

UNAPPROVED/OFF-LABEL USE DISCLOSURE

The EOCME requires CME faculty to disclose to the participants:

1. When products or procedures being discussed are off-label, unlabelled, experimental, and/or investigational (not US Food and Drug Administration [FDA] approved); and
2. Any limitations on the information presented, such as data that are preliminary or that represent ongoing research, interim analyses, and/or unsupported opinions. Faculty may discuss information about pharmaceutical agents that is outside of FDA-approved labelling. This information is intended solely for CME and is not intended to promote off-label use of these medications. If you have any questions, contact the medical affairs department of the manufacturer for the most recent prescribing information.

TO ENROLL

To enroll in the *Neuroimaging Clinics of North America* Continuing Medical Education program, call customer service at 1-800-654-2452 or sign up online at http://www.theclinics.com/home/cme. The CME program is available to subscribers for an additional annual fee of USD 265.00.

METHOD OF PARTICIPATION

In order to claim credit, participants must complete the following:

1. Complete enrolment as indicated above.
2. Read the activity.
3. Complete the CME Test and Evaluation. Participants must achieve a score of 70% on the test. All CME Tests and Evaluations must be completed online.

CME INQUIRIES/SPECIAL NEEDS

For all CME inquiries or special needs, please contact elsevierCME@elsevier.com.

NEUROIMAGING CLINICS OF NORTH AMERICA

SERIES OF RELATED INTEREST

Advances in Clinical Radiology
Available at: Advancesinclinicalradiology.com
MRI Clinics of North America
Available at: MRI.theclinics.com
PET Clinics
Available at: https://www.pet.theclinics.com/
Radiologic Clinics of North America
Available at: Radiologic.theclinics.com

Contributors

CONSULTING EDITOR

SURESH K. MUKHERJI, MD, MBA, FACR
Clinical Professor, Marian University, Director
of Head and Neck Radiology, ProScan
Imaging, Regional Medical Director, Envision
Physician Services, Carmel, Indiana

EDITORS

PRASHANT RAGHAVAN, MBBS
Associate Professor, Neuroradiology,
Department of Diagnostic Radiology and
Nuclear Medicine, University of Maryland
School of Medicine, Baltimore, Maryland

ROBERT E. MORALES, MD
Assistant Professor, Neuroradiology, Director,
Diagnostic Neuroradiology Fellowship,

Department of Diagnostic Radiology and
Nuclear Medicine, University of Maryland
School of Medicine, Baltimore, Maryland

SUGOTO MUKHERJEE, MD
Professor of Neuroradiology, Department of
Radiology and Medical Imaging, University
of Virginia Health System, Charlottesville,
Virginia

AUTHORS

JENNIFER C. ALYONO, MD
Assistant Professor, Department of
Otolaryngology–Head and Neck Surgery,
Stanford University, Stanford, California

YOSHIMI ANZAI, MD, MPH
Professor, Department of Radiology and
Imaging Sciences, University of Utah School of
Medicine, Salt Lake City, Utah

NAFI AYGUN, MD
Division of Neuroradiology, Department of
Radiology and Radiological Science, Johns
Hopkins Hospital, Baltimore, Maryland

J. RAJIV BAPURAJ, MD
Professor, Neuroradiology Division, Radiology,
Michigan Medicine, Ann Arbor, Michigan

KRISTEN L. BAUGNON, MD
Associate Professor, Department of Radiology
and Imaging Sciences, Division of
Neuroradiology, Head and Neck Imaging,
Emory University, Atlanta, Georgia

ZOE P. BERMAN, MD
Hansjörg Wyss Department of Plastic
Surgery, NYU Langone Health, New York,
New York

PARAAG R. BHATT, MD
Neuroradiology Fellow, Department of
Radiology, Stanford University, Stanford,
California

DAVID DREIZIN, MD
Associate Professor, Trauma and Emergency
Radiology, Department of Diagnostic
Radiology and Nuclear Medicine, R Adams
Cowley Shock Trauma Center, University of
Maryland School of Medicine, Baltimore,
Maryland

NANCY J. FISCHBEIN, MD
Professor, Department of Radiology, and, by
courtesy, of Neurology, Neurosurgery, and
Otolaryngology–Head and Neck Surgery,
Stanford University, Stanford, California

DANIEL T. GINAT, MD, MS
Department of Radiology, Section of
Neuroradiology, University of Chicago,
Chicago, Illinois

MICHAEL GUNSON, DDS, MD
Private Practice in Oral and Maxillofacial
Surgery, Santa Barbara, California

**GLORIA J. GUZMÁN PÉREZ-CARRILLO,
MD, MSc, MPH**
Assistant Professor of Radiology,
Neuroradiology Section, Co-Director,
Advanced Neuro-Imaging Clinical Service,
Director, Office of Diversity, Equity and Justice,
Mallinckrodt Institute of Radiology,
Washington University School of Medicine, St
Louis, Missouri

MARI HAGIWARA, MD
Department of Radiology, NYU Langone
Health, New York, New York

JEFFREY D. HOOKER, MD
Clinical Fellow, Neuroradiology, Department of
Radiology and Medical Imaging, University of
Virginia Health System, Charlottesville, Virginia

JASON HOSTETTER, MD
Assistant Professor, Department of Radiology,
University of Maryland School of Medicine,
Baltimore, Maryland

JANA IVANIDZE, MD, PhD
Assistant Professor of Radiology, Divisions of
Molecular Imaging and Therapeutics, and
Neuroradiology, Department of Radiology,
Weill Cornell Medicine, New York, New York

MARK J. JAMESON, MD
Associate Professor, Department of
Otolaryngology–Head and Neck Surgery,
University of Virginia Health System,
Charlottesville, Virginia

DAVID JOYNER, MD
Assistant Professor of Neuroradiology,
Department of Radiology and Medical Imaging,
University of Virginia Health System,
Charlottesville, Virginia

TUBA KALELIOGLU, MD
Clinical Instructor of Neuroradiology,
Department of Radiology and Medical Imaging,

University of Virginia Health System,
Charlottesville, Virginia

REMY LOBO, MD
Assistant Professor, Neuroradiology Division,
Radiology, Michigan Medicine, Ann Arbor,
Michigan

JOSE MATTOS, MD, PhD
Assistant Professor, Department of
Otolaryngology–Head and Neck Surgery,
University of Virginia Health System,
Charlottesville, Virginia

ROBERT E. MORALES, MD
Assistant Professor, Neuroradiology, Director,
Diagnostic Neuroradiology Fellowship,
Department of Diagnostic Radiology and
Nuclear Medicine, University of Maryland
School of Medicine, Baltimore, Maryland

SUGOTO MUKHERJEE, MD
Professor of Neuroradiology, Department of
Radiology and Medical Imaging, University of
Virginia Health System, Charlottesville,
Virginia

ROHINI NARAHARI NADGIR, MD
Division of Neuroradiology, Department of
Radiology and Radiological Science, Johns
Hopkins Hospital, Baltimore, Maryland

GOPI K. NAYAK, MD
Department of Radiology, NYU Langone
Health, New York, New York

LAKIR D. PATEL, MD
Resident, Department of Diagnostic Radiology
and Nuclear Medicine, University of Maryland
School of Medicine, Baltimore, Maryland

SOHIL H. PATEL, MD
Associate Professor of Neuroradiology,
Department of Radiology and Medical Imaging,
University of Virginia Health System,
Charlottesville, Virginia

MRUDULA PENTA, MD
Assistant Professor, Department of Radiology,
Stanford University, Stanford, California

PRASHANT RAGHAVAN, MBBS
Associate Professor, Neuroradiology,
Department of Diagnostic Radiology and

Nuclear Medicine, University of Maryland School of Medicine, Baltimore, Maryland

KALEN RILEY, MD, MBA
Assistant Professor of Clinical Radiology and Imaging Sciences, Department of Radiology and Imaging Sciences, Indiana University School of Medicine, Indianapolis, Indiana

TANVIR RIZVI, MD
Assistant Professor of Neuroradiology, Department of Radiology and Medical Imaging, University of Virginia Health System, Charlottesville, Virginia

EDUARDO D. RODRIGUEZ, MD, DDS
Hansjörg Wyss Department of Plastic Surgery, NYU Langone Health, New York, New York

ELANA B. SMITH, MD
Assistant Professor, Trauma and Emergency Radiology, Department of Diagnostic Radiology and Nuclear Medicine, R Adams Cowley Shock Trauma Center, University of Maryland School of Medicine, Baltimore, Maryland

ASHOK SRINIVASAN, MD, FACR
Professor and Division Director, Neuroradiology Division, Radiology, Michigan Medicine, Ann Arbor, Michigan

DANIA TAMIMI, BDS, DMSc
Private Practice in Oral and Maxillofacial Radiology, Orlando, Florida

SEVCAN TURK, MD
Fellow, Neuroradiology Division, Radiology, Michigan Medicine, Ann Arbor, Michigan

KALPESH VAKHARIA, MD, MS
Associate Professor, Chief of Facial Plastic and Reconstructive Surgery, Department of Otorhinolaryngology–Head and Neck Surgery, R Adams Cowley Shock Trauma Center, University of Maryland School of Medicine, Baltimore, Maryland

MATTHEW E. WITEK, MD, MS
Associate Professor, Department of Radiation Oncology, University of Maryland School of Medicine, Medical Director, Maryland Proton Treatment Center, Baltimore, Maryland

JEFFREY XI YANG, MD
Division of Neuroradiology, Department of Radiology and Radiological Science, Johns Hopkins Hospital, Baltimore, Maryland

SANDRINE YAZBEK, MD
Assistant Professor, Department of Radiology, University of Maryland School of Medicine, Baltimore, Maryland

India? Maryland, University of Maryland School of Medicine, Baltimore, Maryland

KALTA RILEY, MD, MBA
Assistant Professor of Clinical Radiology, with Imaging Sciences, Department of Radiology and Imaging Sciences, Indiana University School of Medicine, Indianapolis, Indiana

TANVIR RIZVI, MD
Assistant Professor of Neuroradiology, Department of Radiology and Medical Imaging, University of Virginia Health System, Charlottesville, Virginia

EDUARDO D. RODRIGUEZ, MD, DDS
Hansjörg Wyss Department of Plastic Surgery, NYU Langone Health, New York, New York

ELANA C. SMITH, MD
Assistant Professor, Trauma and Emergency Radiology, Department of Diagnostic Radiology and Nuclear Medicine, R Adams Cowley Shock Trauma Center, University of Maryland School of Medicine, Baltimore, Maryland

ASHOK SRINIVASAN, MD, FACR
Professor and Division Director, Neuroradiology Division, Radiology, Michigan Medicine, Ann Arbor, Michigan

DANIA TAMIMI, BDS, DMSc
Private Practice in Oral and Maxillofacial Radiology, Orlando, Florida

SEVCAN TÜRK, MD
Neuroradiology Division, Radiology, Michigan Medicine, Ann Arbor, Michigan

KAUSTUBH WARAHARIA, MD, MS
Associate Professor, Chief of Facial Plastic and Reconstructive Surgery, Department of Otolaryngology—Head and Neck Surgery, Program Director, Head & Neck Center, University of Maryland School of Medicine, Baltimore, Maryland

MATTHEW E. WITEK, MD, MS
Associate Professor, Department of Radiation Oncology, University of Maryland School of Medicine, Medical Director, Maryland Proton Treatment Center, Baltimore, Maryland

JEFFREY XI YANG, MD
Division of Neuroradiology, Department of Radiology and Radiological Science, Johns Hopkins Hospital, Baltimore, Maryland

SANDRINE YAZBEK, MD
Assistant Professor, Department of Radiology, University of Maryland School of Medicine, Baltimore, Maryland

Contents

American College of Radiology NI-RADS is a surveillance imaging template used to predict residual or recurrent tumor in the setting of head and neck cancer. The lexicon and imaging template provides a framework to standardize the interpretations and communications with referring physicians and provides linked management recommendations, which add value in patient care. Studies have shown reasonable interreader agreement and excellent discriminatory power among the different NI-RADS categories. This article reviews the literature associated with NI-RADS and serves as a practical guide for radiologists interested in using the NI-RADS surveillance template at their institution, highlighting frequently encountered pearls and pitfalls.

The management of neck nodes in head and neck cancer is critical, given a markedly increased poor prognosis in patients with nodal metastasis. The surgical management of neck nodes has undergone radical changes secondary to a paradigm shift from curative surgery to nonsurgical organ and function-preserving options, such as radiation therapy. In the neck after treatment, radiologists should be familiar with imaging findings in various types of neck dissections and post-chemoradiation changes, along with signs of residual or recurrent disease. A multidisciplinary approach is essential with well-designed evidence-based surveillance imaging protocols and standardized reporting.

Cancers of the pharynx and larynx are treated using a combination of chemotherapeutic, radiation, and surgical techniques, depending on the cancer type, biology, location, and stage, as well as patient and other factors. When imaging in the post-surgical setting, the knowledge of the type of tumor, preoperative appearance, and type of surgery performed is essential for accurate interpretation. Surgical anatomic changes, surgical implants/devices, and potential postsurgical complications must be differentiated from suspected recurrent tumors.

Posttreatment imaging evaluation of sinuses encompasses a wide gamut of procedures, ranging from endoscopic procedures for sinonasal inflammatory diseases to markedly radical surgeries for malignant neoplasms (with or without reconstructions), as well as providing access for surgeries involving the anterior and central skull base. Advances in both techniques and devices have expanded the use of endoscopic approaches in managing both benign and malignant lesions, in addition to being the primary surgical method for treating all medically refractive sinonasal inflammatory disorders. Familiarity with the complex anatomy in the sinonasal region and knowledge of the various procedures is indispensable in interpreting these imaging studies.

This review article discusses the basic principles behind the use of flaps and grafts for reconstructive surgery in the head and neck, with a special emphasis on the types of commonly used free flaps, their imaging appearance as well as some frequently encountered postoperative complications. Given the ubiquity and complexity of these reconstructive techniques, it is essential that head and neck radiologists be familiar in distinguishing between the expected evolving findings, complications, and tumor recurrence.

Chemoradiation for head and neck cancer is associated with a variety of early and late complications. Toxicities may affect the aero-digestive tract (mucositis, salivary gland injury), regional osseous and cartilaginous structures (osteoradionecrosis (ORN) and chondronecrosis), vasculature (progressive radiation vasculopathy and carotid blow out syndromes), and neural structures (optic neuritis, myelitis, and brain injury). These may be difficult to distinguish from tumor recurrence on imaging, and may necessitate the use of advanced MRI and molecular imaging techniques to reach the correct diagnosis. Secondary radiation-induced malignancies include thyroid cancer and a variety of sarcomas that may manifest several years after treatment. Checkpoint inhibitors can cause a variety of adverse immune events, including autoimmune hypophysitis and encephalitis.

PET/computed tomography and PET/MR imaging are used to evaluate the post-treatment neck. Although 18F-FDG is helpful in the staging and treatment response assessment of head and neck cancer, recently developed PET radiotracers targeting specific surface markers are promising for applications of diagnostic problem solving and improved extent delineation. Diffusion-weighted MR imaging is helpful in the differential diagnosis of head and neck neoplasms, and improves the sensitivity and specificity for the detection of certain pathologies. Following standardized imaging parameters for PET/computed tomography and diffusion-weighted imaging in PET/MR imaging improves diagnostic accuracy and allows for future research data mining.

Advances in MR and computed tomography (CT) techniques have resulted in greater fidelity in the assessment of treatment response and residual tumor on one hand and the assessment of recurrent head and neck malignancies on the other hand. The advances in MR techniques primarily are related to diffusion and perfusion imaging which rely on the intrinsic architecture of the tissues and organ systems. The techniques exploit the density of the cellular architecture; and the vascularity of benign and malignant lesions which in turn affect the changes in the passage of contrast through the vascular bed. Dual-energy CT and CT perfusion are the major advances in CT techniques that have found significant applications in the assessment of treatment response and tumor recurrence.

The thyroid and parathyroid glands are endocrine structures located in the visceral space of the infrahyoid neck. Imaging plays a critical role in the evaluation of patients with thyroid cancer, both in the pre and posttreatment setting. Disorders of thyroid function, that is, hyperthyroidism and hypothyroidism, are also fairly common, although imaging utilization is less frequent with these conditions. Parathyroid dysfunction results in disordered calcium metabolism. Imaging is frequently applied in the preoperative assessment of these patients undergoing parathyroidectomy; however, routine imaging in the postoperative setting is uncommon. Parathyroid carcinoma is rare; however, imaging may be used in the pre and posttreatment setting.

For pathologic conditions affecting the skull base and cerebellopontine angle, imaging techniques have advanced to assess for residual disease, disease progression, and postoperative complications. Knowledge regarding various surgical approaches of skull base tumor resection, expected postoperative appearance, and common postsurgical complications guides radiologic interpretation. Complexity of skull base anatomy, small size of the relevant structures, lack of familiarity with surgical techniques, and postsurgical changes confound radiologic evaluation. This article discusses the imaging techniques, surgical approaches, expected postoperative changes, and complications after surgery of the skull base, with emphasis on the cerebellopontine angle, anterior cranial fossa, and central skull base regions.

Evaluation of the postoperative temporal bone can be difficult given the complex anatomy of this region and the myriad surgical approaches for management of a variety of conditions. This article provides an understanding of common postsurgical changes of the temporal bone and their typical imaging appearances. Ultimately, greater radiologist knowledge of postoperative temporal bone imaging findings will help to serve patients and referring clinicians with prompt diagnosis and recognition of expected postintervention changes compared with postoperative complications and/or disease recurrence.

There is a plethora of surgical procedures that are performed in the eye and orbit. The consequences of these procedures can often be observed on diagnostic imaging through the presence of various implants and altered anatomy. The expected postoperative changes in the eye and orbit, the impact of implants on image quality and safety, and potential associated complications are reviewed in this article. Conventional computed tomography and MR imaging scans are useful for the postoperative assessment of the eye and orbit. The computed tomography and MR imaging findings related to the postoperative eye and orbit are reviewed in this article.

Surgical procedures in the oral cavity and maxillofacial complex are diverse and involve multiple tissues unique to this region. These procedures are used to remove pathology and infection, restore function, optimize occlusal relationships, prosthetically replace teeth and temporomandibular joints, improve esthetics, and increase upper respiratory tract dimensions. Procedures in the oral cavity are often complicated by infection stemming from the naturally occurring oral flora, but can also be complicated iatrogenically. This article explores the more commonly encountered surgical procedures through examination of the indications, anatomy to consider, and the radiographic imaging of success and failure of these procedures.

In order for a radiologist to create reports that are meaningful to facial reconstructive surgeons, an understanding of the principles that guide surgical management and the hardware employed is imperative. This article is intended to promote efficient and salient reporting by illustrating surgical approaches and rationale. Hardware selection can be inferred and a defined set of potential complications anticipated when assessing the adequacy of surgical reconstruction on postoperative computed tomography for midface, internal orbital, and mandible fractures.

Pre- and postoperative imaging is increasingly used in plastic and reconstructive surgery for the evaluation of bony and soft tissue anatomy. Imaging plays an important role in preoperative planning. In the postoperative setting, imaging is used for the assessment of surgical positioning, bone healing and fusion, and for the assessment of early or delayed surgical complications. This article will focus on imaging performed for the surgical reconstruction of the face, including orthognathic surgery, facial feminization procedures for gender dysphoria, and face transplantation.

Foreword
Imaging of the Post Treatment Head and Neck

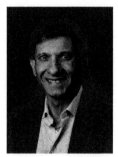

Suresh K. Mukherji, MD, MBA, FACR
Consulting Editor

I am convinced from my 25+ years of practice that one of the main reasons many radiologists choose not to take vacation is because their partners, who loathe interpreting posttreatment neck studies, would "save" these studies as punishment for the vacationing radiologist! I am certainly in the minority of those who enjoy interpreting the posttreatment neck. I have always found these studies challenging and fun, albeit some of you may have a different definition of "fun."

This is a very comprehensive issue, which covers all aspects of the posttreatment neck. The articles are devoted to the postoperative neck, grafts and flaps, thyroid and parathyroid, eye and orbit, sinuses, facial bones, temporal bone, and skull base. There are also articles focused on advanced techniques and surveillance imaging.

I have had the good fortune of knowing Drs Raghavan, Morales, and Mukherjee for many years and was delighted when these talented and renowned neuroradiologists agreed to use their passion and experience to create such a great issue. I also want to thank this extraordinarily talented group of authors for their wonderful contributions in these extremely challenging times. Thank you again to all for creating such a clear and comprehensive issue that I am sure our readers with find both informative and fun!

Suresh K. Mukherji, MD, MBA, FACR
Marian University
Head and Neck Radiology
ProScan Imaging
Carmel, IN, USA

E-mail address:
sureshmukherji@hotmail.com

Neuroimag Clin N Am 32 (2022) xv
https://doi.org/10.1016/j.nic.2021.10.001
1052-5149/22/© 2021 Published by Elsevier Inc.

Preface

Imaging of the Post Treatment Head and Neck

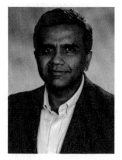
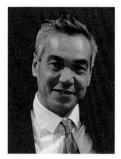
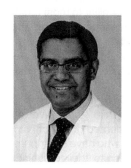

Prashant Raghavan, MBBS   Robert E. Morales, MD   Sugoto Mukherjee, MD

Editors

Treatment for congenital, traumatic, and neoplastic diseases of the head and neck may result in radical alterations in already complex anatomy, with structures removed either in part or in their entirety or reconstructed with hardware or grafts derived from elsewhere in the body. Expected changes in anatomy may mimic or mask recurrence of the disease treated. These procedures may result in complications that may be serious in their own right. It is no surprise then, that there is perhaps no imaging study that radiologists approach with more trepidation than cross-sectional examinations of the posttreatment head and neck. This issue of the *Neuroimaging Clinics* attempts to demystify interpretation of these studies by assembling an array of review articles written by an expert group of neuroradiologists, oncologists, and otolaryngologists.

The issue begins with a discussion on the use of NI-RADS to assess residual or recurrent head and neck squamous cell carcinoma in general. Separate articles devoted to cervical node dissection and surgery for sinonasal, skull base,

aerodigestive tract, and thyroid and parathyroid cancer discuss the clinical principles behind these procedures and expected postoperative imaging findings and provide tips for detection of complications and recurrent cancer. The use of grafts and flaps in head and neck cancer reconstruction is also addressed in a separate article. The article on imaging after chemoradiation provides an oncologist's perspective in addition to a comprehensive overview of the complications that may ensue. The use of advanced CT, MR imaging, and metabolic imaging in detecting recurrent head and neck cancer is addressed across two articles, which also include recommendations for imaging protocols that may be incorporated into routine practice.

Reviews of imaging after surgery on the temporal bones, skull base, and cerebellopontine angle, an area where neurosurgical and otolaryngologic practices intersect, span the gamut from simple procedures, such as tympanostomy, to craniofacial resection. A nuanced and detailed review of the complex topic of imaging after craniofacial

Neuroimag Clin N Am 32 (2022) xvii–xviii
https://doi.org/10.1016/j.nic.2021.09.004
1052-5149/22/© 2021 Published by Elsevier Inc.

neuroimaging.theclinics.com

trauma repair provides a wealth of clinical information that is vital to the precise interpretation of the studies. Reviews of imaging of the postoperative eye and orbit and after dentoalveolar surgical procedures provide an overview of procedures that are more commonly performed than one is given to understand but remain unfamiliar to most radiologists. A separate review describes imaging after facial reconstruction, including gender reaffirmation surgery and face transplantation, procedures that are being increasingly performed in recent years.

We would like to thank Dr Suresh Mukherji for inviting us to guest edit this issue. We are immensely thankful to the talented group of rising stars and experts in the field who have contributed their time and expertise despite their crushingly busy schedules. Thanks also go to John Vassallo and Karen Solomon at Elsevier without whose support and patience this issue would not have been possible. We would like to dedicate this issue to our families, the patients behind the stories and images that form the foundation of this issue, and also our fellow health care workers at the frontlines of the battle against COVID-19.

Prashant Raghavan, MBBS
Diagnostic Radiology and Nuclear Medicine
University of Maryland School of Medicine,
Baltimore, MD, USA

Robert E. Morales, MD
Diagnostic Radiology and Nuclear Medicine
University of Maryland
Baltimore, MD, USA

Sugoto Mukherjee, MD
Department of Radiology and Medical Imaging
University of Virginia Health System
1215 Lee Street
PO Box 800170
Charlottesville, VA 22908-1070, USA

E-mail addresses:
Prashant.raghavan@gmail.com (P. Raghavan)
rmorales@umm.edu (R.E. Morales)
sm5qd@virginia.edu (S. Mukherjee)

NI-RADS to Predict Residual or Recurrent Head and Neck Squamous Cell Carcinoma

Kristen L. Baugnon, MD*

KEYWORDS

- NI-RADS • Surveillance • Head and neck cancer • Head and neck squamous cell carcinoma

KEY POINTS

- NI-RADS is a helpful surveillance imaging template that standardizes interpretations and communication with referring physicians.
- NI-RADS scores provide a level of suspicion for recurrence of head and neck cancer with linked management recommendations.
- ACR NI-RADS templates are available for CECT, MR imaging, and PET/CT.
- NI-RADS lexicon and scores have been linked with outcomes and shown to provide discriminatory power in detection of head and neck cancer recurrence.
- Use of NI-RADS templates allows the radiologist to add value in patient care.

INTRODUCTION/BACKGROUND

The American College of Radiology (ACR) published its first Reporting and Data System (RADS) for breast imaging in 1993 and, since that time, there have been several additional ACR-endorsed RADS systems that have emerged, including computed tomography (CT) colonography, coronary artery disease, liver imaging, lung, neck imaging (NI-RADS), adnexal masses, prostate imaging, and thyroid imaging.[1] These RADS systems are devised by a consensus group of experts, and help to[1]:

- Provide a standardized terminology, report organization, and assessment classification, typically used when there is a binary outcome for the interpretation of the study (ie, is there cancer or not).
- Reduce ambiguity in reports, linking management recommendations with an assessment classification, which provides an actionable report for the referring provider.
- Simplify communication, clearly directing management via a multidisciplinary approach.
- Facilitate radiologic-pathologic correlation for quality improvement.
- Foster evidence-based practice by providing data-minable reports for future studies.
- Add value to the radiologist, because they help to move patient-centered care forward.

NI-RADS was first introduced in 2015 as a novel surveillance imaging template for head and neck cancer.[2] Head and neck primary malignancies recur in up to 15% to 50% of cases, most commonly in the first 2 to 3 years after treatment, and therefore surveillance imaging is important during that time frame to attempt to identify recurrence as early as possible, allowing for increased options for salvage treatment.[3] Post-treatment changes to the already complex anatomy of the

Department of Radiology and Imaging Sciences, Division of Neuroradiology, Head and Neck Imaging, Emory University, 1364 Clifton Road, Atlanta, GA 30322, USA
* 2666 Redding Road, Northeast, Brookhaven, GA 30319.
E-mail address: kmlloyd@emory.edu
Twitter: @KLBaugnon (K.L.B.)

Neuroimag Clin N Am 32 (2022) 1–18
https://doi.org/10.1016/j.nic.2021.08.003
1052-5149/22/© 2021 Elsevier Inc. All rights reserved.

head and neck can complicate the interpretation of post-treatment imaging, and in the setting of free text reporting, can lead to a varied and suboptimal interpretation, which often depends on the preferences and experience level of the interpreting radiologist. NI-RADS standardized reporting templates provide a standard nomenclature and approach for interpreting these complex examinations, allowing for improved communication between radiologists and their referring clinicians, and standardization across institutions.

This article serves as a practical guide to using the NI-RADS approach and system for interpreting these complex post-treatment head and neck cancer studies. We review the different templates and legends for the different imaging modalities, providing case-based examples for guidance on assigning categories, and highlighting important commonly encountered pearls and pitfalls.

IMAGING TECHNIQUE/ALGORITHM

There are few evidence-based guidelines and standards regarding the optimal timing and modality of imaging surveillance. The National Comprehensive Cancer Network recommends baseline post-treatment imaging "within 6 months of treatment" for advanced head and neck primary cancers but does not officially recommend imaging for asymptomatic patients after 6 months.[4] However, 79% of surveyed head and neck surgeons admit to using imaging surveillance on asymptomatic patients.[5] PET combined with contrast-enhanced CT (CECT) has been shown to have good sensitivity and moderate specificity for detecting recurrent or persistent disease in the post-treatment setting; however, the optimal timing and frequency has not been standardized.[6,7] Beyond the initial baseline examination, there are few studies demonstrating a clear benefit or survival advantage for universal surveillance imaging. However, a recent study used NI-RADS data to look back at asymptomatic recurrence rates and determined that more than one-third of recurrences detected on imaging were clinically occult, and 80% of those occurred beyond the 6-month post-treatment timepoint.[8] Given the high recurrence rates and frequent difficulty clinically assessing the primary site and neck for recurrence caused by post-treatment changes, most institutions have adopted a routine surveillance protocol for advanced head and neck cancers. Developing a consensus surveillance imaging algorithm at your institution with the stakeholders involved is important before using the NI-RADS imaging template. Standardizing the approach and the template also helps to study optimal

imaging protocols for certain high-risk patient populations in the future.

In the NI-RADS white paper published by the *Journal of the American College of Radiology* in 2018, the ACR NI-RADS committee suggested the following baseline surveillance imaging regimen for head and neck squamous cell carcinomas:

- Baseline post-treatment PET/CECT at 8 to 12 weeks after completion of definitive therapy (has been shown to have a high negative predictive value at this timepoint).[9]
- If the initial study is negative, CECT of the neck alone (or PET/CECT) 6 months later.
- If this is negative, repeat CECT of the neck alone 6 months later.
- If second follow-up study is negative, then CECT of the neck and chest performed 12 months later.[10]

If there are suspicious findings on imaging (NI-RADS scores 2 or higher, as discussed later), more frequent imaging or intervention may be necessary.[11] Because 95% of asymptomatic recurrences occur within the first 24 months after treatment, routine PET/CT surveillance after this time may be of limited value.[7,9] Although NI-RADS was initially developed for use with PET and CECT imaging, the ACR committee recommends the use of templates for MR imaging as well, because MR imaging is often best for assessing intracranial, perineural, and/or orbital disease in patients with certain primary tumors, including sinonasal, nasopharyngeal, orbital, or parotid malignancies, or other skull base tumors with propensity for perineural tumor spread. Finally, although most head and neck primary malignancies requiring surveillance imaging are certainly squamous cell carcinoma, this template can be adopted and applied to any head and neck primary malignancy.

NECK IMAGING REPORTING AND DATA SYSTEM TEMPLATE AND LEGEND

The post-treatment neck imaging templates are streamlined and efficient to use (Box 1). The radiologist enters the initial stage, subsite, human papilloma virus status, and prior treatment completion dates in the Clinical Indication section. The technique can be prepopulated, and dates of comparisons added. The body of the report includes sections devoted to postsurgical change, if applicable, and postradiation changes (ie, laryngeal mucosal edema, subcutaneous stranding, and thickening of the skin), and a section dedicated to the primary site and to the neck, looking for local residual or recurrent disease or for imaging does exist and will become available for comparison).

- Category 1: No evidence of recurrence. Linked management recommendation is for routine follow-up.
- Category 2: Low suspicion, ill-defined areas of abnormality, with only mild enhancement or mild fluorodeoxyglucose (FDG) uptake. Linked management recommendation is for direct inspection of superficial or mucosal abnormalities, or short interval follow-up of deeper abnormalities with imaging.
- Category 3: High suspicion, discrete, new, or enlarging lesion with marked enhancement and/or intense focal FDG uptake. Linked management recommendation is for biopsy.
- Category 4: Definitive recurrence, either pathologically proven or definite radiologic or clinical progression.

Reporting templates, including the legends with management recommendations included at the end of the report, are slightly different for CECT/MR imaging and PET (**Box 2** and **3**). Current lexicons are specific for CECT and PET findings; however, MR imaging lexicon verbiage has been suggested in the literature[12,13] and will likely be published by the ACR NI-RADS committee in the future. If there are findings that are worthy of the impression beyond the assessment of the primary site or nodal basin (ie, lung nodules suspicious for metastasis, severe atherosclerotic disease, or bone metastasis), additional findings are added at the bottom of the impression.

NECK IMAGING REPORTING AND DATA SYSTEM CATEGORIES

The specific categories with their imaging description, lexicon for image interpretation, and pearls and pitfalls are discussed in detail below. In the report template, a category is assigned separately for the primary and the neck.

NECK IMAGING REPORTING AND DATA SYSTEM CATEGORY 0: INCOMPLETE ASSESSMENT
Primary Site

A NI-RADS 0 designation is made for the primary site when there are post-treatment changes on a new baseline study, with no prior imaging available for comparison; however, there is knowledge that prior examinations do exist and could potentially become available for review at a later time, at which point an addendum with an updated score/management recommendation should be provided. This score should be used rarely, and

metastatic cervical lymphadenopathy, prepopulated with normal findings. Thus, in a routine study, with no suspicious findings for recurrence, which is a default for the template, it is quick for the radiologist to tab through the sections and quickly finalize the report. In the setting of suspicious findings, it is easy for the radiologist to modify the respective section to add specific findings.

In the Impression section, the primary site and the neck are each individually assigned a category from 0 to 4, based on the radiologist's level of suspicion regarding the possibility of recurrence. There is a legend at the bottom of the report linking the category of the primary site and the neck to a management recommendation, based on literature-based best practices and consensus opinion of the ACR NI-RADS committee.[10] The categories are as follows:

- Category 0: New baseline study. Need prior imaging for comparison to score (if prior

---

Box 2
CECT or MR imaging Surveillance Legend

Primary

1. No evidence of recurrence: routine surveillance

2. Low suspicion

   a. Superficial abnormality (skin, mucosal surface): direct visual inspection

   b. Ill-defined deep abnormality: short interval follow-up[a] or PET

3. High suspicion (new or enlarging discrete nodule/mass): biopsy

4. Definitive recurrence (path proven, clinical or definitive imaging progression): no biopsy needed

Nodes

1. No evidence of recurrence: routine surveillance

2. Low suspicion: (enlarging lymph node without morphologically abnormal features): short-interval follow-up or PET

3. High suspicion (new or enlarging lymph node with morphologically abnormal features): biopsy if clinically needed

4. Definitive recurrence (path proven, clinical or definitive imaging progression): no biopsy needed

[a]Short-interval follow-up: 3 mo at our institution

From ACR NI-RADS. Available at https://www.acr.org/-/media/ACR/Files/RADS/NI-RADS/CECT-or-MRI-Surveillance-Legend.txt Accessed July 2021, reprinted with permission.

---

in most settings with post-treatment changes, but no suspicious features, the radiologist should feel confident giving an NI-RADS 1. However, there are instances when this assessment is helpful. In the author's institutional experience, this category is most commonly assigned in the setting of post-treatment MR imaging NI-RADS assessments of sinonasal, nasopharyngeal, or any other tumor with skull base or perineural involvement, where there is persistent abnormal soft tissue, and it is difficult to determine if it represents sterile treated tumor versus persistent or progressive active disease (**Fig. 1**). Additionally, this denotation is helpful in the setting of unusual tumors or in follow-up MR imaging to obtain the pretreatment imaging to determine if abnormalities are similar to the pretreatment appearance of tumor.

Neck

This category is helpful in the setting of post-treatment changes in treated lymph nodes, when there is persistent CT or PET imaging abnormality, but no prior post-treatment or pretreatment imaging available. Obtaining prior imaging can obviate sooner follow-up or further work-up with biopsy (**Fig. 2**).

Pearls and Pitfalls

Occasionally it is difficult to acquire prior imaging. If the prior studies are unable to be acquired and one cannot assign an NI-RADS 0 category, it may be necessary to perform short-term interval follow-up of abnormalities, or PET imaging to further evaluate anatomic post-treatment change, and assign an NI-RADS 2 category, rather than NI-RADS 3 category, unless the finding is highly suspicious. Biopsy, particularly fine-needle aspiration, in the setting of post-treatment change can be confusing for the pathologist, because treated metastatic lymph nodes can demonstrate atypical squamous cells in a background of keratin debris when they involute, leading to false-positive studies and potentially unnecessary neck dissections.

NECK IMAGING REPORTING AND DATA SYSTEM CATEGORY 1: NO EVIDENCE OF RECURRENCE

This category reflects no imaging evidence of recurrence, with a linked management recommendation of routine surveillance. Most scans fall into this category (approximately 85% in one study), and the NI-RADS 1 category has been associated with an approximately 1% to 4% risk of recurrent disease.[14,15]

Primary Site

Lexicon/imaging appearance

- Expected post-treatment changes with non-mass-like distortion of soft tissues
- Low density submucosal edema (ie, postradiation edema)
- Hypoenhancing effacement of fat planes
- Linear diffuse mucosal enhancement
- No abnormal FDG uptake; includes diffuse curvilinear mucosal enhancement or FDG uptake (ie, benign postradiation mucositis)[10]

Evaluation of the primary site should include distortion of soft tissues without masslike enhancement or focal FDG uptake. After radiation, it is not uncommon to see findings of radiation mucositis, with diffuse linear enhancement and FDG uptake in the treatment field (**Fig. 3**). After surgical resection of tumor, particularly in the oral cavity, there are common PET pitfalls and false positives one can encounter, described later. In the setting of an unknown primary, the Primary category can be removed, can just be listed as Unknown, or given an "X." A recent publication suggests NI-RADS MR imaging lexicon should include non-mass-like T2-weighted hyperintensity, and facilitated diffusion (absence of diffusion restriction), along with other NI-RADS 1 lexicon criteria to assist with NI-RADS 1 scoring at the primary site.[13]

Neck

Lexicon/imaging appearance

- Nodal soft tissue with no FDG uptake

Evaluation of the neck with post-treatment baseline imaging (typically PET/CECT) is important in the setting of definitive chemoradiation therapy (CRT), because often the imaging determines the necessity of a post-treatment salvage neck dissection. Several studies, including a large prospective randomized controlled trial, have shown that imaging surveillance with a negative PET/CT can spare a patient with initial advanced nodal disease (stage N2 or N3) a salvage post-treatment neck dissection after definitive CRT, with equivalent survival outcomes.[16] It is common in patients with significant lymphadenopathy pretreatment, i.e. initial stage N2 or N3 disease, to have persistent nodal soft tissue on subsequent post-treatment studies. However, no FDG uptake within a lymph node on a baseline PET/CECT completed 8 to 12 weeks post-therapy has been associated with a 90% to 100% negative predictive value in several studies, with higher specificities and negative predictive value with more delayed imaging, 12 to 16 weeks or greater after treatement.[9] Thus, with a small amount of residual nonenhancing nodal tissue with no FDG uptake, the radiologist can confidently score the neck a NI-RADS 1, and the patient is recommended to undergo routine surveillance (**Fig. 4**).

Pearls and Pitfalls

Postsurgical and post-treatment pitfalls are common. It is not uncommon to have enhancement or FDG uptake in the post-treatment setting, and it does not always indicate recurrent tumor. When one encounters questionable suspicious findings on a post-treatment imaging study, it is even more important to review the medical record, determining if there were negative surgical margins, or if there are worrisome findings on physical examination or clinical history (ie, worsening pain). If the surgeon had negative surgical margins, it would be less likely to be recurrence on the first baseline post-treatment imaging study, unless the patient was immunocompromised or had high-risk features, such as extensive perineural and lymphovascular invasion on pathology. Additionally, if the patient was unable to complete the entire course of radiation or chemotherapy, the patient may be at increased risk for failure and persistent disease on the initial post-treatment baseline examination.

One commonly encountered pitfall is in the setting of postsurgical PET imaging of the oral cavity. Tongue fasciculations after glossectomy can often cause ipsilateral or contralateral focal FDG uptake; however, the absence of associated focal masslike enhancement should allow

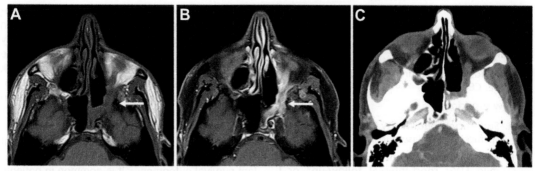

Fig. 1. NI-RADS 0, primary site. T1-weighted precontrast (*A*) and postcontrast (*B*) MR images of a patient establishing care at our institution with history of advanced sinonasal malignancy with perineural tumor spread, treated at outside institution with surgical resection followed by adjuvant radiation therapy (XRT), completed 3 years earlier. Surveillance MR imaging shows abnormal enhancing soft tissue in the depths of the surgical bed extending into the left pterygopalatine fossa and foramen rotundum (*arrows*). Because there were no prior studies available for comparison, but knowledge that prior studies existed and able to be obtained, the primary site was initially assigned a NI-RADS 0 score. (*C*) CECT from 1 year earlier was submitted for comparison demonstrating stability of the findings, thought to most likely represent sterile treated perineural tumor. The original report was addended and NI-RADS score of 1 was assigned.

one to differentiate post-treatment change from tumor and assign a NI-RADS 1 score at the primary site (**Fig. 5**). Muscular portions of the flap and vascular pedicles can also often enhance differentially, and are confused with tumor. Additionally, in the setting of tumor involvement of the skull base, either directly or via perineural spread, often the imaging features never return to normal. In this setting, it is often prudent to assign a NI-RADS 2 score, until stability is ensured on short-term follow-up studies, and the patient can then be downgraded to an NI-RADS 1, keeping in mind that progression of perineural tumor can sometimes develop slowly over time, necessitating comparison with multiple prior examinations to completely ensure stability.

In the neck, in the setting of persistent enlarged nodal lesions on the first post-treatment baseline examination, if there is no significant FDG uptake at 12 weeks post-treatment, yet there are persistent worrisome morphologic features on CECT or MR imaging, such as persistent necrosis, heterogeneous enhancement, or significant enlargement, even if there is not significant FDG uptake, CECT could be considered discordant with the PET, and a NI-RADS 2 category can be assigned (see next).

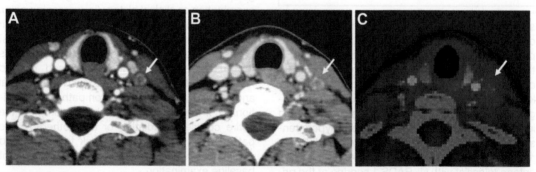

Fig. 2. NI-RADS 0, neck. (*A*) CECT of a patient with a history of left tonsillar squamous cell carcinoma (SCCA) status post chemoradiation therapy at an outside institution, establishing care at our institution, shows a peripherally enhancing left level 4 lymph node (*arrow*). Without prior imaging or metabolic imaging, it is difficult to determine if the lymph node represented treated or active disease, and thus the neck was assigned a score of NI-RADS 0. Subsequently, a CECT (*B*) and PET (*C*) that had been obtained previously for the patient's first baseline post-treatment scan showed the node to be similar in appearance, and without any significant FDG uptake. An addendum was then made to the initial CECT, assigning a NI-RADS score of 1.

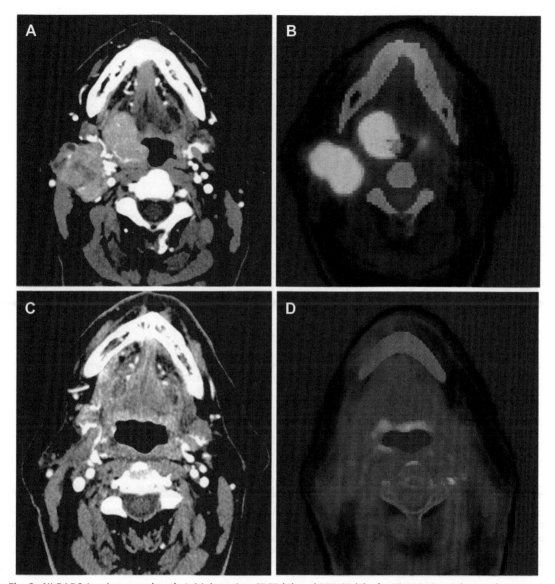

Fig. 3. NI-RADS 1, primary and neck. Initial staging CECT (*A*) and PET/CT (*B*) of a T2N1 P16+ right oropharynx primary SCCA. Baseline post-treatment follow-up CECT (*C*) and PET/CT (*D*) showing post-treatment changes with mild diffuse mucosal enhancement and FDG uptake, and minimal residual soft tissue in the neck without enhancement or FDG uptake, compatible with response to therapy. No evidence of recurrence at the primary site or in the neck: NI-RADS 1.

NECK IMAGING REPORTING AND DATA SYSTEM CATEGORY 2: LOW SUSPICION FOR RECURRENCE

This category reflects a low suspicion for recurrence, with linked management of direct visual inspection for mucosal lesions, and short-term follow-up imaging (ie, in 3 months) or PET imaging for deeper lesions (if the study was a CECT or MR imaging alone). Approximately 10% of studies are scored in this category, and overall, the NI-RADS 2 category has been associated with an approximately 5% to 17% risk of recurrent disease, highest for the mucosal lesions.[14,15]

Primary Site

Lexicon/imaging appearance

- Focal mucosal enhancement
- Ill-defined soft tissue with only mild differential enhancement
- No discrete nodule or mass
- Mild FDG uptake

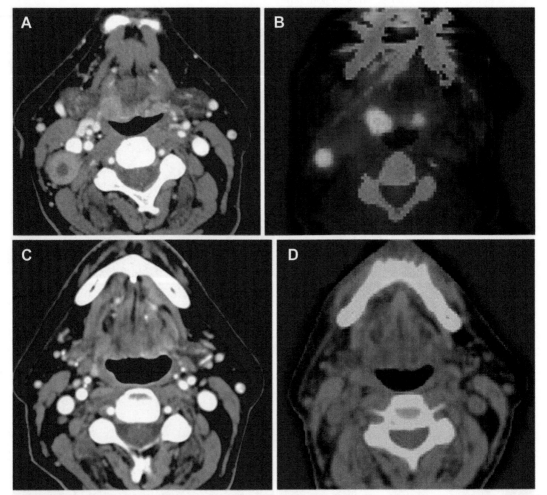

Fig. 4. NI-RADS 1, primary site and neck. CECT (*A*) and PET (*B*) showing the initial staging images of a patient with a T1N1 P16 + SCCA of the right base of tongue. Post-treatment CECT (*C*) and PET (*D*) images showing resolution of the abnormal enhancement at the primary site with mild residual diffuse linear enhancement and only minimal residual nodal soft tissue without significant FDG uptake. No evidence of recurrence at the primary site or in the neck: NI-RADS 1.

- Mismatch or discordance between CECT and PET/CT

Evaluation of the primary site is separated into mucosal abnormalities and deep soft tissue abnormalities, because they are associated with different management recommendations. Superficial mucosal lesions should be ascribed a category 2a, and the recommendation is direct visual inspection, because they should be easily clinically inspected, and biopsy could be obtained at the discretion of the surgeon. Mucosal injury is common after radiation, and in the setting of focal mucosal enhancement (rather than diffuse linear enhancement), or enhancement associated with ulceration, this could represent either radiation injury or recurrent tumor. Thus, in the early post-treatment setting, even if the findings are concordant, a NI-RADS score of 2a should be assigned, because the superficial mucosal lesion should be amenable to direct inspection (Fig. 6). Additionally, in the setting of mucosal abnormalities, particularly if there are discordant findings, such as focal FDG uptake without a definite mucosal enhancing lesion on CECT, a score of NI-RADS 2a should be assigned (Fig. 7). In one paper, NI-RADS 2a lesions were associated with a 7% chance of recurrence.[15]

Deep soft tissue lesions at the primary site in which there is ill-defined or only mildly enhancing soft tissue, without discrete nodule or mass, or soft tissue with only mild FDG uptake, are indeterminate lesions, and should be categorized as NI-RADS 2b lesions, with the recommendation for

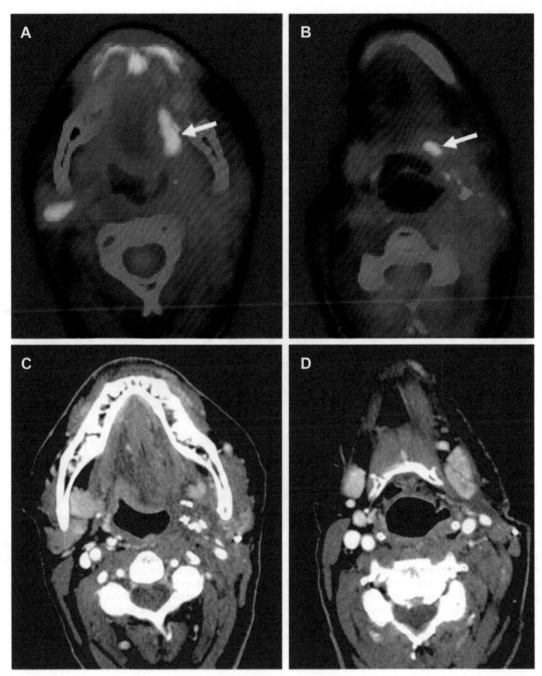

Fig. 5. NI-RADS 1, primary site, tongue fasciculations. Patient with left oral tongue SCCA status post left partial glossectomy and neck dissection followed by adjuvant XRT. Baseline post-treatment PET/CT (*A, B*) showing linear FDG uptake along the course of the hyoglossus muscle on the left extending down to the hyoid bone (*arrow*). (*C, D*) CECT does not demonstrate any abnormal enhancement in the region, compatible with FDG uptake caused by tongue fasciculations. No evidence of recurrence at the primary site: NI-RADS 1.

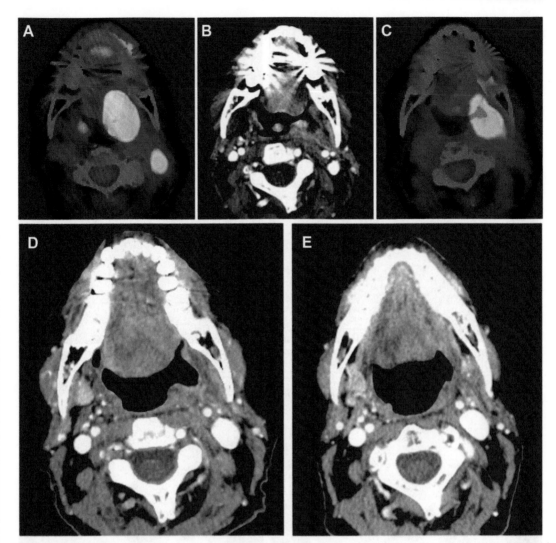

Fig. 6. NI-RADS 2a, mucosal uptake. (A) Initial staging PET/CT showing large left tonsillar SCCA with ipsilateral nodal metastasis. (B, C) Baseline post-treatment CECT and PET/CT 12 weeks after completion of therapy shows large ulceration with masslike enhancement posteriorly and significant focal FDG uptake. Given early post-treatment setting and superficial nature of the lesion, this was assigned an NI-RADS 2a for the primary site. Surgeon examined the patient, but decided to follow up short term instead of biopsy. (D) Short-term follow-up CECT shows persistent ulceration and heaped up enhancing mucosa posteriorly. This was again given an NI-RADS 2a. Biopsy was performed and was negative for malignancy. (E) Follow-up CECT shows improvement and near resolution of the abnormality. No evidence of disease clinically: NI-RADS 1.

short-term interval follow-up, or PET/CT, if the initial study was only a CECT or MR imaging, at which point PET/CT can help either downgrade or upgrade the finding (Fig. 8). In one paper, NI-RADS 2b lesions were associated with a 5.6% chance of recurrence.[15]

Also, another recent publication suggests that the NI-RADS MR imaging lexicon should also include T2-weighted signal and diffusion restriction into the grading criteria, and the presence of intermediate T2 signal and diffusion restriction at the primary site should upgrade one stage from the NI-RADS assignment based on the other NI-RADS lexicon criteria. Thus, if the score was an NI-RADS 1 based on the enhancement characteristics, then the presence of soft tissue with intermediate T2 signal and diffusion restriction would upstage to an NI-RADS 2b, and if already an NI-RADS 2b, then the presence of both of those criteria would upstage to an NI-RADS 3.[13] A specific MR imaging lexicon has not yet been released by the ACR NI-RADS committee.

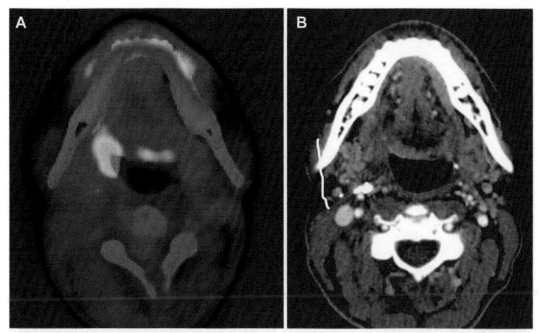

Fig. 7. NI-RADS 2a, mucosal uptake. Status post transoral robotic surgery and right neck dissection followed by adjuvant XRT for right tonsillar SCCA. Early post-treatment PET/CECT with focal uptake in the right glossotonsillar sulcus (*A*), which does not show significant enhancement on CECT (*B*). Although findings are most likely post-treatment in nature, findings are discordant and mucosal, therefore an NI-RADS 2a score was assigned, with the recommendation for direct inspection.

Neck

- Residual lymph node tissue post-treatment with mild FDG uptake
- Mismatch or discordance between CECT and PET/CT
- Enlarging lymph node, with otherwise normal morphologic features

Persistent nodal soft tissue after CRT is common, and although the negative predictive value of PET/CT at 12 weeks is high, if there is residual FDG uptake within the nodal tissue, the examination is therefore indeterminate, and should be scored an NI-RADS 2 (Fig. 9). Additionally, if there are discordant features, such as persistent enlargement, necrosis, or heterogeneous enhancement on CECT, and/or mild to no uptake on FDG/PET, those patients can also be scored an NI-RADS 2, recommending a short-term follow-up to ensure resolution of the suspicious findings (Fig. 10). Finally, at any point after treatment, it is not uncommon to see nodal enlargement without otherwise abnormal morphologic features, such as necrosis, which can be early disease recurrence, or simply reactive lymphadenopathy. In this setting, it is appropriate to score the neck as an NI-RADS 2 and recommend short-term follow-up or PET/CT to further evaluate these findings.

Pearls and Pitfalls

To summarize, if there are indeterminate findings, or any discordant findings between cross-sectional CECT or MR imaging and PET imaging, at either the primary site or the neck, that site should be classified as NI-RADS 2 and recommended either direct visualization or short-term follow-up imaging. If there are concordant findings, and there is a discrete biopsy target, the NI-RADS score should be a 3, as discussed in the next section. The exception to that rule is in the early post-treatment setting, because it is not uncommon for radiation injury to demonstrate focal enhancement and FDG uptake, and therefore the recommendation in that setting is direct visualization of the abnormality, allowing the surgeon to decide on biopsy. One additional potential pitfall is in the setting of abnormalities in the post-treatment larynx and hypopharynx, because direct visualization of the larynx and cross-sectional imaging are difficult to interpret after CRT. Therefore, PET/CT is often extremely helpful in the setting of surveillance imaging of the larynx to help guide direct clinical inspection. Finally, at the author's institution, we have found it extremely helpful to work backward in the setting of challenging cases. If there is a questionable abnormality, but it is not

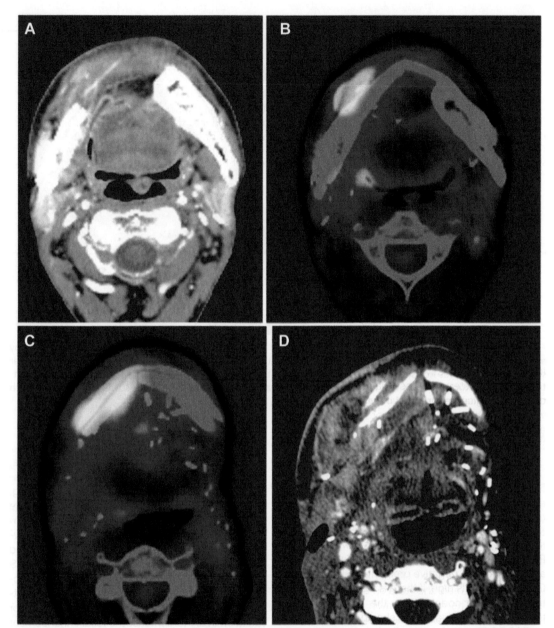

Fig. 8. NI-RADS 2b, deep lesion at primary site. Patient with history of T4aN0 right mandibular alveolar ridge SCCA, status post composite resection, with osteocutaneous flap reconstruction, with postoperative adjuvant XRT. Negative margins, and no perivascular or lymphovascular invasion in the pathologic specimen. Postoperative course complicated by wound infection, status post incision and drainage. (A-C) Initial baseline post-treatment PET/CECT shows abnormal amorphous enhancing and hypermetabolic soft tissue in the surgical bed. Given the early postsurgical and post-treatment imaging and history of infection, this was scored an NI-RADS 2b. (D) Subsequent short-term follow-up CECT shows extensive recurrence in the surgical bed. NI-RADS 3, because the surgeon needs pathologic confirmation before treatment.

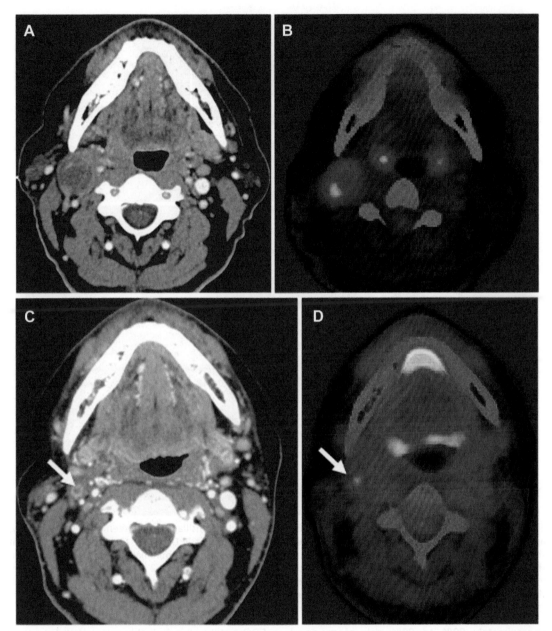

Fig. 9. NI-RADS 2, neck. T1N1 P16+ right tonsillar SCCA. (*A, B*) Initial staging PET/CECT with large necrotic right level IIA nodal mass with FDG uptake. (*C, D*) Initial baseline post-treatment PET/CECT 12 weeks after completion of therapy with focal peripheral enhancement centrally within the nodal mass, with persistent FDG uptake (*arrows*), compatible with an NI-RADS 2 in the neck.

discrete or focal enough to target for a biopsy, then it is likely prudent to wait and score the lesion as an NI-RADS 2 to reimage. Usually, waiting 3 months or waiting until a PET/CT is obtained does not change the patient's salvage options, and helps the lesion declare itself, allowing for a better biopsy target, or, as the literature shows in most cases, resolving in the interval.

NECK IMAGING REPORTING AND DATA SYSTEM CATEGORY 3

This category reflects a high suspicion for recurrence, with linked management recommendation of biopsy. The minority of scans fall into this category (approximately 5% in one study), and NI-RADS 3 category has been associated with an

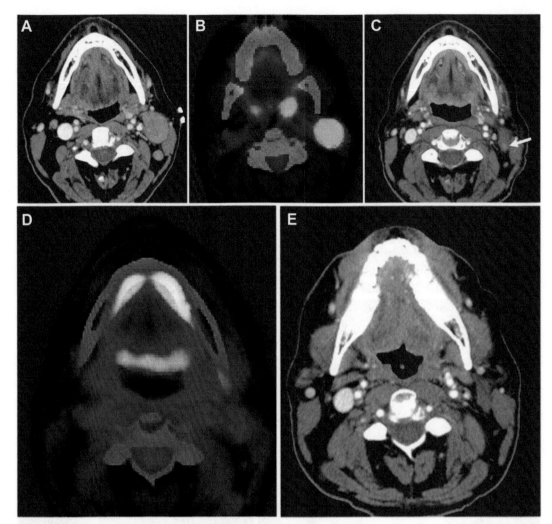

Fig. 10. NI-RADS 2, neck. (*A, B*) Initial staging PET/CECT showing a left tonsillar primary (seen on PET images only) and ipsilateral level II lymphadenopathy. (*C, D*) Baseline post-treatment PET/CECT at 12 weeks post-treatment showing residual nodal soft tissue with focal enhancement (*arrow*), but with minimal to no FDG uptake. Given the focal enhancement, this was considered discordant and scored as a NI-RADS 2 in the neck, with the recommendation for short-term follow-up. (*E*) Follow-up examination showed resolution of residual enhancement and slight continued decrease in size of residual nodal soft tissue: NI-RADS 1.

approximately 60% to 80% risk of recurrent disease.[14,15]

Primary Site

Lexicon/imaging appearance

- New or enlarging discrete nodule or mass with intense differential contrast enhancement
- Intense focal FDG uptake
- Concordant/matched findings on CECT/MR imaging and PET

When evaluating the primary site and encountering new or enlarging focal masslike enhancing soft tissue, particularly if it demonstrates intense focal FDG uptake, this is highly suspicious for recurrence, and should be assigned a NI-RADS 3, with the recommendation for biopsy (**Fig. 11**). On MR imaging, if this lesion is also associated with intermediate signal on T2-weighted images similar to the original tumor and restricted diffusion, those are additional highly suspicious features.[13]

Neck

- Morphologically abnormal lymph node with necrosis or extranodal extension of tumor
- Enlarging lymph node with intense FDG uptake

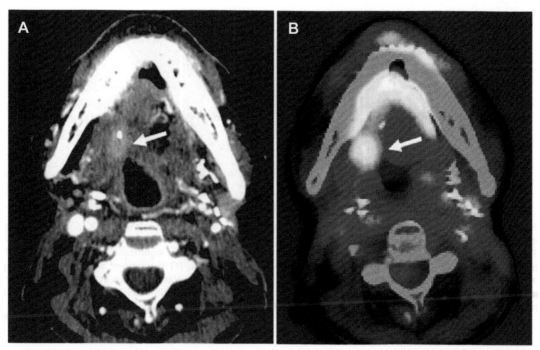

Fig. 11. NI-RADS 3, primary site. Patient with history of recurrent advanced laryngeal SCCA status post laryngectomy. (*A, B*) Surveillance post-treatment PET/CECT shows focal enhancing soft tissue and concomitant FDG uptake within the soft tissues of the base of tongue at the superior margin of the anastomosis (*arrows*). NI-RADS 3, highly suspicious for recurrent disease and recommend biopsy. This was ultimately biopsied via CT guidance and confirmed to be recurrent disease.

If one encounters a new or enlarging morphologically abnormal lymph node, with necrosis, extranodal extension of tumor, and/or intense FDG uptake, one should assign an NI-RADS 3 category and recommend biopsy.

Pearls and Pitfalls

Biopsy of mucosal recurrences is at the discretion of the referring surgeon, so some may advocate for assigning a NI-RADS 2a category to all mucosal abnormalities, allowing the surgeon to decide, because historically, radiologists are not "mucosal doctors." Additionally, the false positives in this category most often occur in the setting of radiation necrosis. However, if the abnormality develops later after the first baseline post-treatment examination, and is a new discrete abnormality, a NI-RADS 3 category is assigned, indicating to the surgeon the radiologist's high level of suspicion. For submucosal or neck recurrences, often the radiologist is involved in image-guided biopsy of abnormalities, and, as such, invested in assigning a NI-RADS 3 category to those lesions that would be a potential target for biopsy. Finally, occasionally it is challenging to determine whether to assign a NI-RADS 3, for

high suspicion versus a NI-RADS 4, definitive recurrence (eg, in the setting of a patient who is already on palliative chemotherapy for pulmonary metastasis, in the setting of development of a new, yet definitively pathologic-appearing lymph node). In that situation, talking with the referring clinician is helpful to determine if a biopsy would be necessary to determine further treatment. If that is the case, one can assign the neck a NI-RADS 3, but if it would not change management, a NI-RADS 4 score could also be assigned. In that scenario, another alternative is to assign an NI-RADS 3 score, with the recommendation for biopsy if it would change clinical management (**Fig. 12**).

NECK IMAGING REPORTING AND DATA SYSTEM CATEGORY 4

This category reflects definitive recurrence, with linked management recommendation of clinical management and treatment of known disease. NI-RADS 4 category either represents pathologically proven recurrence or definitive radiologic and/or clinical progression of disease, and is associated with a 100% risk of recurrent disease.[14,15]

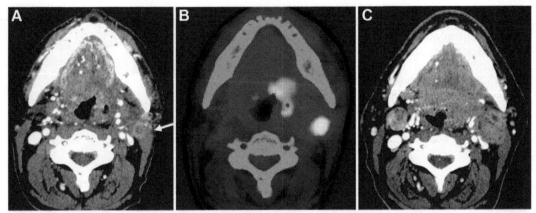

Fig. 12. NI-RADS 3, neck. (*A, B*) Patient with history of left tonsillar SCCA. Post-treatment PET/CECT demonstrates enhancing ulcerated soft tissue at the primary site, with mild FDG uptake, scored NI-RADS 2a at the primary site. There is also focal peripherally enhancing nodal soft tissue with concordant significant FDG uptake in the left level II nodal station (*arrow*). This was scored a NI-RADS 3 in the neck. (*C*) The patient was lost to follow-up and then returned with another CECT demonstrating significant progression of disease at the left oropharynx primary site, and now bilateral pathologic and necrotic lymphadenopathy. NI-RADS 3 at the primary site and neck, with recommendation for biopsy if it would change clinical management.

Primary Site and Neck

Lexicon/imaging appearance/diagnostic criteria

- Pathologic confirmation
- Unequivocal radiographic appearance

This category was originally created for those patients who have already been diagnosed with pathologically proven recurrence, and are either undergoing evaluation before salvage treatment, or on a chemotherapy trial, which requires surveillance imaging. However, it has been modified to include those patients with definitive recurrence on imaging that may not require tissue confirmation before further treatment (**Fig. 13**).

Pearls and Pitfalls

Often patients with recurrent tumor who may not have been eligible for treatment with a curative intent (ie, not a candidate for further surgical resection or radiation therapy) may be treated with a palliative intent with a chemotherapy or immunotherapy trial. As more experience and expertise with these newer chemotherapy and immunotherapy agents is gained, we are seeing more patients experience a significant response to therapy, and it can then become difficult to determine how to score them. As the imaging improves on subsequent surveillance imaging studies, the scores can be downgraded to lower scores, occasionally going from an NI-RADS 4 to a NI-RADS 2, and sometimes all the way to a NI-

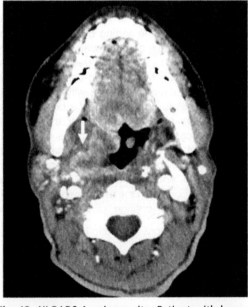

Fig. 13. NI-RADS 4, primary site. Patient with known recurrent disease on chemotherapy trial who presents for surveillance imaging with extensive recurrence and disease progression along the right oropharynx extending into the right parapharyngeal space soft tissues (*arrow*). This was pathologically proven recurrent disease, and unequivocal recurrence on imaging, compatible with NI-RADS 4

RADS 1 if the findings completely resolve. However, some may advocate that the NI-RADS template only applies to those patients being treated with a curative intent.

DISCUSSION/OUTCOMES/FUTURE DIRECTIONS

Several studies have shown moderate to strong interreader and intrareader reliability assigning NI-RADS categories, even using readers with different experience levels coming from different institutions, with significantly increased interrater agreement compared with using prose description of findings and impression without assigning NI-RADS categories.[12,17–19] A recent survey of referring physicians and radiologists after implementing NI-RADS at their institution found that 100% of referring providers and most (88%) surveyed radiologists preferred using NI-RADS over free-form dictations, because it improved consistency of reporting, and helped to provide clear, direct, actionable reports that helped to guide clinical management.[20] Future studies need to focus around applying NI-RADS categories to MR imaging examinations, and using NI-RADS to help determine the most cost-effective and appropriate surveillance imaging algorithms for different head and neck cancer types and subsites.

SUMMARY

NI-RADS is a practical tool that can help to streamline interpretation of complex post-treatment head and neck surveillance imaging studies in predicting residual and recurrent head and neck cancer, and ultimately improves patient care.

CLINICS CARE POINTS

- Neck Imaging Reporting and Data System (NI-RADS) is a novel surveillance imaging template for head and neck cancer, which has moderate to strong interrater reliability and excellent discriminatory power for helping to predict recurrent or residual disease in the post-treatment setting.
- The templates are user-friendly and preferred to free-form dictations by referring providers and radiologists alike after integration into practice.

DISCLOSURE

The author is part of the group that initiated NI-RADS and serves on the ACR NI-RADS committee.

REFERENCES

1. An JY, Unsdorfer KML, Weinreb JC, et al. TI-RADS: Reporting and Data Systems. Radiographics 2019; 39:1435–6.
2. Aiken AH, Farley A, Baugnon KL, et al. Implementation of a novel surveillance template for head and neck cancer: Neck Imaging Reporting and Data System (NI-RADS). J Am Coll Radiol 2016;13(6): 743–6.
3. Cahng J, Wu C, Yuan K, et al. Locoregionally recurrent head and neck squamous cell carcinoma: incidence, survival, prognostic factors, and treatment outcomes. Oncotarget 2017;8(33):55600–12.
4. Wierzbicka M, Napierala J. Updated National Comprehensive Cancer Network. Head and neck cancers, version 2.2014: clinical practice guidelines for treatment of head and neck cancers 2010-2017. Otolaryngol Pol 2017;21:1–6.
5. Roman BR, Patel SG, Wang MB, et al. Guideline familiarity predicts variation in self-reported use of routine surveillance PET/CT by physicians who treat head and neck cancer. J Natl Compr Canc Netw 2015;13:69–77.
6. Branstetter BF, Blodgett TM, Zimmer LA, et al. Head and neck malignancy: is PET/CT more accurate than PET or CT alone? Radiology 2005;235:580–6.
7. Beswick DM, Gooding WE, Johnson JT, et al. Temporal patterns of head and neck squamous cell carcinoma recurrence with positron-emission tomography/computed tomography monitoring. Laryngoscope 2012;122:1512–7.
8. Gore A, Baugnon KL, Beitler JJ, et al. Posttreatment imaging in patients with head and neck cancer without clinical evidence of recurrence: should surveillance imaging extend beyond 6 months? AJNR Am J Neuroradiol 2020;41(7):1238–44.
9. Voichita Bar-Ad, Mishra M, Ohri N, et al. Positron emission tomography for neck evaluation following definitive treatment with chemoradiotherapy for locoregionally advanced head and neck squamous cell carcinoma. Rev Recent Clin Trials 2012;7(1): 36–41.
10. Aiken AH, Rath TJ, Anzai Y, et al. ACR Neck Imaging Reporting and Data Systems (NI-RADS): a White Paper of the ACR NI-RADS Committee. J Am Coll Radiol 2018;15:1097–108.
11. Wangaryattawanich P, Branstetter BF, Hughes M, et al. Negative predictive value of NI-RADS category 2 in the first posttreatment FDG-PET? CT in head

and neck squamous cell carcinoma. Am J Neuroradiol 2018;39(10):1884–8.

12. Elsholtz FHJ, Erxleben C, Bauknecht HC, et al. Reliability of NI-RADS criteria in the interpretation of contrast-enhanced magnetic resonance imaging considering the potential role of diffusion-weighted imaging. Eur Radiol 2021;31(8):6295–304.

13. Ashour MM, Darwish EAF, Fahiem RM, et al. MRI posttreatment surveillance for head and neck squamous cell carcinoma: proposed MR NI-RADS criteria. Am J Neuroradiol 2021;42:1123–9.

14. Krieger D, Hudgins PA, Nayak GK, et al. Initial performance of NI-RADS to predict residual or recurrent head and neck squamous cell carcinoma. Am J Neuroradiol 2017;38(6):1193–9.

15. Dinkelborg P, Ro SR, Shnayien S, et al. Retrospective evaluation of NI-RADS for detecting postsurgical recurrence of oral squamous cell carcinoma on surveillance CT or MRI. AJR Am J Roentgenol 2021; 217:198–206.

16. Mehanna H, Wong WL, McConkey CC, et al. PET-CT surveillance versus neck dissection in advanced head and neck cancer. N Engl J Med 2016;374: 1444–54.

17. Hsu D, Rath TJ, Branstetter BF, et al. Interrater reliability of NI-RADS on posttreatment PET/contrast enhanced CT scans in head and neck squamous cell carcinoma. Radiol Imaging Cancer 2021. https://doi.org/10.11148/ryca2021200131.

18. Abdelazia TT, Razk AAKA, Ashour MMM, et al. Inter-reader reproducibility of the Neck Imaging Reporting and Data System (NI-RADS) lexicon for the detection of residual/recurrent disease in treated head and neck squamous cell carcinoma. Cancer Imaging 2020;20:6†.

19. Elsholtz FHJ, Ro SR, Shnayeien S, et al. Impact of double reading on NI-RADS diagnostic accuracy in reporting oral squamous cell carcinoma surveillance imaging: a single center study. Dentomaxillofac Radiol 2021. https://doi.org/10.1259/dmfr.20210168.

20. Bunch PM, Meegalla NT, Abualruz AR, et al. Initial referring physician and radiologist experience with Neck Imaging Reporting and Data System. Laryngoscope 2021. https://doi.org/10.1002/lary.29765.

Lymph Node Dissection
Principles and Postoperative Imaging

David Joyner, MD[a], Tanvir Rizvi, MD[a], Tuba Kalelioglu, MD[a], Mark J. Jameson, MD[b], Sugoto Mukherjee, MD[a],*

KEYWORDS

- Lymph node • Neck dissection • Post treated neck • Head and neck cancer • NI-RADS
- Surveillance imaging

KEY POINTS

- The management of metastatic nodal disease is a key part of treatment of head and neck cancers.
- The neck can be managed with a variety of surgical methods, as well as by radiation with or without chemotherapy.
- Knowledge of the typical methods and extent of nodal dissections (as well as the related understanding of the typical nodal basins involved for different primary tumor sites) aids interpretation of post-treatment imaging and further treatment planning.
- To decrease variability, reporting methodology from the Neck Imaging and Reporting Data System should be used for post-treatment surveillance imaging.

INTRODUCTION AND HISTORY

Metastatic lymph node spread of squamous cell carcinomas of head and neck portends poor prognosis and survival. Neck dissection in its different forms comprises the bulwark of surgical treatment for clinical and subclinical metastatic neck cancer. Although neck dissections have been performed for the past 200 years, the major underlying principles of neck dissection surgeries are based on seminal works of George Washington Crile and Hayes Martin in the early and mid-20th century. Martin in his landmark article titled "Neck Dissection" in 1951 emphasized that the spinal accessory nerve, internal jugular vein, and the sternocleidomastoid muscle should be removed in the presence of cervical lymph node metastasis.[1] This approach was the norm for head and neck surgeons until the latter part of the twentieth century, when modifications of the radical dissection technique started being accepted.

The morbidity associated with radical neck dissection (RND) especially related to shoulder function resulted in modifications, resulting in various conservative surgeries also referred to as functional neck dissections. The concept of selective nodal dissection was introduced by Byers in 1985.[2] The present classification of neck nodal surgeries is based on Shah's landmark article from 1990, where he classified the deep lymph nodes of the neck into 5 different levels assigned Roman numerals from I through V.[3] In 2002, the current standard classification of neck dissections was proposed by the American Head and Neck Society and the American Academy of Otolaryngology–Head and Neck Surgery,[4] which classifies and describes radical neck dissection, extended neck dissection, modified radical neck dissection and selective neck dissection.[4]

Four major changes over the last 40 years have led to a continued refinement and evolution of the

[a] Department of Radiology and Medical Imaging, University of Virginia Health System, Charlottesville, VA 22903, USA; [b] Department of Otolaryngology–Head and Neck Surgery, University of Virginia Health System, Charlottesville, VA 22903, USA
* Corresponding author. Department of Radiology and Medical Imaging, University of Virginia Health System, PO Box 800170, 1215 Lee Street, Charlottesville, VA 22908-0170.
E-mail address: sm5qd@virginia.edu

Neuroimag Clin N Am 32 (2022) 19–36
https://doi.org/10.1016/j.nic.2021.09.001

neck dissections. The first of these was the advent of cross-sectional imaging, including computed tomography (CT), MR imaging, and PET studies, which have led to more accurate preoperative assessment of neck disease and subsequent increase in selective nodal dissections. Second, the shift in thinking from the resection of tumors and wound closure to an increased emphasis on establishing normal function and appearance has led to newer techniques and advances in head and neck reconstructive surgery. A third major change has involved the remarkable improvements in radiotherapy (RT) over the past few decades, which has now led to a large subset of patients with head and neck cancer undergoing RT as their primary treatment or as adjuvant therapy after surgery, which has led to a gradual shift toward nonsurgical management. Last, the exponential increase in human papillomavirus (HPV)–associated oropharyngeal cancers involving a younger subset of patients, who also have better outcomes, has led to a fundamental rethinking of the role of surgery. As a consequence of all these improvements, a paradigm shift has taken place from curative primary surgery to function–preservation RT and other nonsurgical options in many patients.

IMAGING IN THE POST-TREATMENT HEAD NECK

Imaging in the post-treatment neck depends on the early versus late stage presentation of the head and neck cancer, which dictates management as well as the extent of the disease. Typically, early stage head and neck cancers are treated with either RT or surgery. Locally advanced head and neck cancers without distant metastasis require multimodal treatment, which usually consists of a combination of curative surgery followed by adjuvant RT, with or without chemotherapy. The overall imaging appearance in the treated neck depends on effects of RT, surgery for the primary site (with or without reconstruction) and the type of neck dissection (radical neck dissection, selective neck dissection, etc).

Early post-RT changes include reticulation of the subcutaneous fatty tissues; thickening of the skin, fascial tissues, and platysma; thickening with increased enhancement of the pharyngeal walls and mucosal surfaces; and hyperenhancement of the major salivary glands (Fig. 1). Later findings include loss of neck fat, atrophy of the salivary glands, and thickening of fascia, platysma, and constrictor muscles (see Fig. 1).

Expected changes after RT in the neck nodes include decreased size of pathologic nodes, development of irregular nodal margins, increased perinodal fat reticulation, and edema in the adjacent superficial and deep neck spaces along, with thickening of the adjacent fasciae (Fig. 2). The decreased size of the larger pathologic neck nodes on a contrast-enhanced CT scan alone is not a reliable predictor of residual disease, and an accompanying PET scan with fluorine-18-2-fluoro-2-deoxy-D-glucose (FDG-PET) scan may be essential in excluding residual nodal disease (see Fig. 2).

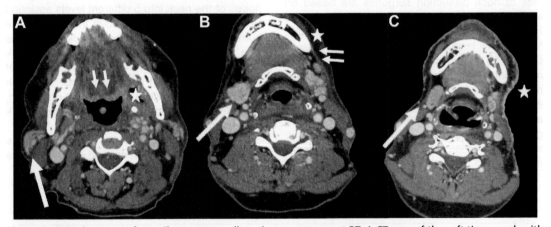

Fig. 1. Post-RT changes. Left tonsil squamous cell carcinoma status post RT. A CT scan of the soft tissue neck with contrast axial section (A) at the tonsillar level shows hyperenhancement of both parotid glands (solid white arrow), enhancement of tongue base/pharyngeal mucosa (white double arrows) and partially necrotic left tonsillar mass (white star). Further inferior axial section (B) shows reticulation of the subcutaneous fatty tissues (white star), thickening of the skin, fascial tissues, and platysma (white double arrows) and hyper enhancement of the submandibular glands (solid white arrow). Follow-up CT scan of the soft tissue neck 1 year later (C) shows delayed postradiation changes with loss of neck fat, thickening of the skin (white arrow), and atrophy of the submandibular glands (solid white arrow).

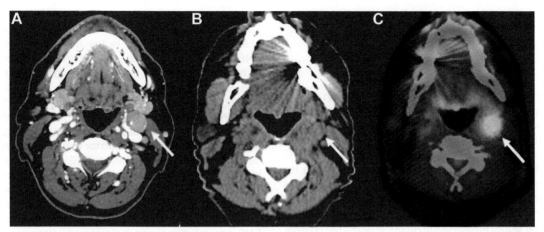

Fig. 2. Post-RT changes in neck lymph node. A p16+, cT0pN1M0 squamous cell carcinoma status post biopsy of the left oropharynx. A CT scan of the soft tissue neck with contrast (*A*) shows a pathologic left level IIA node without extranodal extension (*solid white arrow*). Noncontrast CT status post radiation to the left oropharynx and unilateral regional lymph node area shows a decreased size of the enlarged left neck lymph node (*solid white arrow*) (*B*). A decrease in the in size of the lymph node is not a reliable predictor for predicting residual disease, and FDG-PET scan (*C*) shows uptake (*solid white arrow*), representing residual nodal disease.

The post-treatment appearance at the primary tumor location after surgery depends on the site and size of the primary defect, as well as the type of reconstruction performed. The changes after RT and complex neck reconstructions are covered in further details in separate articles elsewhere in this issue. The major types of neck dissection, the underlying principles and their imaging appearance are discussed elsewhere in this article.

In the post-treatment setting, both contrast-enhanced CT scans and contrast-enhanced MR imaging are relatively insensitive in identifying residual or recurrent nodal disease, with PET/CT scans having much greater sensitivity and specificity. Conventional imaging criteria for recurrent or residual nodal disease in a post-treatment neck include an increase in size (typically using similar size thresholds as those on staging scans), necrosis, abnormal morphology, or evidence of extranodal extension (ENE). A combined FDG-PET/contrast-enhanced CT scan represents the best imaging modality to exclude residual/recurrent cancers, especially in the early post-RT setting, and has the highest negative predictive value.[5]

If the diagnosis is unclear on a CT scan or MR imaging, or tissue confirmation is necessary, most cervical nodes are readily accessible via fine needle aspiration. Ultrasound guidance is sufficient for most nodal groups, although some deeper nodes (ie, retropharyngeal) may require CT guidance.

PRINCIPLES OF NECK DISSECTION SURGERY

Squamous cell carcinomas of the head and neck commonly metastasize to cervical lymph **nodes;** even in patients without clinical or imaging evidence of nodal disease, occult metastases are often present. The management of the lymph nodes is a key part of improving survival, and can be accomplished by surgical resection or RT. For non–HPV-related disease, stages I and II suggest a small primary lesion without nodal disease, whereas stages III and IV include larger primary lesions with invasion of adjacent structures and/or lymph node metastasis.

Owing to the prevalence of occult nodal disease, elective neck dissections are often performed in patients who clinically have N0 disease and are undergoing surgical resection of the primary tumor. Early nodal disease (N1/2a) is also managed with selective neck dissection when the primary is treated surgically. In patients who present with locoregionally (N2b/2c/3) advanced disease who are being treated primarily with surgery, neck dissections (possibly radical or modified radical) are performed for treatment of the nodal disease as well as for staging.

Alternatively, in patients for whom the primary tumor is being treated with RT with or without chemotherapy, the neck may also be managed initially via (chemo)radiation with neck dissection deferred for use as salvage therapy if there is evidence of residual or recurrent nodal disease on clinical examination or imaging.

NODAL STAGING AND CHANGES IN THE AMERICAN JOINT COMMITTEE ON CANCER/UNION FOR INTERNATIONAL CANCER CONTROL CANCER STAGING MANUAL, EIGHTH EDITION

From an imaging perspective, a thorough understanding of the various radiologic landmarks, which are used as boundaries, is essential in accurate staging of lymph node groups[6] (**Fig. 3**). These boundaries have been summarized in **Table 1**. Although a complete review of nodal staging for head and neck cancer is beyond the scope of this article, it is worthwhile to review some of the important changes made to the nodal staging in the eighth edition of the American Joint Committee on Cancer's Cancer Staging Manual.[7,8]

One of the major changes involves introduction of different clinical and pathologic N classifications for staging regional lymph node metastasis. Both clinical TNM (cTNM) and pathologic (pTNM) classifications have different purposes. The cTNM classification applies to all patients whether they undergo surgery or nonsurgical therapy. The pTNM classifications provides additional information (high-risk histopathological features of the primary site, ENE, volume of nodal disease, etc),

which is only available after surgery and allows for additional adjuvant treatment.

Another major change is the introduction of ENE, which is now a part of N classification for all head and neck sites other than nasopharyngeal and HPV-associated oropharyngeal cancers. Although imaging findings may suggest or support ENE (irregular margin, infiltration of adjacent fat planes or other soft tissue structures), imaging findings alone are not sufficient for the designation as ENE positive[9] (**Fig. 4**). Clinical ENE is defined as invasion of skin, muscle infiltration, tethering or fixation to adjacent structures, or cranial nerve, brachial plexus, sympathetic trunk, or phrenic nerve invasion with dysfunction[10]; alternatively, ENE can be diagnosed histologically after neck dissection.

A change in the prognostic significance of T and N stages of oropharyngeal cancer over time[11] in part led to the adoption of a new staging system for HPV-associated (p16-positive) oropharyngeal cancers. The clinical nodal staging for HPV-associated oropharyngeal cancer in the eighth edition is based on node laterality and size, as summarized in **Table 2**. Pathologic staging for HPV-associated oropharyngeal cancer, in contrast, is based on the number of nodes involved, as detailed in **Table 3**. The clinical nodal staging for all non-HPV, non–Epstein-Barr virus squamous cell cancers is summarized in **Table 4**. Last, nasopharyngeal carcinomas, which are usually Epstein-Barr virus related, and are often nonkeratinizing carcinomas, have a modified nodal staging, which is summarized in **Table 5**.

NECK DISSECTION CLASSIFICATION

The classification system for cervical lymph nodal dissection, which is currently in most widespread use, was defined in a 2001 proposal by the American Head and Neck Society and the American Academy of Otolaryngology–Head and Neck Surgery.[4] In this classification, the core categories of neck dissections are radical neck dissection, modified radical neck dissection, selective neck dissection, and extended neck dissection (**Table 6**).

Radical Neck Dissection

A radical neck dissection removes all lymph nodes from levels I to V ipsilateral to the tumor. The ipsilateral internal jugular vein, sternocleidomastoid muscle, and spinal accessory nerve are sacrificed (**Fig. 5**). Of note, a radical dissection does not include all nodal groups; for example, the suboccipital, periparotid, buccinator, retropharyngeal, and

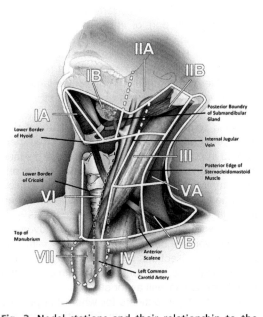

Fig. 3. Nodal stations and their relationship to the relevant anatomic landmarks for an imaging-based classification. (*From* Mukherjee S, Jameson MJ, Wintermark M, Raghavan P. Lymph Nodes. In: Raghavan P, Mukherjee S. Jameson MJ. Wintermark M, editors. Manual of Head and Neck Imaging, pp.29-52. with permission. (Fig 3 and Box 1 in original).)

Table 1
Imaging-based nodal classification

Levels	Boundaries				
	Superior	Inferior	Anterior (Medial)	Posterior (Lateral)	
IA Submental group	Symphysis of mandible	Body of hyoid	Anterior belly of contralateral digastric muscle	Anterior belly of ipsilateral digastric muscle	
IB Submandibular group	Body of mandible	Posterior belly of digastric muscle	Anterior belly of digastric muscle	Stylohyoid muscle	
IIA Upper jugular group nodes	Skull base	Horizontal plane defined by the inferior border of hyoid bone	Stylohyoid muscle	Vertical plane defined by the spinal accessory nerve	
IIB Upper jugular group nodes	Skull base	Horizontal plane defined by the inferior border of hyoid bone	Vertical plane defined by the spinal accessory nerve	Lateral border of the sternocleidomastoid muscle	
III Mid jugular group	Horizontal plane defined by the inferior border of hyoid bone	Horizontal plane defined by the inferior border of cricoid cartilage	Lateral border of the sternohyoid muscle	Lateral border of the sternocleidomastoid muscle or sensory branches of the cervical plexus	
IV Lower jugular group	Horizontal plane defined by the inferior border of cricoid cartilage	Clavicle	Lateral border of the sternohyoid muscle	Lateral border of the sternocleidomastoid muscle or sensory branches of the cervical plexus	
VA Posterior triangle group	Apex of the convergence of sternocleidomastoid and trapezius muscles	Horizontal plane defined by the inferior border of the cricoid cartilage	Lateral border of the sternocleidomastoid muscle or sensory branches of the cervical plexus	Anterior border of the trapezius muscle	
VB Posterior triangle group	Horizontal plane defined by the inferior border of cricoid cartilage	Clavicle	Lateral border of the sternocleidomastoid muscle or sensory branches of the cervical plexus	Anterior border of the trapezius muscle	

(continued on next page)

Table 1
(continued)

| Levels | Boundaries | | | |
	Superior	Inferior	Anterior (Medial)	Posterior (Lateral)
VI Central or anterior group	Hyoid bone	Top of manubrium	Common carotid artery	Common carotid artery
VII Superior mediastinal group	Top of manubrium	Inominate vein	Common carotid artery	Common carotid artery

Note: Other superficial nodal groups continue to be referred to by their anatomic names including parotid, facial, post auricular, etc. lymph nodes.
Modified from Mukherjee S, Jameson MJ, Wintermark M, Raghavan P. Lymph Nodes. In: Raghavan P, Mukherjee S. Jameson MJ. Wintermark M, editors. Manual of Head and Neck Imaging, pp.29 to 52.

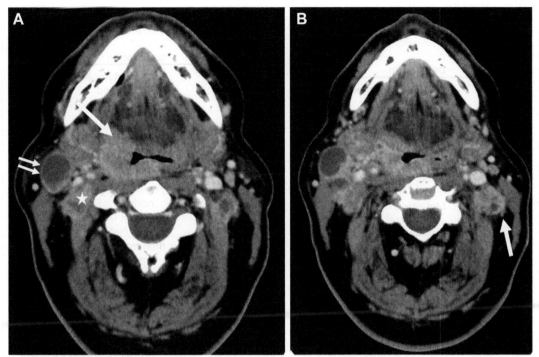

Fig. 4. Extracapsular nodal extension: CT soft tissue neck axial section (*A*) in a case of right tonsil squamous cell carcinoma shows a poorly defined right tonsillar enhancing primary mass (*solid white arrow*). Multiple enlarged, and necrotic bilateral cervical lymph nodes are present including a predominantly cystic right level IIA lymph node (*white double arrows*). Another more posterior necrotic right level II lymph node (*white star* in *A*) also shows extracapsular extension, with loss of adjacent fat places. Further inferior axial section (*B*) shows a left level II node which also shows extracapsular extension with irregular margins (*white solid arrow*) with subtle infiltration of adjacent fat planes.

Table 2
Clinical nodal staging for HPV-related oropharyngeal squamous cell cancers

Stage	Description
Nx	Regional lymph nodes cannot be assessed
N0	No regional lymph node metastasis
N1	One or more ipsilateral lymph nodes, none larger than 6 cm
N2	Contralateral or bilateral lymph nodes, none >6 cm
N3	Lymph node(s) >6 cm

Modified from Lydiatt WM, Patel SG, O'Sullivan B, Brandwein MS, Ridge JA, Migliacci JC, Loomis AM, Shah JP. Head and Neck cancers-major changes in the American Joint Committee on cancer eighth edition cancer staging manual. CA Cancer J Clin. 2017 Mar;67(2):122 to 137.

Table 3
Pathologic assessment of regional lymph nodes (pN) in HPV-related (p16-positive) oropharyngeal cancers

Stage	Description
pNX	Regional lymph nodes cannot be assessed
pN0	No regional lymph node metastasis
pN1	Metastasis in ≤4 lymph nodes
pN2	Metastases in >4 lymph nodes

Modified from Lydiatt WM, Patel SG, O'Sullivan B, Brandwein MS, Ridge JA, Migliacci JC, Loomis AM, Shah JP. Head and Neck cancers-major changes in the American Joint Committee on cancer eighth edition cancer staging manual. CA Cancer J Clin. 2017 Mar;67(2):122 to 137.

Table 4
Clinical nodal staging for all non-HPV, non–Epstein-Barr virus squamous cell cancers

Stage	Description
Nx	Regional lymph nodes cannot be assessed
N0	No regional lymph node metastasis
N1	Metastasis in a single ipsilateral lymph node ≤3 cm in greatest dimension and ENE−
N2a	Metastasis in a single ipsilateral lymph node >3 cm but ≤6 cm in greatest dimension and ENE−
N2b	Metastasis in multiple ipsilateral nodes, none >6 cm in greatest dimension and ENE−
N2c	Metastasis in bilateral or contralateral lymph node(s), none >6 cm in greatest dimension and ENE−
N3a	Metastasis in a lymph node >6 cm in greatest dimension and ENE−
N3b	Metastasis in any node(s) with clinically overt ENE+ (ENEc)

Modified from Lydiatt WM, Patel SG, O'Sullivan B, Brandwein MS, Ridge JA, Migliacci JC, Loomis AM, Shah JP. Head and Neck cancers-major changes in the American Joint Committee on cancer eighth edition cancer staging manual. CA Cancer J Clin. 2017 Mar;67(2):122 to 137.

Table 5
Nodal staging for nasopharyngeal carcinomas

Stage	Description
NX	Regional lymph nodes cannot be assessed
N0	No regional lymph node metastasis
N1	Unilateral metastasis in cervical lymph node(s) and/or unilateral or bilateral metastasis in retropharyngeal lymph node(s), ≤6 cm, above the caudal border of cricoid cartilage
N2	Bilateral metastasis in cervical lymph node(s), ≤6 cm, above the caudal border of cricoid cartilage
N3	Unilateral or bilateral metastasis in cervical lymph node(s), >6 cm, and/or extension below the caudal border of cricoid cartilage

Modified from Lydiatt WM, Patel SG, O'Sullivan B, Brandwein MS, Ridge JA, Migliacci JC, Loomis AM, Shah JP. Head and Neck cancers-major changes in the American Joint Committee on cancer eighth edition cancer staging manual. CA Cancer J Clin. 2017 Mar;67(2):122 to 137.

anterior compartment nodes are typically excluded.[4]

Modified Radical Neck Dissection

A modified radical neck dissection also removes all ipsilateral lymph nodes from levels I to V, but spares at least one of the internal jugular vein, sternocleidomastoid, or spinal accessory nerve; commonly all 3 structures are spared (**Fig. 6**).

Although a radical neck dissection is considered the basic procedure from which other neck dissection methods are derived,[4] it is less commonly performed in current clinical practice. Radical neck dissection is associated with greater morbidity, particularly related to shoulder pain and dysfunction resulting from spinal accessory nerve sacrifice. In addition, if bilateral neck dissections are necessary, sacrifice of the bilateral internal jugular veins may result in severe facial swelling[12] or

other vascular complications. The modified radical neck dissection addresses the morbidity associated with the radical neck dissection by preserving structures that are uninvolved by tumor. A radical neck dissection is now often reserved for patients with extensive nodal disease, particularly with involvement of the spinal accessory nerve and/or internal jugular vein.

Selective Neck Dissection

Selective neck dissection spares at least 1 nodal group that would typically be removed in a radical dissection (**Fig. 7**). The most likely drainage routes of the primary tumor site are selected for removal; a tumor is unlikely to have skip metastases in more distant nodal groups without involvement of the more proximal nodal basins.

An earlier classification system from 1991 included designations of supraomohyoid, lateral, posterolateral, and anterior neck dissections; for clarity, the 2001 classification recommends naming these as selective neck dissection followed by the levels/groups removed in parentheses. Some examples of typical selective dissections can be seen in **Table 7**.

Table 6
Neck dissection classification

Type of Neck Dissection	Lymph Node Levels Removed	Nonlymphatic Structures Removed
Radical neck dissection	I, II, III, IV, V	Sternocleidomastoid muscle, internal jugular vein, spinal accessory nerve
Modified radical neck dissection Type I Type II Type III	I, II, III, IV, V I–V I–V I–V	Sparing ≥1 of the following: Sternocleidomastoid muscle, internal jugular vein, spinal accessory nerve Ipsilateral SCM and internal jugular vein removed, spinal accessory preserved Ipsilateral SCM removed, internal jugular vein and spinal accessory preserved Ipsilateral SCM, internal jugular vein and spinal accessory preserved
Selective neck dissection	Preservation of one or more lymph node stations compared with radical neck dissection	SCM, internal jugular vein, and spinal accessory preserved
Extended neck dissection (END)	I, II, III, IV, V and additional nodal stations	Structures removed in radical neck dissection and additional structures such as carotid artery, overlying skin, strap and paraspinal muscles, platysma, hypoglossal and vagus nerves.
Central compartment neck dissection	VI, pre- and paratracheal, precricoid (Delphian) and perithyroidal Can be unilateral or bilateral	Total thyroidectomy or thyroid lobectomy

A selective dissection of level II may or may not involve both the IIA and IIB groups; removal of IIB nodes carries increased morbidity compared with IIA owing to manipulation of the spinal accessory nerve. Level IIB is more commonly involved in oropharyngeal cancers and thus commonly included in a selective neck dissection for this site, although it may be left out of selective neck dissection for oral cavity or laryngeal tumors.

A selective neck dissection (VI) (sometimes referred to as a central compartment dissection) involves the removal of all lymph nodes from level VI, including the paratracheal, precricoid, and perithyroidal nodes. Level VI dissection may be unilateral or bilateral and is frequently combined with total thyroidectomy or lobectomy for differentiated thyroid cancers (**Fig. 8**).

Selective neck dissections can be used in cases of limited neck disease without evidence of infiltration of nonlymphatic structures; selective neck dissection is also used in staging of the neck in patients who are negative clinically for nodal disease and are being managed primarily by surgery, particularly when the risk of occult metastasis is high.

If a primary tumor is initially managed with radiation with or without chemotherapy, this procedure may be followed by either planned or salvage neck dissection. A planned dissection usually occurs 1 to 2 months after RT and may be performed to assess residual disease in the setting of extensive nodal metastases at initial presentation. Alternatively, if the initial nodal disease burden is low, the patient may be observed after initial RT, with neck dissection reserved as a salvage therapy if there is evidence of persistent or recurrent disease.

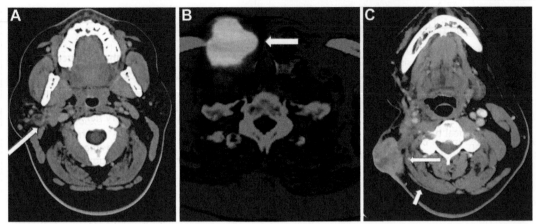

Fig. 5. Radical neck dissection with recurrence and trapezius atrophy. Adenocarcinoma of the right parotid gland with intraparotid lymphadenopathy (*arrow*) (*A*). Three years after right parotidectomy and right radical neck dissection (levels IIB, IIA, III, IV, and VA), with concomitant chemotherapy and RT, the patient presented with large right supraclavicular metastatic lesion with a maximum standardized uptake value of 26 on a PET scan (*arrow*) (*B*). Subsequent recurrence in the posterior cervical space (*long arrow*), 8 months after right radical neck dissection, right thyroid lobectomy, right clavicle resection, central neck dissection, right axillary dissection, and creation of a skin rotation–advancement flap. Right trapezius muscle denervation atrophy changes secondary to sacrificed right spinal accessory nerve (*short arrow*) (*C*).

Extended Neck Dissection

Extended neck dissection refers to removal of at least 1 additional nodal group (eg, retropharyngeal or buccinator nodes) or nonlymphatic structure

(eg, carotid artery or hypoglossal nerve), which is not removed as a part of a standard radical neck dissection.

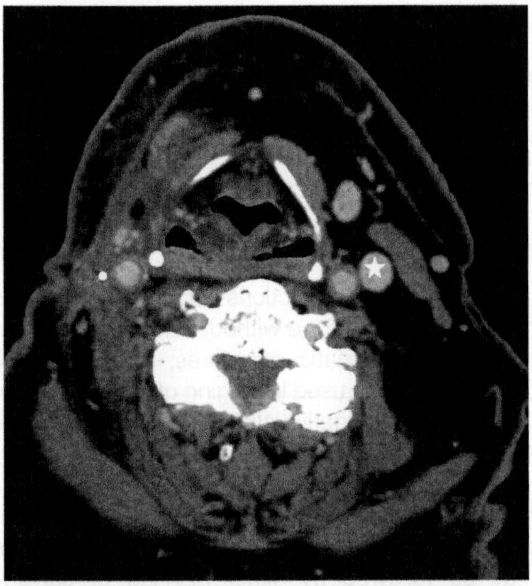

Fig. 6. Modified radical neck dissection. The right internal jugular vein is absent (compare with the *star* on left), but the sternocleidomastoid and spinal accessory nerve were preserved in this patient. There are typical postoperative and postradiation changes present on the right, including a loss of fat planes, amorphous soft tissue, subcutaneous reticulation, and platysma thickening, as well as surgical clips from the previous nodal dissection.

Sentinel Node Biopsy

Although not included in the 2001 classification schema, sentinel node biopsy is commonly performed for melanoma and has also been studied for some mucosal primary tumor sites in the neck, particularly early stage oral cavity cancers. Many patients with head and neck cancer who are negative clinically for nodal disease undergo elective neck dissections, but a significant portion of these will be negative for metastases meaning that the resection may not have been necessary. Sentinel node biopsy is an alternate technique that potentially could identify early sites of nodal involvement, leading to less extensive neck dissections and, as a result, decreased morbidity. Sentinel node biopsy involves the injection of a radiopharmaceutical, dye, or both at the site of a tumor, followed by removal of the initial node or group of nodes to take up the agent (**Fig. 9**). These sentinel nodes are then examined for the presence of tumor to determine whether further nodal treatment is warranted. Although routinely used for breast cancer and melanoma, sentinel node biopsy is not yet common in noncutaneous head and neck cancers. There is increasing evidence that sentinel node biopsy is promising in early stage oral cancer with clinical N0 staging, with

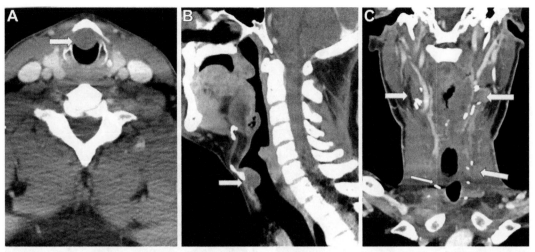

Fig. 7. Bilateral selective neck dissections in a case of adenoid cystic carcinoma of the subglottis. A hypoenhancing nodule arising from the anterior wall of the subglottis with moderate narrowing of the airway (*long arrow*) (*A, B*). Status post total laryngectomy and bilateral selective neck dissections (left IIA, IIB, III, IV; right IIA, III, IV). Surgical clips of bilateral selective neck dissections (*arrows*) (*C*).

decreased morbidity compared with elective dissection and potentially similar outcomes.[13–15]

Salvage Neck Dissection

The management of residual neck nodes after chemoradiation, especially in locally advanced head and neck cancers, may require salvage neck dissection. Given the poor outcomes of neck salvage surgery in these patients, careful evaluation of the residual/recurrent neck disease, comorbid conditions, and the post-RT neck

Table 7	
Selective neck dissection levels	

Site of Primary	Typical selective Dissection Levels
Oral cavity	I–III (bilateral if midline structures involved)
Oropharynx, hypopharynx, larynx	II–IV
Midline anterior lower neck	VI
Cutaneous posterior scalp/upper neck	II–V, postauricular, suboccipital
Cutaneous preauricular, anterior scalp, temporal	II–III, VA, external jugular, parotid, facial
Cutaneous anterior/ lateral face	I–III, parotid, facial

fibrosis is required. The role of imaging and image-guided biopsy is critical in detecting residual/recurrent diseases and planning the extent of surgery. In addition to selective nodal dissection, the term superselective nodal dissection has gained vogue in these scenarios, providing better functional outcomes. Superselective nodal dissections refers to compartmental removal of lymph nodes, and all fibrofatty tissue contents within the defined boundaries of 1 or 2 contiguous nodal levels.[16] Superselective neck dissection can be used both in the elective treatment of a clinical N0 neck (as an alternative to sentinel node biopsy), salvage treatment of persistent lymph node disease after (chemo)RT, and in residual nodal disease in papillary thyroid carcinomas.[17]

RECONSTRUCTION AFTER NECK DISSECTION

Reconstruction after neck dissection depends primarily on the oncological defect related to the resection, and reconstruction needs of the primary site. Most modern head and neck reconstructions use either surgical flaps or grafts, which are distinguished by the presence of their own blood supply (in flaps) versus neoangiogenesis (in grafts). These are covered in detail in a separate article in this issue. Imaging evaluation in this complex setting requires a careful analysis of the presurgical imaging and review of the operative notes. Assessment of the post-treatment imaging requires a thorough evaluation of the primary site, which includes inspection of the flap itself and its margins with the resection site, as well as the rest of the neck soft tissues.[18] Knowledge of flap complications both

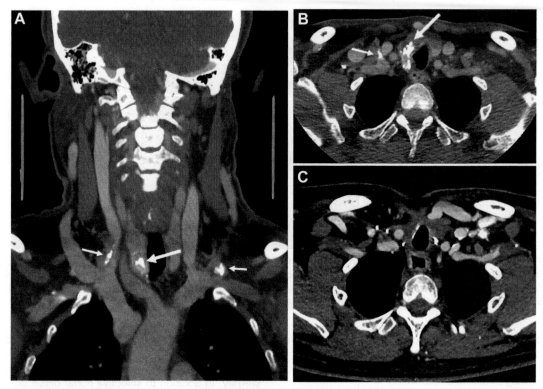

Fig. 8. Selective neck dissection in a case of papillary thyroid carcinoma. Coronal (*A*) and axial (*B*) CT images at the time of initial presentation demonstrate a calcified mass in the right thyroid (*thick arrows*) with metastatic involvement of multiple bilateral cervical lymph nodes (*thin arrows*) (*A, B*). After undergoing thyroidectomy and extensive neck dissection (including central compartment nodal dissection), a follow-up CT scan (*C*) shows surgical clips and amorphous soft tissue, but no residual enhancing thyroid tissue.

in the immediate setting (such as ischemia or infarctions) as well as in a delayed setting (such as dehiscence, fistulas, infections, or necrosis) is essential. In many cases, the presence of baseline imaging is critical. Head and neck radiologists should be prepared for nodal recurrences at the expected drainage pathways, as well as in unusual locations owing to altered anatomy after resection and reconstruction. The primary site should be assessed for tumor recurrence particularly at the flap tissue or resection cavity margins, looking for mass-like lesions with enhancement, similar to the original tumor.[19]

COMPLICATIONS OF NECK DISSECTION SURGERY

A radical neck dissection necessitates the sacrifice of the spinal accessory nerve, commonly leading to shoulder pain and dysfunction. This particular complication was a major factor in adoption of the modified radical neck dissection as an alternative method of neck management.

In addition, other nerves can potentially be injured, including the facial nerve, marginal mandibular nerve, phrenic nerve, vagus nerve, hypoglossal nerve, lingual nerve, greater auricular nerve, or sympathetic chain.[20]

Sacrifice of the internal jugular vein may lead to facial or laryngeal edema, intracranial pressure elevation, stroke, or blindness[20]; alternatively, if the internal jugular vein is preserved, thrombosis or hemorrhage can occur after surgery.

Carotid artery rupture is associated with a high mortality rate. Risk factors include tumor involvement of the arterial wall, wound breakdown, pharyngocutaneous fistula, and infection.[21] Endovascular repair has decreased mortality compared with open surgical repair for carotid blowout.[22] Endovascular methods for controlling carotid rupture include carotid occlusion, embolization or covered stent placement[21] (**Fig. 10**).

Chyle leak may occur, particularly if there is injury to the thoracic duct or, less commonly, the right lymphatic duct.

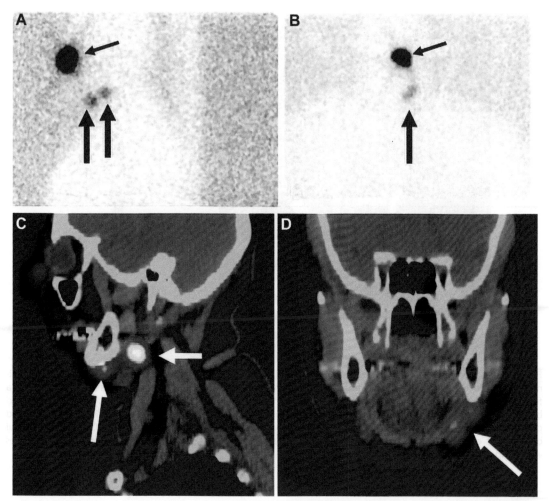

Fig. 9. Sentinel node imaging. A patient with a left cheek melanoma undergoing sentinel node mapping with technetium-99m–labeled sulfur colloid. Left lateral (*A*) and anterior (*B*) planar images demonstrate uptake at the injection site (*thin arrows*) as well as left level IB and II lymph nodes (*thick arrows*). Corresponding sagittal and coronal SPECT/CT images (*C* and *D*, respectively) confirm the localization (*thick arrows*) and provide increased anatomic detail for surgical planning.

NECK IMAGING AND REPORTING DATA SYSTEM AND IMAGING SURVEILLANCE

Post-treatment surveillance imaging in head and neck cancer represents a multifactorial challenge. This is due to a combination of inherent overlap of imaging findings in recurrent disease and post-treatment findings as well as lack of standardized imaging protocols, management recommendations and reporting templates. The Neck Imaging Reporting and Data Systems (NI-RADS) attempts to address all these issues along with the added objectives of improving patient communication and building an easily referable standardized database for future research. NI-RADS is also now part of the ACR Reporting and Data Systems (RADS) which provide standardized imaging terminology,

report organization, assessment structure and classification for reporting and data collection in patient imaging and is referred to as ACR-NI-RADS.[23]

For the purposes of this article, we will focus on the NI-RADS as it applies to regional nodes in the post-treatment setting. A separate article in this same issue is dedicated entirely to NI-RADS. The ACR-NI-RADS lexicon, categories and management recommendations are summarized in **Table 8**. The NI-RADS lexicon for lymph nodes uses the morphologic appearance of the residual nodal tissue (margins, necrosis), its evolving size (stable or increasing) and FDG uptake (none, mild or intense) (**Figs. 11** and **12**).

Surveillance imaging in the first 6 months after treatment has been a source of concern owing to

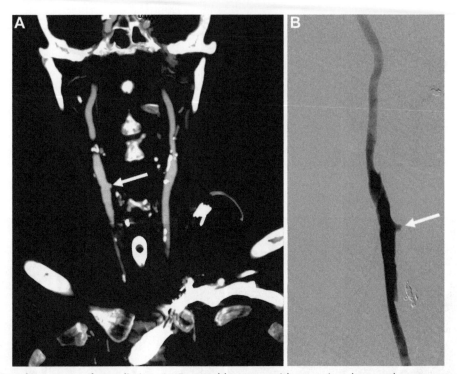

Fig. 10. Pseudoaneurysm after radiation. A 47-year-old woman with a previous laryngeal squamous cell carcinoma. She developed a pharyngocutaneous fistula and retropharyngeal abscess 10 years after treatment; a few days after drainage of her abscess, she returned to the emergency department with profuse bright red bleeding from the fistula site after coughing. CT Angiography of the neck (*A*) showed a right common carotid pseudoaneurysm (*thick arrow*), which was subsequently confirmed by catheter angiography (*B*). After a successful balloon test occlusion of the right internal carotid artery, the right distal common and internal carotid arteries were embolized with coils.

a lack of standardization, more so in asymptomatic patients who fall under NI-RADS category 1. The only available guideline from the National Comprehensive Cancer Network recommends imaging within the first 6 months. A consensus surveillance imaging algorithm as discussed in the ACR-NI-RADS White Paper suggests a FDG-PET/contrast-enhanced CT scan at 8 to 12 weeks after completion of definitive therapy as a baseline, followed by another contrast-enhanced CT or FDG-PET/contrast-enhanced CT scan 6 months later, if negative. If 2 consecutive FDG-PET/contrast-enhanced CT scans are negative, then surveillance imaging can be stopped. If only contrast-enhanced CT scanning is being done, another contrast-enhanced CT scan of the neck is recommended at 6 months, which is followed by a contrast-enhanced CT scan of the neck and chest 12 months later if the second contrast-enhanced CT scan is negative.[23]

As an added caveat, combined FDG-PET/contrast-enhanced CT scanning is more accurate than either PET or a contrast-enhanced CT scan alone and has a high negative predictive value in head and neck cancer surveillance, as it provides metabolic information as well as high-resolution anatomic detail.[5] This modality should be the imaging choice after head and neck squamous cell carcinoma treatment whenever possible. MR imaging with or without a PET scan should be added for tumors with skull base, intraorbital, intracranial, or perineural involvement.

Table 8
NI-RADS categories for neck/lymph nodes

Category	Neck	Imaging Findings	Management
Incomplete	0	New baseline study without any prior imaging available AND knowledge that prior imaging exists and will become available as comparison	Assign score in addendum after prior imaging examinations become available
No evidence of recurrence	1	Expected post-treatment changes. If residual nodal tissue, no FDG uptake or enhancement	Routine surveillance
Low suspicion	2	Mild/moderate FDG in residual nodal tissue or persistent areas of heterogeneous enhancement. Enlarging or new lymph node without definitive abnormal morphologic features. Any discordance between PET and contrast-enhanced CT scan: enlarging lymph node but little to no FDG uptake	Short interval follow-up (3 mo) or PET if scoring on contrast-enhanced CT scan alone
High suspicion	3	Residual nodal tissue with intense FDG. New enlarged lymph node or enlarging lymph node with abnormal morphologic features on contrast-enhanced CT only or focal intense FDG uptake if PET available	Image guided or clinical biopsy if clinically indicated
Definitive recurrence	4	Pathologically proven or definite radiologic and clinical progression	Clinical Management

Morphologically abnormal features that are definitive include new necrosis or gross ENE, as evidenced by invasion of adjacent structures.

Residual nodal tissue refers to a node that was abnormal and identified on a pretreatment scan. In these cases, hypo-enhancement and irregular borders are not unexpected and are likely a sign of treatment response, especially if there is no FDG uptake.

New or enlarging node is a node that develops during surveillance (not on a pretreatment scan). In these nodes, irregular borders or necrosis are abnormal features.

Abbreviation: FDG, fluorine-18-2-fluoro-2-deoxy-D-glucose.

Modified from Aiken AH, Rath TJ, Anzai Y, Branstetter BF, Hoang JK, Wiggins RH, Juliano AF, Glastonbury C, Phillips CD, Brown R, Hudgins PA. ACR Neck Imaging Reporting and Data Systems (NI-RADS): A White Paper of the ACR NI-RADS Committee. J Am Coll Radiol. 2018 Aug;15(8):1097 to 1108.

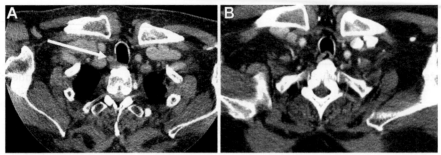

Fig. 11. NI-RADS 2. A patient with squamous cell carcinoma, with an unknown primary site, status post modified radical right neck dissection. A contrast-enhanced neck CT scan (*A*) demonstrates an enlarging right paratracheal node (*arrow* in *A*) compared with earlier examination (*B*), without central necrosis or evidence of extranodal extension. This entity should be further assessed by either a PET/CT scan or 3-month follow-up neck CT scan.

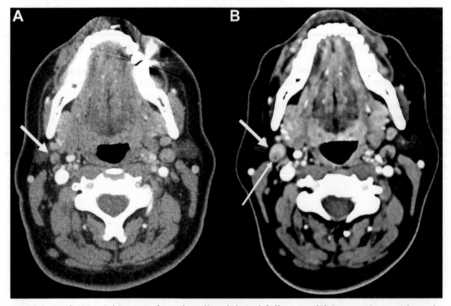

Fig. 12. NI-RADS 3. Neck CT axial images from baseline (*A*) and follow-up (*B*) in a patient with oral cavity squamous cell carcinoma show an enlarging right level IIA node (*large arrow*) with a new area of internal necrosis (*small arrow* in *B*). Fine needle aspiration in this patient confirmed nodal recurrence.

SUMMARY

Management of the neck is a key component of treating head and neck cancer as metastasis to cervical lymph nodes are common and portend poor prognosis. Lymph node dissections are performed to treat nodal metastatic disease, as well as to provide pathologic staging information. Increasing numbers of patients are now treated initially with radiation and chemotherapy, with neck dissections performed as salvage therapy; patients who are being surgically managed initially will routinely undergo neck dissections at the time of primary tumor resection. When imaging the postoperative neck, familiarity with the types of neck dissections performed is necessary to understand which nodes and other structures are typically removed (and, conversely, which nodal groups are typically left). Signs of nodal recurrence include new, enlarging, or morphologically abnormal lymph nodes on a CT scan, or abnormal FDG uptake on a PET scan.

CLINICS CARE POINTS

- Radiologists should work with clinicians in setting up a evidence-based baseline and surveillance imaging protocols.
- Staging patients accurately requires awareness of the current AJCC staging and upcoming changes, and a collaborative approach with radiologists, pathologists, and head and neck surgeons.
- Reporting in the postsurgical setting requires careful review of clinical history of primary tumor, surgical notes and treatment plan, including awareness of structures removed or reconstructed, while looking for imaging pitfalls, as well as new or recurrent cancers.
- NI-RADS reporting should be used to standardize interpretation, reporting and management.

DISCLOSURE

The authors have nothing to disclose.

REFERENCES

1. Martin H, del Valle B, Ehrlich H, et al. Neck dissection. Cancer 1951;4(3):441–99.

2. Byers RM. Modified neck dissection. A study of 967 cases from 1970 to 1980. Am J Surg 1985;150(4):414–21.

3. Shah JP. Patterns of cervical lymph node metastasis from squamous carcinomas of the upper aerodigestive tract. Am J Surg 1990;160(4):405–9.

4. Robbins KT, Clayman G, Levine PA, et al. Neck dissection classification update: revisions proposed by the American Head and Neck Society and the American Academy of Otolaryngology–Head and Neck Surgery. Arch Otolaryngol Neck Surg 2002;128(7):751.

5. Branstetter BF, Blodgett TM, Zimmer LA, et al. Head and neck malignancy: is PET/CT more accurate than PET or CT alone? Radiology 2005;235:580–6.

6. Som PM, Curtin HD, Mancuso AA. Imaging-based nodal classification for evaluation of neck metastatic adenopathy. Am J Roentgenol 2000;174(3):837–44.

7. Zanoni DK, Patel SG, Shah JP. Changes in the 8th Edition of the American Joint Committee on Cancer (AJCC) staging of head and neck cancer: rationale and implications. Curr Oncol Rep 2019;21(6):52.

8. Glastonbury CM, Mukherji SK, O'Sullivan B, et al. Setting the stage for 2018: How the changes in the American joint committee on cancer/Union for International Cancer Control cancer staging manual eighth edition impact radiologists. Am J Neuroradiol 2017;38(12):2231–7.

9. Lydiatt W, O'Sullivan B, Patel S. Major Changes in Head and Neck Staging for 2018. Am Soc Clin Oncol Educ Book 2018;(38):505–14.

10. Edge SB, Edge SB, American Joint Committee on Cancer. AJCC cancer staging manual. 8th edition. Springer.; 2017.

11. Keane FK, Chen Y-H, Neville BA, et al. Changing prognostic significance of tumor stage and nodal stage in patients with squamous cell carcinoma of the oropharynx in the human papillomavirus era. Cancer 2015;121(15):2594–602.

12. Ronen O, Samant S, Robbins KT. Neck Dissection, . Cummings Otolaryngology: head and neck surgery. 7th ed. Elsevier; 2021. p. 1806–30.

13. Schilling C, Stoeckli SJ, Haerle SK, et al. Sentinel European Node Trial (SENT): 3-year results of sentinel node biopsy in oral cancer. Eur J Cancer 2015;51(18):2777–84.

14. Garrel R, Poissonnet G, Moyà Plana A, et al. Equivalence Randomized Trial to Compare Treatment on the Basis of Sentinel Node Biopsy Versus Neck Node Dissection in Operable T1-T2N0 Oral and Oropharyngeal Cancer. J Clin Oncol 2020;38(34):4010–8.

15. Hasegawa Y, Tsukahara K, Yoshimoto S, et al. Neck dissections based on sentinel lymph node navigation versus elective neck dissections in early oral

cancers: a randomized, multicenter, non-inferiority trial. J Clin Oncol 2019;37(15_suppl):6007.

16. Robbins KT, Shannon K, Vieira F. Superselective neck dissection after chemoradiation: feasibility based on clinical and pathologic comparisons. Arch Otolaryngology Head Neck Surg 2007;133(5): 486–9.

17. Verma A, Chen AY. Indications and outcomes of superselective neck dissection: a review and analysis of the literature. Laryngoscope Investig Otolaryngol 2020;5(4):672–6.

18. McCarty JL, Corey AS, El-Deiry MW, et al. Imaging of surgical free flaps in head and neck reconstruction. Am J Neuroradiol 2019;40(1):5–13.

19. Lall C, Tirkes TA, Patel AA, et al. Flaps, slings, and other things: CT after reconstructive surgery–

expected changes and detection of complications. AJR Am J Roentgenol 2012;198:W521–33.

20. Mydlarz WK, Eisele DW. Complications of neck surgery. In: Cummings Otolaryngology: head and neck surgery. 7th edition. Elsevier; 2021. p. 1831–9.

21. Suárez C, Fernández-Alvarez V, Hamoir M, et al. Carotid blowout syndrome: modern trends in management. Cancer Manag Res 2018;10:5617–28.

22. Lu H-J, Chen K-W, Chen M-H, et al. Predisposing factors, management, and prognostic evaluation of acute carotid blowout syndrome. J Vasc Surg 2013;58(5):1226–35.

23. Aiken AH, Rath TJ, Anzai Y, et al. ACR Neck Imaging Reporting and Data Systems (NI-RADS): a White Paper of the ACR NI-RADS Committee. J Am Coll Radiol 2018;15(8):1097–108.

Postoperative Pharynx and Larynx

Jason Hostetter, MD*, Sandrine Yazbek, MD

KEYWORDS

- Head and neck cancer • Pharyngectomy • Laryngectomy • Laryngoplasty

KEY POINTS

- The complex functional anatomy of the pharynx and larynx necessitates multiple surgical techniques depending on tumor location and extent.
- Knowledge of surgical approaches to laryngeal and pharyngeal cancers is key to differentiating expected post-operative changes from complications.
- Post-surgical changes may confound interpretation when evaluating for recurrent disease, and common false-positive and false-negative appearances should be understood.

INTRODUCTION

Cancers of the pharynx and larynx comprise 3.5% of all newly diagnosed cancers in the United States with more than 66,000 new cases each year and almost 4000 deaths.[1] Most of these, more than 95%, are squamous cell carcinomas.[2] These cancers are treated using a combination of chemotherapeutic, radiation, and surgical techniques, depending on the cancer type, biology, location, and stage, as well as patient and other factors. When imaging in the postsurgical setting, the knowledge of the type of tumor, preoperative appearance, and type of surgery performed is essential for accurate interpretation. Surgical anatomic changes, surgical implants/devices, and potential postsurgical complications must be differentiated from suspected recurrent tumors.

Imaging protocols

Cross-sectional CT, PET, and MRI are the mainstays of pharynx and larynx cancer diagnostic and surveillance imaging. After definitive therapy, whether surgical or nonsurgical, imaging is performed primarily to evaluate local persistent or recurrent disease as well as regional or distant metastasis.[3] Imaging may also be performed to evaluate for posttreatment complications, and the modality and protocol should be tailored to the specific indication.

Surveillance imaging is primarily performed with CT, MRI, combined PET/CT or PET/MRI, and ultrasound. CT, MRI, and PET are the mainstays, with a relatively high sensitivity ranging from 50% to 100% and specificity ranging from 33% to 100%.[4,5] PET has been shown to have the highest sensitivity for primary and recurrent disease, and as a result, is the modality of choice for most referring clinicians for surveillance.[5] Surveillance imaging timelines and algorithms vary widely among radiation oncologists and surgeons, and recommendations vary depending on tumor location, size, and presence of regional metastases. Most patients will undergo imaging within 6 months posttreatment; however, the benefit of continued surveillance imaging beyond 6 months in asymptomatic patients is unclear.[5,6] The National Comprehensive Cancer Network guidelines have no specific imaging follow-up recommendations beyond 6 months posttreatment in asymptomatic patients.[7] The American College of Radiology (ACR) NI-RADS whitepaper recommends an extended timeline to approximately 2 years posttreatment, a period during which 95% of asymptomatic recurrences are detected.[8] The ACR surveillance algorithm includes PET/CT at 8 to 12 months after the completion of definitive

Department of Radiology, University of Maryland School of Medicine, 655 W Baltimore St S, Baltimore, MD 21201, USA
* Corresponding author.
E-mail address: jason.hostetter@som.umaryland.edu

Neuroimag Clin N Am 32 (2022) 37–53
https://doi.org/10.1016/j.nic.2021.08.009
1052-5149/22/© 2021 Elsevier Inc. All rights reserved.

therapy for baseline, CT, or PET/CT 6 months later if negative, CT alone 6 months later if negative, and finally, if imaging remains negative, CT 12 months later.[8] The use of this extended algorithm has shown the ability to detect recurrences beyond 6 months and before clinical signs are evident in 81% of asymptomatic patients.[6]

In symptomatic patients, in the setting of a suspected surgical complication, or suspected recurrence, imaging should be tailored to the clinical scenario. If there is suspicion for recurrent disease, PET/CT or PET/MRI should be considered for greatest sensitivity for active disease and to provide both functional and anatomic detail. If there is a suspected surgical complication such as infection or hemorrhage, CT, MRI, or ultrasound may be preferred to evaluate anatomy without the added radiation dose and time conferred by a PET examination.

EXPECTED POSTOPERATIVE FINDINGS OF THE PHARYNX AND LARYNX
Nasopharyngectomy

Nasopharyngectomy is most often used as a salvage treatment for recurrent or residual nasopharyngeal carcinoma (NPC) after definitive radiation therapy.[9] Tumors will recur either locally or regionally in approximately 10% of patients, and in these radioresistant tumors, surgery is often recommended.[10] NPC is uncommon cancer, representing 0.7% of all cancers diagnosed in 2018, with more than 70% of cases occurring in east and southeast Asia, and showing an association with Epstein–Barr virus infection.[10]

Salvage surgical resection of recurrent NPC results in 5-year survival of 30% to 52%, and gives less morbidity than reirradiation.[11] Given the deep location of the nasopharynx and many high-risk structures in close proximity, surgical access presents a challenge. Traditional open approaches provide excellent access to and visualization of tumors; however, they are technically complicated and associated with a relatively high risk of morbidity, including nerve injury, cosmetic and functional deficits, and vascular injury, among others.[9,11,12] Minimally invasive endoscopic techniques have been developed to help mitigate these issues, including transnasal and transoral approaches[9,11,12] (Fig. 1).

For a transnasal endoscopic approach, operative exposure of the tumor is important and may be maximized by the removal of the posterior bony septum (vomer) and inferior turbinates. More extensive exposure by ethmoidectomy, middle and superior turbinectomies, and medial maxillectomy may be performed depending on the tumor extent.[11,13] For small centrally located tumors limited to the posterior nasopharyngeal wall, the resection can spare the Eustachian tube laterally and extend posteriorly through the longus capitis muscles to the ventral clivus periosteum with the drilling of the clivus. For tumors that extend to the roof of the nasopharynx, the resection may include the floor and anterior wall of the sphenoid sinus as well as the superior turbinates. For tumors that extend laterally to obtain adequate exposure a complete ethmoidectomy, medial maxillectomy (possibly including the lateral *pyriform* aperture), unroofing of the pterygopalatine fossa, and removal of the medial pterygoid plate may be performed. The resection then may include the lateral nasopharyngeal wall with the removal of the cartilaginous Eustachian tube up to the bony junction.[11,14] The surgical resection can also be extended to the middle cranial fossa if necessary. In the event of tumor involvement of the parapharyngeal internal carotid artery (ICA), the ICA may also be partially resected endoscopically provided that the ICA was preoperatively sacrificed.[11] Surgical defects of the middle or posterior cranial fossae, or exposed ICA may be covered with a nasoseptal mucoperiosteal flap, a tunneled temporoparietal fascia flap, or free allograft.[13,15]

When tumors extend beyond the field easily exposed and accessed via an endoscopic transnasal approach, for example, inferior to the plane of the hard palate in the parapharyngeal space, laterally into the infratemporal fossa beyond the pterygoid musculature, or posterior–inferior involvement of the ICA, an open transmaxillary or infratemporal fossa approach may be necessary for adequate visualization. More recently, an endoscopic transoral approach has been described for these tumors, allowing adequate visualization of more inferiorly and laterally extensive tumors by improving cosmesis and morbidity than open approaches.[9]

As the operative approach and resection extent can vary dramatically, comparison with preoperative imaging is critical when interpreting postoperative imaging studies. In general, expected findings in the immediate postoperative setting will include nonmass-like enhancement at the margins of the resection, with or without blood, gas, and surgical material. As these operations are most often performed in the setting of prior radiation therapy, a background of postradiation changes will often be seen, including poor delineation of normal fat planes, fibrosis, ill-defined enhancement, and bone marrow edema or fatty replacement. Postoperative enhancement and marrow edema may be difficult to differentiate from postradiation changes, previously treated nonviable tumor, or residual viable tumor particularly in the parapharyngeal

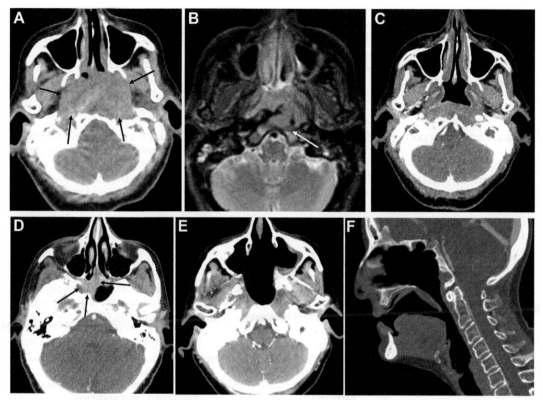

Fig. 1. Nasopharyngectomy for recurrent nasopharyngeal carcinoma. Low-dose localizing CT from a PET/CT examination (*A*) with a large soft tissue mass centered in the nasopharynx and extending to the clivus and skull base (*black arrows*). Fat-suppressed T2 image (*B*) demonstrating invasion of the clivus (*white arrow*). Axial CT after chemotherapy and radiation (*C*) shows a marked decrease in size of the soft tissue mass. Follow-up CT approximately 7 months later (*D*) demonstrates recurrent disease centered along the floor of the sphenoid sinus (*black arrows*). Transnasal nasopharyngectomy is performed, with axial (*E*) and sagittal (*F*) CT images showing medial maxillectomies, turbinectomies, septectomy, ethmoidectomy, and partial resection of the sphenoid and clivus. The midline nasopharyngeal mucosa is removed.

space, pterygopalatine fossa, orbits, and skull base.[16] Comparison with preoperative imaging, stability over time, and concurrent PET/CT or PET/MRI is very helpful in distinguishing posttreatment changes from viable tumor as further described in later sections.

Laryngectomy

Laryngeal cancers comprise approximately 20% of all head and neck cancers, with the vast majority being squamous cell carcinomas.[1] Treatment may involve any combination of chemotherapy, radiotherapy, and surgery, depending on tumor and patient characteristics. For surgical management, the type of resection depends on the extent of the primary tumor as well as the presence and extent of regional or distant metastases (**Table 1**).

The larynx is subdivided into 3 regions: the supraglottic, glottic, and subglottic larynx. The supraglottic larynx is bordered superiorly by the lingual surface of the epiglottis and the

hyoepiglottic ligament, laterally by the laryngeal surfaces of the aryepiglottic folds, anteriorly by the thyrohyoid ligament and inferiorly by the laryngeal ventricles. The glottis extends from the laryngeal ventricles superiorly to include the true vocal cords (comprised of the epithelium, superficial lamina propria, vocal ligament, and vocalis muscle), the anterior commissure, the vocal processes of the arytenoid cartilages, and ending 1 cm below the plane of the vocal cords. The subglottic larynx extends inferiorly from the glottis to the inferior border of the cricoid cartilage. The interarytenoid space and posterior wall of the cricoid cartilage form the posterior border of the glottic and subglottic larynx, whereas the thyroid cartilage, cricoid cartilage, and cricothyroid membrane form the anterior border.[16,17]

The goal of surgery in laryngeal cancer is to remove the tumor by preserving as much function of the larynx and pharynx as possible. Multiple techniques may be used depending on tumor extent to maximize functional and oncologic outcomes.

Table 1
Types of laryngectomy, indications, and contraindications

Laryngectomy Type	Indications	Contraindications
Endoscopic Cordectomy	Unilateral true vocal cord lesion	Spread outside of true cord, that is, the anterior commissure, paraglottic space, arytenoid cartilage
Vertical Partial Laryngectomy	True cord lesion involving anterior commissure or arytenoid cartilage	Invasion of the thyroid cartilage or posterior commissure, cord fixation, or transglottic spread
Supraglottic Laryngectomy	Supraglottic lesion with normal cord mobility and no involvement of the ventricles	Spread to the glottis, thyroid cartilage, cricoid cartilage, or postcricoid area, cord fixation, spread to the base of tongue or apex of the pyriform sinus
Supracricoid Laryngectomy	Supraglottic, glottic, or transglottic lesions with cord fixation or other contraindications to partial or supraglottic laryngectomy	Invasion of the hyoid, arytenoid cartilage fixation, extension to subglottic larynx or base of tongue, massive preepiglottic or paraglottic space invasion, invasion of thyroid cartilage outer perichondrium, extralaryngeal spread of tumor
Near Total Laryngectomy	Unilateral laryngeal or pyriform sinus lesion with the involvement of the cricoid cartilage	Invasion of the interarytenoid or postcricoid regions, involvement of bilateral vocal cord, and arytenoid involvement
Total Laryngectomy	Extensive laryngeal tumors with cartilage invasion, cricoid involvement, salvage surgery after failed radiation or partial laryngectomy	Metastasis, synchronous tumor, invasion of the prevertebral fascia, encasement of the common or internal carotid arteries

Partial laryngectomy

For small tumors contained to the true vocal cord unilaterally, without the involvement of the anterior commissure or paraglottic space, and without the impairment of vocal cord mobility, endoscopic cordectomy with carbon dioxide laser may be performed.[18] The true vocal cord and vocalis muscle only are resected, and after healing and regeneration of the vocal cord, imaging may seem normal.[18]

For tumors that involve either the anterior commissure or arytenoid cartilage, vertical partial laryngectomy may be performed either by frontolateral partial laryngectomy or hemilaryngectomy. In frontolateral partial laryngectomy, a vertical segment of the thyroid cartilage anterior to the tumor is removed, and the involved vocal cord, ipsilateral laryngeal ventricle and false cord, anterior commissure, and anterior-most portion of the contralateral vocal cord are removed (Fig. 2). The ipsilateral arytenoid cartilage may or may not be removed. The contralateral vocal cord mucosa is repaired primarily and the ipsilateral resection site heals by secondary intention.[18] In hemilaryngectomy, the ipsilateral thyroid cartilage lamina is removed along with the ipsilateral true vocal cord up to one-third of the anterior contralateral vocal cord, the ipsilateral arytenoid cartilage, and the mucosa of the ipsilateral aryepiglottic fold (Fig. 3).[18] Postoperative imaging may show scarring of the resected vocal cord and paraglottic space resulting in a dense, "pseudo-cord" appearance, as well as surgical defects of the thyroid lamina and absence of the ipsilateral arytenoid cartilage.[18,19]

For supraglottic laryngeal cancers in which there is no involvement of the glottis, laryngeal ventricles, cartilage invasion, **pyriform** sinus apex, or base of tongue, a supraglottic laryngectomy may be performed.[18] This procedure involves the removal of the epiglottis, aryepiglottic folds, false vocal cords, and laryngeal ventricles, as well as the upper third of the thyroid cartilage and thyrohyoid membrane. A thyrohyoidopexy is then performed, raising the remaining lower two-thirds of the thyroid cartilage and attaching it to the

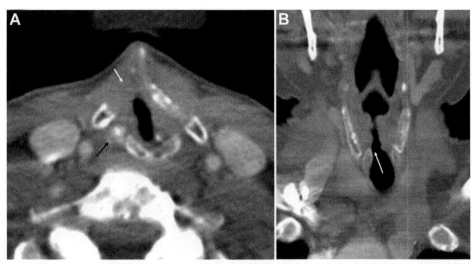

Fig. 2. Right frontolateral partial laryngectomy. Axial contrast enhanced CT image (*A*) with partial resection of the right thyroid cartilage lamina (*white arrow*), and preservation of the ipsilateral arytenoid cartilage (*black arrow*). Coronal image (*B*) with surgical absence of the ipsilateral vocal cord (*white arrow*).

underside of the hyoid.[18] Postoperative imaging will show the foreshortened larynx, absence of the epiglottis, an air-filled cavity in the supraglottic region, and approximation of the hyoid and remaining thyroid cartilage with an otherwise normal-appearing glottic and subglottic larynx (Fig. 4).[18,19] Variations of the supraglottic laryngectomy include the extended supraglottic laryngectomy with the removal of one arytenoid cartilage, the base of the tongue, or the pyriform sinus, and the three-quarters laryngectomy with the removal of the ipsilateral true vocal cord and arytenoid cartilage in addition to the usual supraglottic structures in the event of spread to the

glottis on one side, provided there is no cord fixation or cartilage invasion.[18]

In tumors that involve the supraglottic larynx, glottic larynx, or both and in which supraglottic laryngectomy or partial laryngectomy cannot be performed, supracricoid laryngectomy provides an alternative to total laryngectomy. Supracricoid laryngectomy involves the removal of the supraglottic and glottic larynx, including the thyroid cartilage, thyrohyoid membrane, aryepiglottic folds, true vocal cords, and paraglottic space, with sparing of one or both arytenoid cartilages and the subglottic larynx. In more advanced tumors involving the paraglottic or preepiglottic

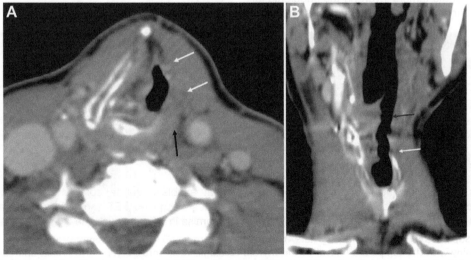

Fig. 3. Left vertical hemilaryngectomy. Axial (*A*) and coronal (*B*) images showing the removal of the left thyroid lamina and true vocal cord (*white arrows*), the ipsilateral arytenoid cartilage (*black arrow*), and the ipsilateral aryepiglottic fold (*red arrow*).

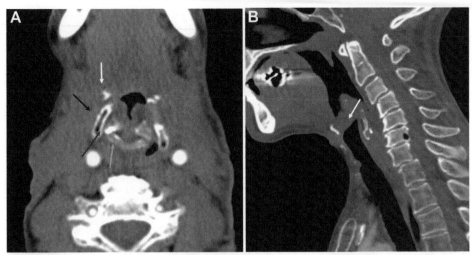

Fig. 4. Supraglottic laryngectomy. Axial (*A*) and sagittal (*B*) CT images showing resection of the upper third of the thyroid cartilage, laryngeal ventricles, aryepiglottic folds, and epiglottis with thyrohyoidopexy. Axial image (*A*) shows the hyoid (*white arrow*), remaining thyroid cartilage (*black arrow*), arytenoid cartilage (*red arrow*), and cricoid cartilage (*green arrow*) in close approximation. Sagittal image (*B*) shows the preserved glottis (*white arrow*) and absent epiglottis with foreshortening of the larynx.

spaces, or invading the thyroid cartilage, the epiglottis, preepiglottic space, and entire thyroid cartilage are removed. In earlier tumors involving the anterior commissure, both vocal cords, or with impaired cord mobility, the epiglottis is spared. The resection is then followed by either cricohyoidopexy or cricohyoidoepiglottopexy depending on whether the epiglottis was removed, in which the cricoid cartilage is raised and attached to the hyoid/epiglottis to reconstruct the larynx (**Fig. 5**).[18,20]

Total and near-total laryngectomy

In transglottic tumors involving the subglottic larynx or laryngeal cartilages in which supracricoid laryngectomy cannot be performed, total or near-total laryngectomy may be performed. Total laryngectomy may also be performed as a salvage surgery after radiation or partial laryngectomy with recurrence. In total laryngectomy, the entire larynx is removed from the hyoid bone superiorly through the cricoid cartilage inferiorly, possibly also including upper tracheal cartilage rings depending on the extent of tumor. The thyroid cartilage, epiglottis, hyoid bone, and glottic structures are all removed, as is part of the thyroid. A permanent tracheostomy is created and a mucosa-lined neopharynx is created connecting the trachea to the pharynx. If one side of the glottis is uninvolved, a voice-preserving near-total laryngectomy may be

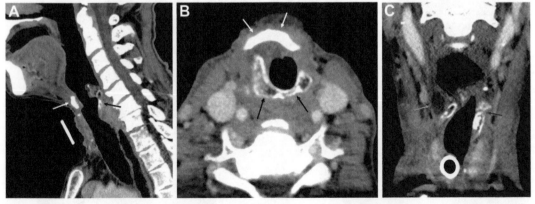

Fig. 5. Supracricoid laryngectomy. Sagittal (*A*), axial (*B*) and coronal (*C*) CT images demonstrate supracricoid laryngectomy with the complete removal of the thyroid cartilage, vocal cords, aryepiglottic folds, and epiglottis. Cricohyoidopexy is seen with the hyoid (*white arrows*) immediately abutting the cricoid cartilage (*black arrows*) and visible in the same plane on axial images (*B*). Both cricoarytenoid joints are preserved (*red arrows*). An incidental postoperative laryngocele is present on the right (*green arrow*).

performed, wherein the recurrent laryngeal nerve, arytenoid cartilage, part of the thyroarytenoid muscle, and parts of the thyroid and cricoid cartilages contralateral to the tumor are preserved.[18,21] Following the removal of the laryngeal structures, the esophagus takes a more anterior position and a more rounded configuration, in contrast to the normally posteriorly flattened appearance (**Fig. 6**).[18,19]

Transoral robotic surgery

Robot-assisted surgery using the da Vinci surgical system (Intuitive Surgery, Sunnyvale, Ca)

allows surgeons to use a minimally invasive, transoral approach to upper aerodigestive tract cancers rather than by traditional open approaches.[22] The robotic system gives the operating surgeon improved visualization via magnified 3D views, better depth perception, as well as the increased dexterity and precision of the robotic surgical implements over other minimally invasive and open techniques. TORS is primarily used in treating squamous cell carcinoma of the oropharynx; however, other sites are also well suited for robotic surgery, such as for lingual tonsillectomy, supraglottic partial laryngectomy, and hypopharyngectomy.

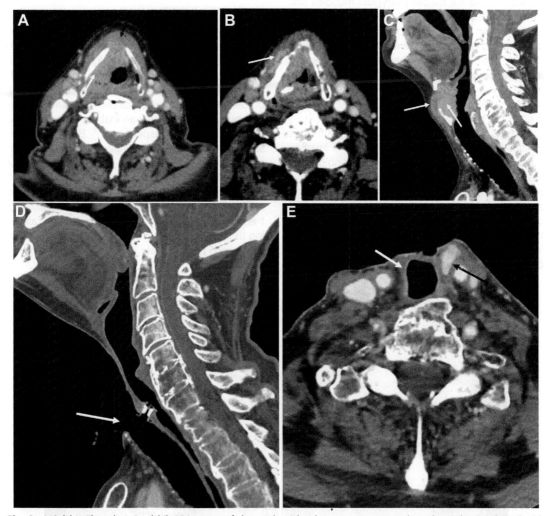

Fig. 6. Axial (*A, B*) and sagittal (*C*) CT images of the neck with a large mass centered on the right vocal cord with involvement of the paraglottic space (*A, white arrow*), anterior commissure and contralateral vocal cord (*A, black arrow*), extension through the thyroid cartilage (*B, white arrow*), involvement of the pre-epiglottic space and extension through the thyrohyoid membrane (*C, white arrows*). Sagittal (*D*) and axial (*E*) CT images after total laryngectomy showing the removal of the hyoid bone and all laryngeal structures with a permanent tracheostomy (*D, white arrow*). Rounded, anterior configuration of the upper esophagus/neopharynx (*E, white arrow*). Thyroid remnant (*E, black arrow*), not to be confused for enhancing tumor.

General contraindications to TORS include unresectable nodal metastases, retropharyngeal course of the internal carotid arteries posterior to the constrictor muscles, tumor invasion of the mandible, skull base, pterygoid plates, Eustachian tube orifice, or pterygomandibular raphe, involvement of the prevertebral muscles or precervical fascia, involvement of the extrinsic tongue muscles of the floor of mouth or mylohyoid muscle, tumor crossing the midline of the tongue.

A lateral oropharyngectomy performed by TORS involves the removal of the tonsil, anterior and posterior tonsillar pillars, portions of the soft palate, tongue base, and posterior pharyngeal wall. Postoperative imaging may show distortion of fat planes around the medial pterygoid muscles and pterygomandibular raphe in the weeks following surgery, with subsequent progressive retraction of the lateral oropharyngeal wall due to the formation of scar (Fig. 7).[22] This may produce the appearance of tilting of the soft palate and uvula toward the site of surgery. Similarly, tongue base tumors resected via TORS will show retraction of the tongue base at the surgical bed.

Patients with T1 and T2 (and select T3) tumors confined to the supraglottis without the involvement of the laryngeal ventricles or arytenoid cartilages are candidates for TORS supraglottic partial laryngectomy. The epiglottis and preepiglottic space, both aryepiglottic folds and false vocal cords are resected, and in contradistinction to the open approach, the thyroid cartilage is left intact. Postoperative imaging may show redundant mucosa covering the arytenoid cartilages, with surgically absent supraglottic structures and intact glottis.[22] Contraindications include cartilage invasion, invasion of the anterior or posterior glottic commissures, and tongue base involvement within 1 cm of the circumvallate papillae.[22]

Transoral partial laryngopharyngectomy can also be performed for patients with T1, T2, and some T3 tumors of the pyriform sinuses or posterior hypopharyngeal wall. The pyriform sinus, aryepiglottic fold, and possibly the ipsilateral arytenoid cartilage are resected. Contraindications include the involvement of the postcricoid region, extension across the midline or to the apex of the pyriform sinus, or abutment/encasement of the carotid artery.

Vocal cord augmentation

Vocal cord paralysis occurs due to injury to the ipsilateral vagus or recurrent laryngeal nerve, which can occur in many settings, including malignancy, trauma, posttreatment, and others. Unilateral paralysis leads to inadequate apposition of the vocal cords, which not only causes problems with phonation but also may cause an inability to protect the airway and resulting aspiration.[23,24] Bilateral paralysis may also disturb phonation; however, most often manifests as dyspnea and biphasic stridor due to the inability to lateralize the cords and open the glottis.[23] Surgical interventions for vocal cord paralysis primarily intend to permanently alter the paralyzed cord size, position, or stiffness, allowing the patient to better approximate the opposing vocal cord and phonate, and to better protect the airway from aspiration.

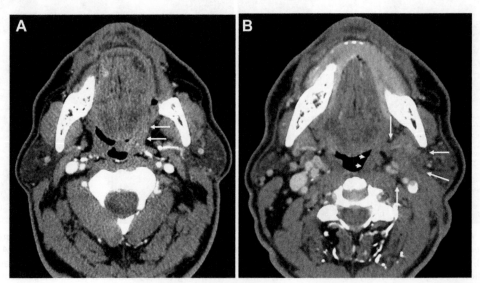

Fig. 7. Axial CT images showing a left tonsillar mass (*arrows, A*), and postoperative images after TORS (*B*). Postoperative images show edema and loss of normal fat planes in the left parapharyngeal space (*arrows*) as well as thickening of the left oropharyngeal wall (*arrowheads*) consistent with postsurgical changes.

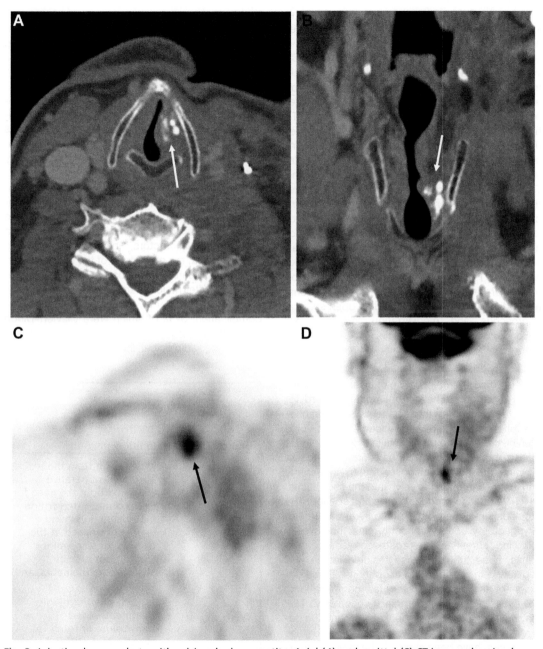

Fig. 8. Injection laryngoplasty with calcium hydroxyapatite. Axial (*A*) and sagittal (*B*) CT images showing hyperattenuating calcium hydroxyapatite injectable material in the left vocal cord and paraglottic space (*white arrows*), with appropriate medialization of the left vocal cord. Calcium hydroxyapatite laryngoplasty is known to be PET avid, as seen on corresponding axial (*C*) and coronal (*D*) PET images (*black arrows*).

Various methods may be used to augment a paralyzed vocal cord. The oldest form of treatment is injection laryngoplasty, wherein a biocompatible material is directly injected into the affected true vocal cord or paraglottic space under endoscopic visualization, resulting in the medialization of the cord-free edge.[23,24] Various materials have been used, including paraffin as early as 1911, now replaced by multiple temporary and permanent materials. Temporary materials include hyaluronic acid gel, collagen, and bovine gelatin. Permanent and long-lasting materials currently used include calcium hydroxyapatite and autologous fat.[23–25] Polytetrafluoroethylene (PTFE) (Teflon; DuPont,

Wilmington, Del) was historically used and is no longer in use due to problems with foreign body reactions and migration from the injection site.[24]

The postinjection appearance by MRI and CT varies depending on the material used. Hyaluronic acid gels may persist between 4 and 12 months and have imaging characteristics similar to water on both CT and MRI, with hypoattenuation, T1 hypointensity, T2 hyperintensity, and minimal peripheral enhancement on postcontrast T1 images.[23] Collagen-based injectables persist for up to 11 months, and seem hyperintense on T1 and T2-weighted images.[23,26] Calcium hydroxyapatite, the mineral component of bone, has a texture closer to that of soft tissue in the injectable formulation, seems hyperattenuating on CT, and lasts for approximately 18 months postinjection.[23,27] Calcium hydroxyapatite may show increased uptake of FDG on PET examinations, and should not be misinterpreted as tumor (**Fig. 8**).[23] Additional methods of laryngoplasty, including open surgical approaches and medialization implants, are beyond the scope of this article.

Tracheoesophageal voice prosthesis

Loss of voice is a major cause of disability after total laryngectomy. The current gold standard for voice rehabilitation in these patients is with tracheoesophageal puncture and placement of a voice prosthesis.[28–30] The prosthesis is a one-way valve placed between the trachea and esophagus, allowing the patient to cover the tracheostomy and force air through the valve into the esophagus, which vibrates to produce sound and speech. The prosthesis may be placed primarily at the time of laryngectomy or secondarily in the weeks following surgery. The prostheses seem as a dense, short tubular device residing in the wall separating the trachea and esophagus. These devices are associated with very few complications; however, patients undergoing secondary TEP may have a reduced risk of leakage around the device, and patients who have undergone 2 courses of radiation have been shown to have higher rates of TEP failure, most often due to an enlarging tracheoesophageal fistula.[29,30] TEP devices can also occasionally dislodge and may be aspirated. CT chest should be performed when there is suspicion for an aspirated prosthesis, as these small devices may not be well seen on plain radiograph.[31]

UNEXPECTED POSTOPERATIVE FINDINGS OF THE PHARYNX AND LARYNX

Follow-up imaging after pharyngeal or laryngeal surgery most commonly seeks to (a) evaluate for residual or recurrent disease, (b) establish a baseline postoperative appearance for future follow-up examinations, or (c) evaluate for potential surgical or other treatment-related complications.

Surgical complications

The Clavien–Dindo classification system for surgical complications, first proposed in 1992, has been used widely for general surgical, urologic and orthopedic procedures, and more recently used in head and neck surgical literature.[32–34] The system, updated in 2004, grades complications from I (any deviation from the normal postoperative course, without the need for intervention) to V (death)[35] (**Table 2**). Complications arise due to a combination of factors, including pre-existing comorbidities, the magnitude of the surgical intervention, and perioperative care.[34] A study of complications after major head and neck surgery with free-flap repair found 64% of patients had a complication, 32% of which were Clavien–Dindo grade III (complication requiring surgical, endoscopic, or radiological intervention) or higher.[34]

Table 2
Clavien–Dindo classification of surgical complications

Grade	Definition
I	Any deviation from the normal postoperative course without the need for treatment or intervention (not including wound infections opened at the bedside, or some minor medications such as analgesics, antiemetics, and so forth)
II	Requiring pharmacologic treatment, blood transfusion, or total parenteral nutrition
III	Requiring surgical, endoscopic, or radiological intervention
IIIa	Intervention without general anesthesia
IIIb	Intervention with general anesthesia
IV	Life-threatening complication requiring ICU management
IVa	Single organ dysfunction
IVb	Multiorgan dysfunction
V	Death

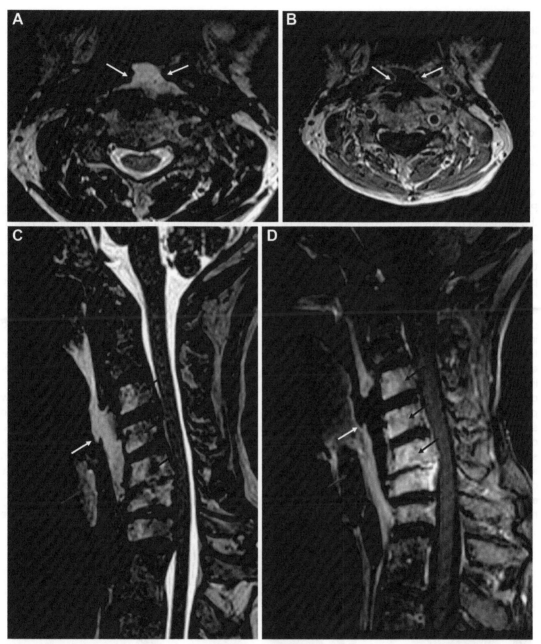

Fig. 9. Abscess after total laryngectomy. Axial (*A*) and sagittal (*C*) T2, and axial (*B*) and sagittal (*D*) T1 postcontrast MRI images demonstrating a peripherally enhancing fluid collection (*white arrows*) communicating with the reconstructed pharynx, and extending along the cervical vertebral elements. Marrow edema and enhancement (*black arrows*) suggest associated osteomyelitis. Fat component of the partially visualized flap reconstruction noted anteriorly (*red arrows*).

Of the complications occurring at the surgical site, the most common were wound infection (34%), wound dehiscence (20%), loss of skin graft (15%), and hematoma (11%).[34] Surgical site and wound complication risk are also increased by multiple patient factors, including malnutrition, low-performance status, smoking, diabetes, and others. In addition, salvage surgery is often performed in a tissue bed that has been previously irradiated, causing impaired healing and increased risk of tissue and wound breakdown.[36]

Abscess

Purulent infection of a surgical site may result in the formation of a walled-off collection of pus or abscess, classically displayed on cross-sectional imaging as a peripherally enhancing fluid collection. On CT, the collection contents will show complex fluid density, and on MRI will show central restricted diffusion. On CT, an abscess may be difficult to differentiate from a noninfected simple postoperative seroma. Factors favoring infection include a collection appearing in the days to weeks following surgery, growing over time, the presence of gas more than a week from surgery, or increasing surrounding edema and inflammatory change. A fluid collection present on immediate postoperative imaging almost certainly represents seroma, and a thin wall without enhancement, lack of surrounding inflammation, and simple fluid density of the collection contents all favor noninfected seroma. On MRI, the distinction can be easier, as a collection with peripheral enhancement and edema with restricted diffusion of the contents is highly suggestive of abscess (**Fig. 9**). However,

as blood clot within hematomas also restricts diffusion, a sterile postoperative hematoma should not be mistaken for abscess.

Fistula and wound dehiscence

Breakdown of the tissue forming the surgical reconstruction may result in the dehiscence of the surgical wound, fistula formation, and exposure of bone or major vessels. If not promptly diagnosed and treated, this can lead to an array of problems, including soft tissue or bone infection, abscess, or vessel rupture. Prior irradiation of the surgical field and, possibly, prior chemotherapy plays a role in poor postoperative wound healing and the formation of wound complications. Radiation causes injury to the vasculature of the soft tissues leading to fibrosis and decreased responsiveness to angiogenic and vasodilatory mediators.[36] For example, the reported incidence of pharyngocutaneous fistula formation after total laryngectomy varies widely from 3% to 75%; however, the risk is highest in patients undergoing salvage laryngectomy with prior radiation (30%) versus primary laryngectomy (10%) with higher rates of fistula formation associated with higher doses of radiation.[36,37]

Imaging studies may in severe cases show gross dehiscence of the surgical wound with an air-filled defect exposing underlying bone, vessels, or soft tissues. CT may show erosive or irregular lucent and sclerotic changes of exposed bone in the setting of osteomyelitis, and if contrast is administered, any vessels adjacent to the defect should be closely evaluated for evidence of injury or pseudoaneurysm formation (**Fig. 10**). In the

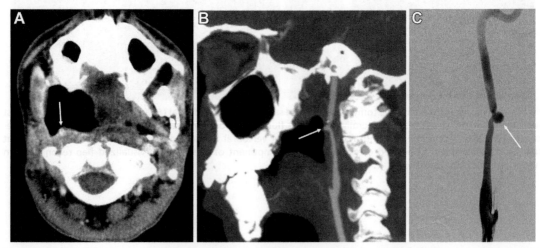

Fig. 10. Deep ulcer with exposed carotid and pseudoaneurysm. Axial CT (*A*), sagittal CTA (*B*), and lateral digitally subtracted angiogram (*C*) in a patient with history of total laryngectomy and radiation demonstrating a deep, air filled ulcer extending into the infratemporal fossa with exposed cervical internal carotid artery (*arrow, A*) and formation of a pseudoaneurysm (*arrows, B, C*).

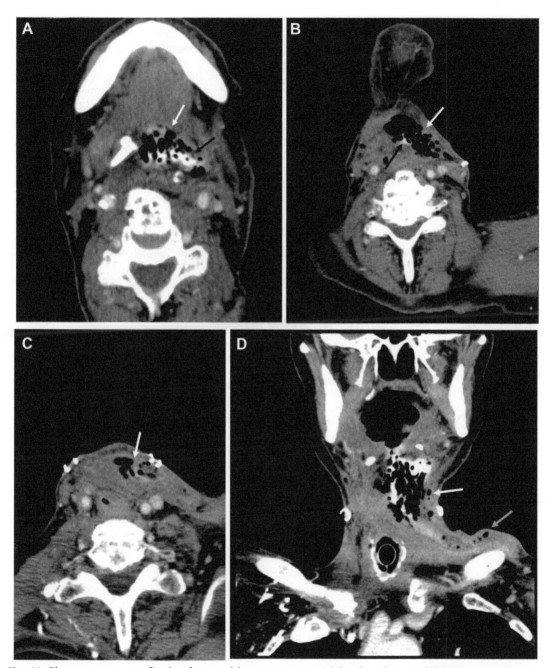

Fig. 11. Pharyngocutaneous fistula after total laryngectomy. Axial (*A–C*) and coronal (*D*) CT images showing extensive soft tissue gas (*white arrows*) as well as oral contrast (*black arrows*) extending from the neopharynx just inferior to the tongue base to the left lower neck skin surface (*green arrow*).

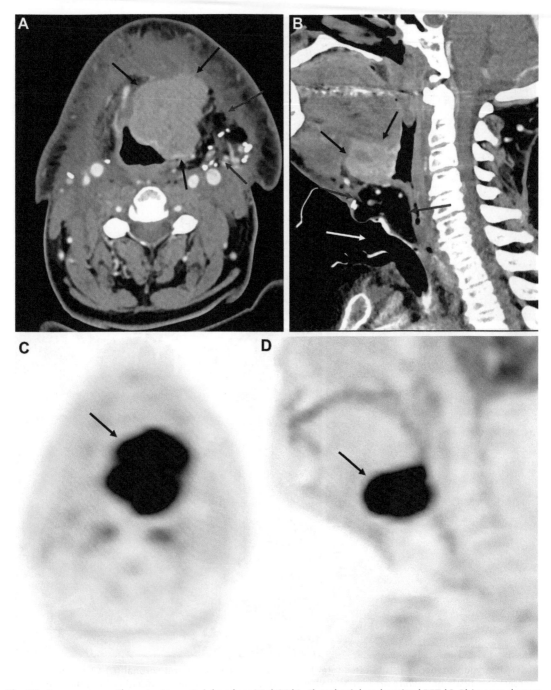

Fig. 12. Recurrence postlaryngectomy. Axial and sagittal CT (*A, B*) and axial and sagittal PET (*C, D*) images demonstrating postoperative changes in total laryngectomy with a tracheostomy (*white arrow*) and flap reconstruction (*red arrows*). An enhancing, PET avid mass is present along the superior anterior margin of the flap reconstruction (*black arrows*) compatible with recurrence.

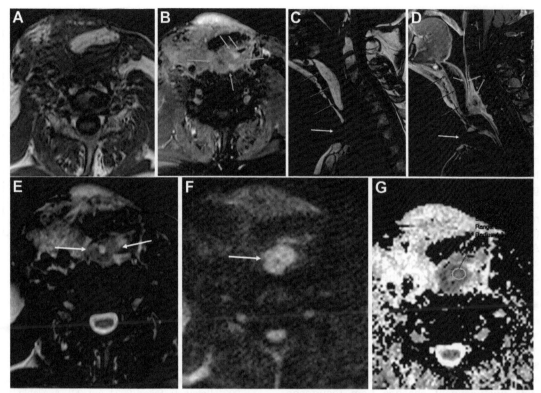

Fig. 13. Recurrence postlaryngectomy. Axial precontrast and fat-suppressed postcontrast T1 (*A, B*), sagittal precontrast and fat-suppressed postcontrast T1 (*C, D*), Axial T2 (*E*), DWI (*F*), and ADC (*G*) images show findings of total laryngectomy with a tracheostomy (*white arrows, C, D*) and absence of the normal laryngeal structures. The fat component of the flap reconstruction shows expected fat signal (*red arrows, A, C, D*). An enhancing mass (*green arrows, B, D*) along the posterior margin of the flap reconstructed neopharynx (*blue arrows, B, D*) shows T2 hyperintensity (*white arrows, E*) and restricted diffusion (*white arrow, F*) with average ADC values of approximately 0.94 x 10-3 (*G*), compatible with recurrent tumors.

event of pharyngocutaneous fistula formation after total laryngectomy, a small fluid and/or gas-filled tract may be seen coursing from the skin surface to the reconstructed neopharynx (**Fig. 11**). Fluid-sensitive, fat-suppressed MRI sequences may be more sensitive for a small fistula.

Recurrence

Imaging remains one of the most important tools in the early detection of recurrent pharyngeal and laryngeal cancers. Up to 25% of early stage and 50% of advanced-stage head and neck cancers show treatment failure in the form of residual or recurrent cancer.[38] In a recent study of patients with recurrent head and neck cancers, more than one-third of recurrences were detected by imaging alone with no clinical evidence of recurrence.[6] In the postsurgical setting, local disease recurrence will usually be found at the margins of the surgical resection, or at the edges of the reconstruction flap if one was used. Comparison with

preoperative imaging allows one to assess the extent of the original tumor and better identify areas that may have been difficult or impossible to fully resect. Comparison to baseline postoperative imaging is also critical, as the normal anatomy will be necessarily distorted after surgery.

Differentiating recurrent tumors from normal postoperative and posttreatment change is one of the primary challenges in interpreting surveillance imaging examinations. NI-RADS has been proposed by the ACR as a standardized reporting system for the surveillance imaging of head and neck cancer to improve the consistency and generalizability of imaging reports,[8] and is further described elsewhere in this issue. New nodular enhancing soft tissue at the margins of the resection or flap with associated increased uptake on FDG-PET imaging is the classic appearance of recurrent disease (**Fig. 12**); however, many cases remain equivocal. Many posttreatment and postsurgical effects can confound interpretation, including false-positive FDG uptake or enhancement related to inflammation, granulation tissue, or early scar, rather than the tumor. CT is primarily useful in assessing morphologic and enhancement characteristics of lesions, with PET adding functional/metabolic data.

MRI provides additional data with which to distinguish posttreatment effects from recurrent disease. For example, the combination of morphologic MRI with diffusion-weighted imaging (DWI) and apparent diffusion coefficient (ADC) maps has been described as a useful adjunct in the post-treatment setting,[2,38] with low ADC values (suggested threshold of 1.22×10^{-3}) favoring recurrent tumors and reflecting high cellularity relative to benign posttreatment changes (Fig. 13). Late scar tissue may also show low ADC values, however, and evaluation must take into account the morphology and signal intensity of the abnormality on other sequences. For example, late scar tissue will show very low T1 and T2 signal with a triangular or linear morphology, as opposed to the intermediate T1 and T2 signal, and mass-like morphology of tumor.[2] As combined PET/MRI becomes more widespread in clinical settings and experience increases, we may see improved ability to discriminate posttreatment changes from recurrence, particularly in challenging cases wherein traditional imaging is equivocal.

SUMMARY

Imaging of the postsurgical pharynx and larynx can be challenging due to the complex anatomy as well as the numerous surgical approaches and techniques used. The expected postsurgical findings, as well as possible superimposed radiation changes, can result in a confusing picture when assessing for recurrent disease or treatment complications. Knowledge of the type and extent of tumor, the surgery performed, and the expected appearance of both common complications and recurrent disease aids in accurate interpretation.

CLINICS CARE POINTS

- Nasopharyngeal carcinoma recurs in approximately 10% of patients, for whom salvage surgery will often be recommended.
- The goal of surgery in laryngeal cancer is to remove the tumor by preserving as much function of the larynx and pharynx as possible.

- Calcium hydroxyapatite laryngoplasty is known to be PET avid, and may cause false-positive uptake on PET/CT studies.
- Tracheoesophageal voice prosthesis devices can occasionally dislodge and may be aspirated. CT chest should be performed when there is suspicion for an aspirated prosthesis, as these small devices may not be well seen on plain radiograph.
- Blood clot within hematomas may restrict diffusion, and a sterile postoperative hematoma should not be mistaken for abscess.
- MRI can be helpful in distinguishing posttreatment effects from recurrent tumor in equivocal cases.

DISCLOSURE

The authors have nothing to disclose.

REFERENCES

1. American Cancer Society, Cancer Facts and Figures 2021 [Internet]. [cited 2021 Apr 20]. Available at: https://www.cancer.org/research/cancer-facts-statistics/all-cancer-facts-figures/cancer-facts-figures-2021.html. Accessed May 21, 2021.
2. Varoquaux A, Rager O, Dulguerov P, et al. Diffusion-weighted and PET/MR Imaging after radiation therapy for malignant head and neck tumors. Radiographics 2015;35(5):1502–27.
3. Manikantan K, Khode S, Dwivedi RC, et al. Making sense of post-treatment surveillance in head and neck cancer: when and what of follow-up. Cancer Treat Rev 2009;35(8):744–53.
4. Anzai Y, Carroll WR, Quint DJ, et al. Recurrence of head and neck cancer after surgery or irradiation: prospective comparison of 2-deoxy-2-[F-18]fluoro-D-glucose PET and MR imaging diagnoses. Radiology 1996;200(1):135–41.
5. Strauss SB, Aiken AH, Lantos JE, et al. Best practices for post-treatment surveillance imaging in head and neck cancer: application of the Neck Imaging Reporting and Data System (NI-RADS). Am J Roentgenol 2021;216(6):1438–51.
6. Gore A, Baugnon K, Beitler J, et al. Posttreatment imaging in patients with head and neck cancer without clinical evidence of recurrence: should surveillance imaging extend beyond 6 months? Am J Neuroradiol 2020;41(7):1238–44.
7. Pfister DG, Spencer S, Adelstein D, et al. Head and neck cancers, version 2.2020, NCCN Clinical Practice Guidelines in Oncology. J Natl Compr Canc Netw 2020;18(7):873–98.

8. Aiken AH, Rath TJ, Anzai Y, et al. ACR Neck Imaging Reporting and Data Systems (NI-RADS): a white paper of the ACR NI-RADS Committee. J Am Coll Radiol 2018;15(8):1097–108.

9. Soriano RM, Rindler RS, Helman SN, et al. Endoscopic transoral nasopharyngectomy. Head Neck 2021;43(1):278–87.

10. Chen Y-P, Chan ATC, Le Q-T, et al. Nasopharyngeal carcinoma. Lancet 2019 Jul;394(10192):64–80.

11. Ong YK, Solares CA, Lee S, et al. Endoscopic nasopharyngectomy and its role in managing locally recurrent nasopharyngeal carcinoma. Otolaryngol Clin North Am 2011;44(5):1141–54.

12. Van Rompaey J, Suruliraj A, Carrau R, et al. Access to the parapharyngeal space: an anatomical study comparing the endoscopic and open approaches: endoscopic anatomy: the parapharyngeal space. Laryngoscope 2013;123(10):2378–82.

13. Al-Sheibani S, Zanation AM, Carrau RL, et al. Endoscopic endonasal transpterygoid nasopharyngectomy. Laryngoscope 2011;121(10):2081–9.

14. Castelnuovo P. Nasopharyngeal endoscopic resection in the management of selected malignancies: ten-year experience. Rhinol J [Internet]. 2010. Available at: http://www.rhinologyjournal.com/abstract.php?id=852. Accessed May 21, 2021.

15. Hadad G, Rivera-Serrano CM, Bassagaisteguy LH, et al. Anterior pedicle lateral nasal wall flap: A novel technique for the reconstruction of anterior skull base defects: anterior pedicle lateral nasal wall flap. Laryngoscope 2011;121(8):1606–10.

16. Seeburg DP, Baer AH, Aygun N. Imaging of patients with head and neck cancer. Oral Maxillofac Surg Clin N Am 2018;30(4):421–33.

17. Mor N, Blitzer A. Functional anatomy and oncologic barriers of the larynx. Otolaryngol Clin North Am 2015;48(4):533–45.

18. Ferreiro-Argüelles C, Jiménez-Juan L, Martínez-Salazar JM, et al. CT findings after laryngectomy. RadioGraphics 2008;28(3):869–82.

19. Mukherji SK, Weadock WJ. Imaging of the post-treatment larynx. Eur J Radiol 2002;12.

20. Sperry SM, Rassekh CH, Laccourreye O, et al. Supracricoid partial laryngectomy for primary and recurrent laryngeal cancer. JAMA Otolaryngol Neck Surg 2013;139(11):1226.

21. D'Cruz AK, Sharma S, Pai PS. Current status of near-total laryngectomy: review. J Laryngol Otol 2012; 126(6):556–62.

22. Loevner LA, Learned KO, Mohan S, et al. Transoral robotic surgery in head and neck cancer: what radiologists need to know about the cutting edge. Radiographics 2013;33(6):22.

23. Vachha BA, Ginat DT, Mallur P, et al. "Finding a voice": imaging features after phonosurgical procedures for vocal fold paralysis. Am J Neuroradiol 2016;37(9):1574–80.

24. Kumar VA, Lewin JS, Ginsberg LE. CT assessment of vocal cord medialization. AJNR Am J Neuroradiol 2006;27(8):1643–6.

25. Mallur PS, Rosen CA. Vocal fold injection: review of indications, techniques, and materials for augmentation. Clin Exp Otorhinolaryngol 2010;3(4):177.

26. Moonis G, Dyce O, Loevner LA, et al. Magnetic resonance imaging of micronized dermal graft in the larynx. Ann Otol Rhinol Laryngol 2005;114(8):593–8.

27. O'Leary MA, Grillone GA. Injection laryngoplasty. Otolaryngol Clin North Am 2006;39(1):43–54.

28. Pun A, Albarki H, Levy S, et al. Radiologic characteristics of voice prostheses and the clinical significance of the missing valve. Aust J Otolaryngol 2020; 3:4. https://doi.org/10.21037/ajo.2020.03.01.

29. Neto JCB, Dedivitis RA, Aires FT, et al. Comparison between primary and secondary tracheoesophageal puncture prosthesis: a Systematic Review. ORL J Otorhinolaryngol Relat Spec 2017;879(4): 222–9.

30. Clancy K. Outcomes of tracheoesophageal puncture in twice-radiated patients. Am J Otolaryngol 2019;40(6):10227.

31. Abia-Trujillo D, Tatari MM, Venegas-Borsellino CP, et al. Misplaced tracheoesophageal voice prosthesis: a case of foreign body aspiration. Am J Emerg Med 2021;41:266.e1-2.

32. Monteiro E, Sklar MC, Eskander A, et al. Assessment of the Clavien-Dindo classification system for complications in head and neck surgery: the Clavien-Dindo Classification System. Laryngoscope 2014; 124(12):2726–31.

33. Clavien PA, Sanabria JR, Strasberg SM. Proposed classification of complications of surgery with examples of utility in cholecystectomy. Surgery 1992; 111(5):518–26.

34. McMahon JD, MacIver C, Smith M, et al. Postoperative complications after major head and neck surgery with free flap repair—prevalence, patterns, and determinants: a prospective cohort study. Br J Oral Maxillofac Surg 2013;51(8):689–95.

35. Dindo D, Demartines N, Clavien P-A. Classification of surgical complications: a new proposal with evaluation in a cohort of 6336 patients and results of a survey. Ann Surg 2004;240(2):205–13.

36. Kwon D, Genden EM, de Bree R, et al. Overcoming wound complications in head and neck salvage surgery. Auris Nasus Larynx 2018;45(6):1135–42.

37. Herranz J, Sarandeses A, Fernandez M, et al. Complications after total laryngectomy in nonradiated laryngeal and hypopharyngeal carcinomas✩. Otolaryngol Head Neck Surg 2000;122(6):892–8.

38. Ailianou A, Mundada P, De Perrot T, et al. MRI with DWI for the detection of posttreatment head and neck squamous cell carcinoma: why morphologic MRI criteria matter. Am J Neuroradiol 2018;39(4): 748–55.

Imaging After Sinonasal Surgery

Jeffrey D. Hooker, MD[a], Sohil H. Patel, MD[a], Jose Mattos, MD, PhD[b], Sugoto Mukherjee, MD[a],*

KEYWORDS

• Sinonasal surgery • FESS surgery • Paranasal sinuses • Endoscopy • Complications
• Sinus imaging • Skull base

KEY POINTS

- Functional endoscopic sinonasal surgery (FESS) is the preferred method for treating medically refractive sinusitis.
- Advances in FESS techniques have expanded the role of FESS surgery in managing benign and malignant masses, as well as becoming the preferred approach in providing access for skull base and pituitary surgeries.
- Familiarity with the various procedures, knowledge of the various causes of surgical failures and complications, and understanding of the complex anatomy in this region, is essential for accurate interpretation.

INTRODUCTION

Modern sinonasal surgery is heavily dependent on endoscopic techniques both for treating mucosal inflammatory conditions and for accessing various benign and malignant sinonasal, skull base, and periorbital lesions. Over the last 2 decades, endoscopic approaches for various sinonasal surgeries have become ubiquitous and have significantly reduced patient morbidity with faster recovery times.

Most sinonasal surgeries come under the umbrella term functional endoscopic sinus surgery (FESS) (Box 1), which is a minimally invasive surgical technique, most often performed for the treatment of chronic sinusitis or sinonasal polyposis. The overall aim is to create or restore patency of the normal anatomic drainage pathways to allow for the clearance of secretions and normal sinus ventilation. Multiple different surgical techniques can be used during a single surgery based on the individual anatomy and specific locations of disease. Advances in technology and increasing familiarity with endoscopic techniques have led to the increasing use of endoscopic approaches for both benign and malignant sinonasal tumors.[1] Open surgeries are still used for more extensive disease or in instances whereby achieving adequate tumor resection is not amenable to endoscopic technique.

Imaging is a critical tool for preoperative planning, diagnostic workup of causes of treatment failure, and for the evaluation of postsurgical complications (Box 2). Imaging for sinonasal malignant and benign tumors is performed for preoperative staging, surgical planning, and postoperative tumor surveillance. Expected imaging findings following endoscopic surgery for both benign and malignant indications are largely site-specific.

[a] Department of Radiology and Medical Imaging, University of Virginia Health System, Charlottesville, VA 22903, USA; [b] Department of Otolaryngology–Head and Neck Surgery, University of Virginia Health System, Charlottesville, VA 22903, USA
* Corresponding author. Department of Radiology and Medical Imaging, University of Virginia Health System, 1215 Lee Street, PO Box 800170, Charlottesville, VA 22908-0170.
E-mail address: sm5qd@virginia.edu

Neuroimag Clin N Am 32 (2022) 55–73
https://doi.org/10.1016/j.nic.2021.08.008
1052-5149/22/© 2021 Elsevier Inc. All rights reserved.

Box 1
Types of sinus surgery

External nose and septum

- Rhinectomy (partial or total, with prosthesis or reconstruction)
- Septoplasty (either primary or for access/approach)

Directed toward anterior osteomeal unit

- Maxillary or middle meatus antrostomy and uncinectomy
- Middle and inferior turbinectomy
- Ethmoidectomy (total or partial)

Directed toward posterior osteomeal unit

- Sphenoidotomy
- Posterior ethmoidectomy

Frontal sinus procedures

- Endoscopic frontal sinusotomy (Draf type I, II, and III [modified Lothrop])

Caldwell–Luc surgery

Approach for orbital procedures

Approach for skull base and pituitary surgeries

Approach for the resection of benign and malignant mass lesions

Surgery for malignant masses

- Maxillectomy (partial/lateral/total), palatectomy (partial), turbinectomy
- Craniofacial resection

Osteoplastic flap frontal sinus obliteration and frontal sinus cranialization

IMAGING TECHNIQUE

Imaging following sinonasal surgery for chronic sinusitis has historically relied on direct imaging in the coronal plane. Multidetector CT now allows for imaging in the axial plane with isotropic voxels and multiplanar reconstruction in the coronal, sagittal, or oblique planes. Thin section axial imaging and multiplanar reconstruction also allow for a reduction in dental amalgam artifacts and the use of imaging data with intraoperative stereotactic guidance systems.[2] Administration of intravenous contrast is usually not necessary for imaging after FESS unless there is a concern for infection.[3] Magnetic resonance imaging (MRI) is usually reserved for cases of suspected intracranial complications or in situations whereby there is diagnostic uncertainty not amenable to direct visual or endoscopic evaluation.[3] Angiography may be used in select cases when there is concern for vascular complication. Computed tomography angiography (CTA), magnetic resonance angiography (MRA), or catheter-based angiography may be used.

Although MRI or CT with intravenous contrast is most commonly used following surgery for the resection of sinonasal tumors, PET/CT is a very useful tool for the evaluation of residual/recurrent disease and nodal involvement. The timing of imaging following surgery for sinonasal malignancy is an important factor to consider. A baseline postoperative MRI or CT is typically performed between 1 and 4 months following surgery to allow the expected postoperative inflammatory changes in subside. Most clinicians then follow the National Comprehensive Cancer Center (NCCN) guidelines for the timing of additional surveillance imaging.[4]

SURGICAL TECHNIQUES AND IMAGING FINDINGS
Septoplasty

Most often, the initial step in endoscopic sinus surgery is septoplasty to provide better surgical access for subsequent surgical techniques. Septoplasty may also be performed to relieve any associated nasal cavity obstruction secondary to a deviated nasal septum and/or any associated bony septal spur. Severe nasal septal deviation or a large spur can also contribute to sinusitis secondary to mass effect on associated osteomeatal unit structures. Imaging findings following septoplasty include a straightened nasal septum, thinned septal mucosa, irregular septal mucosal contour, and absence of any bony spurs.[5,6] In the early postoperative period following septoplasty, nasal stents or packing material may be identified[3,7] Imaging findings of septoplasty are best depicted in the coronal or axial planes(**Fig. 1**).

To help facilitate endonasal approaches to the anterior skull base or sellar region, the posterior nasal septum may be resected. Often, this is conducted in concert with the removal of other structures such as ethmoid septations, one or both middle turbinates, or the superior turbinates. If not resected, the turbinates may be lateralized. These actions are performed to help improve accessibility to the site of interest, improve the manipulation of surgical instruments in the posterior nasal cavity, and to improve visibility. Postsurgical changes from septectomy are best seen in the axial plane.[8]

Rhinectomy

Most malignancies involving the external nose only require limited local surgical excision or radiotherapy.[9] For advanced cases, partial or total

---

Box 2
Complications following FESS surgery

Minor complications

- Recurrent sinusitis and polyposis
- Residual frontal sinus disease
- Lateralized middle turbinates/scarring stenosis or middle meatus
- Adhesions and septations
- Mucus recirculation
- Neo-osteogenesis
- Nasal septal perforations
- Empty nose syndrome

Major complications

Vascular injury

- Hemorrhage
- Pseudoaneurysm

Orbital complications

- Hematoma
- Abscess
- Penetration
- Motility disorder
- Blindness

Intracranial injury

- CSF leak, meningocele, and encephalocele
- Subarachnoid and parenchyma injury with edema and/or hemorrhage
- Infection – abscess/cerebritis

---

rhinectomy may be performed. Reconstruction may be performed with autologous regional or free tissue flaps, although this is a technically difficult procedure and outcomes are often unsatisfactory.[9] Nasal prostheses are currently the reconstruction technique of choice following rhinectomy.[9,10] (**Fig. 2**).

MAXILLARY SINUS SURGERY
Maxillary Antrostomy and Uncinectomy

Following septoplasty, removal of the uncinate process (uncinectomy) may be performed.[11] Uncinectomy allows for greater surgical access to the maxillary ostium, frontal recess, and anterior ethmoid complex,[12] for treating obstruction involving the anterior osteomeatal complex. Next, widening of the maxillary sinus ostium and infundibulum (maxillary antrostomy or middle meatus antrostomy) may be performed (**Fig. 3**). If

present, maxillary polyps, mucosal hypertrophy, or tumors amenable to endoscopic treatment may then be resected (**Fig. 4**). Imaging findings of uncinectomy and maxillary antrostomy include the absence or partial absence of the uncinate process and widening of the maxillary ostium and infundibulum. These findings are typically best depicted in the coronal plane.

Caldwell–Luc Procedure

Several procedures which are no longer commonly performed or performed less frequently than previously for certain indications may sometimes be seen on imaging, particularly in older patients. The Caldwell–Luc procedure involves the external access of the maxillary sinus through a surgically created defect in the buccal mucosal surface of the maxillary bone and passage through the anterior wall of the maxillary sinus.[13] This is usually followed by a middle meatal antrostomy or an inferior nasoantral window or inferior meatal antrostomy, a surgically created defect in the medial wall of the maxillary sinus below the inferior turbinate attachment.[13] The canine fossa puncture has a similar approach to the Caldwell–Luc procedure and is sometimes performed for specific indications related to maxillary sinus disease.[14] Postprocedural changes from Caldwell–Luc procedure are best seen in the axial plane as a defect in the anterior wall of the maxillary sinus (**Fig. 5**). Postsurgical changes from inferior nasalantral window creation or inferior meatus puncture are best seen in the coronal plane as a defect in the medial maxillary wall inferior to the inferior turbinate attachment.

Maxillectomy

Maxillectomy can be partial or total. For tumors centered along the medial maxillary wall or the lateral nasal wall, a medial maxillectomy may be performed. In a medial maxillectomy, the medial maxillary sinus wall/lateral nasal wall is removed, traditionally along with the inferior turbinate and the nasolacrimal duct although the preservation of the inferior turbinate or nasolacrimal duct may be attempted.[15] Depending on tumor extent and/or ability to access the necessary areas, other structures may be resected or manipulated including the middle turbinate or portions of the ethmoid cavity. Depending on tumor extent, partial maxillectomy can involve the lateral wall, or can be extended to include portions of the palate, orbital floor, or other structures (**Fig. 6**). If the palate or orbital floor is resected, one may see palatal prostheses, palatal reconstruction flaps, orbital floor mesh reconstruction hardware, or orbital floor

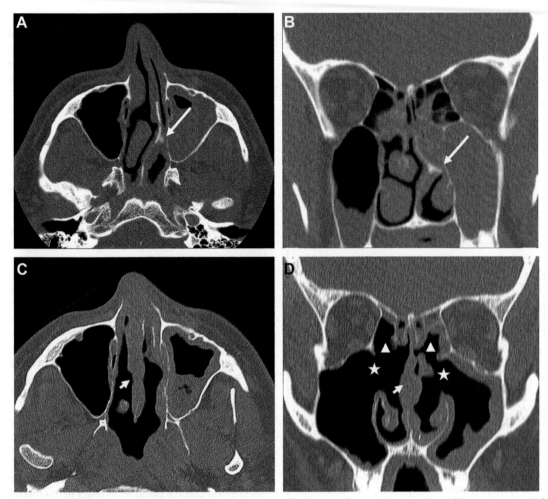

Fig. 1. Septoplasty. Pre (*A, B*) and postoperative images (*C, D*) showing changes in septoplasty (short *arrow* in C,D) for a leftward deviated nasal septum with a large spur (*long arrow* in A and B). This procedure was conducted in combination with other FESS procedures of bilateral maxillary antrostomy (*white star*) and ethmoidectomies (*white triangle*).

reconstruction flaps on postoperative imaging.[16–20] Partial maxillectomy may be performed endoscopically or via an open approach.

Total maxillectomy involves the resection of all of the maxillary sinus walls. Removal of the orbital contents or orbital exenteration may also sometimes be necessary. Because this involves the resection of several tissues and significant alterations in anatomy, flaps, or prosthesis are used to reconstruct the midface for both functional and cosmetic reasons.[21] Free flaps are most commonly used but local pedicled flaps may also be seen.[21]

NASAL TURBINATE SURGERY
Middle Turbinectomy

Middle turbinectomy is commonly performed during FESS and may be performed to allow for greater access during approaches to sinonasal or sellar tumors. The middle turbinate vertical insertion at the skull base is an important surgical landmark during endoscopic sinus surgery.[22] Surgeons generally attempt to stay lateral to the middle turbinate in an effort to avoid inadvertently causing a cerebrospinal fluid (CSF) leak.[12] For this reason, middle turbinectomy is most often partial with a portion of the vertical insertion at the skull base usually intentionally left intact (see **Fig. 3**). The presence or absence of a residual middle turbinate following endoscopic sinus surgery with middle turbinectomy should be noted. To prevent recurrent osteomeatal complex obstruction, following partial middle turbinectomy, the residual middle turbinate may be purposefully fixated to the lateral wall of the nasal septum.[23] (see **Fig. 3**). This is beneficial anatomically and should be noted in the radiology report. Likewise, a lateralized middle

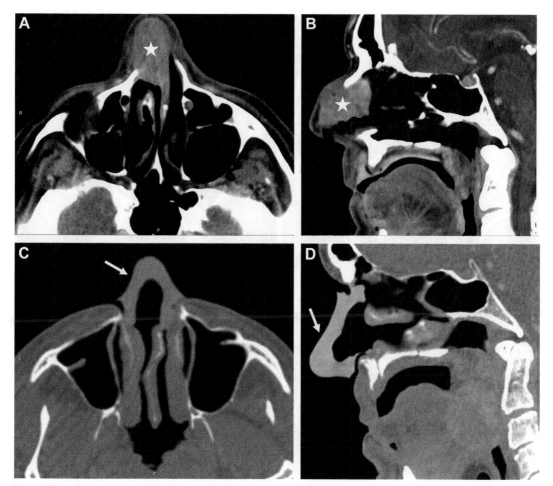

Fig. 2. Rhinectomy with nasal prosthesis. Total rhinectomy with reconstruction using a silicone nasal prosthesis (*white arrow* in *C, D*) in a patient with T4 squamous cell carcinoma of the right nasal cavity (*white star* in *A, B*) with the erosion of the nasal bones.

turbinate on postsurgical imaging is an important finding to identify and communicate as this could be a potential cause for recurrent osteomeatal complex obstruction and sinusitis.[23] Findings of middle turbinectomy are generally easiest to appreciate in the coronal plane.

Inferior Turbinectomy

Inferior turbinate reduction or inferior turbinoplasty may be performed for cases of nasal cavity obstruction secondary to the mucosal inflammation of these structures. Resection can be total or partial. Resection can involve submucosa or bone.[24] Lateralization of the inferior turbinates via out-fracture may be performed.[24] Additionally, various types of ablation (radiofrequency, ultrasound, cryoablation) can be used to produce scarring and subsequent reduction in mucosal volume.[24] On imaging, finding of inferior turbinate

reduction or turbinoplasty includes the partial or complete absence of the inferior turbinate, lateralization of the inferior turbinate, or thinning of the inferior turbinate mucosal structures. These findings are best depicted in the coronal plane.

ETHMOID SINUS SURGERY
Ethmoidectomy

Depending on the extent of disease and patient anatomy, total or partial ethmoidectomy may be performed (**Fig. 7**). If the posterior ethmoid air cells are entered, a portion of the vertical basal lamella of the middle turbinate must be removed. This structure demarcates the anterior from the posterior ethmoid air cells. The presence of residual ethmoid air cells should be noted, especially if disease is present. Residual cells are usually located superiorly near the skull base or posteriorly near the sphenoid sinuses and may be intentionally

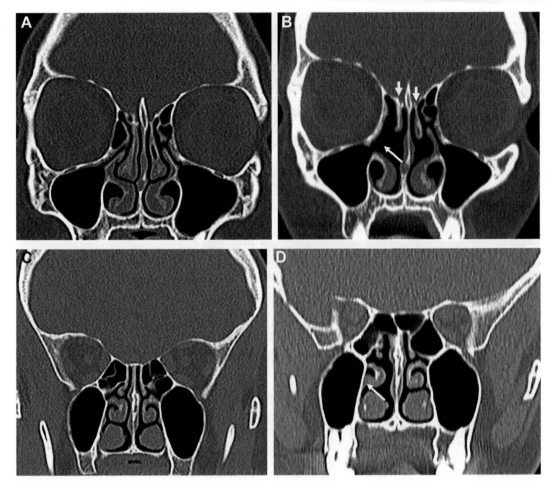

Fig. 3. FESS procedures. Pre (*A*) and postsurgical (*B*) images show FESS procedures changes including right-sided uncinate resection (*long white arrow, B*), ethmoidectomy, right maxillary antrostomy, and bilateral turbinate reductions. Note the preservation of the vertical lamella following middle turbinate reduction surgery (*short white arrow, B*). In another patient, pre (*C*) and postprocedure (*D*) images show the subtle changes in lateralization of the middle turbinate (*white arrow, D*).

left intact to avoid CSF leak or optic nerve injury.[12] A deep olfactory fossa, an asymmetrically low olfactory fossa on one side, or dehiscence of the cribriform plate or ethmoid roof may predispose to iatrogenic injury. Findings of ethmoidectomy are best seen in the axial and coronal planes.

SPHENOID SINUS SURGERY
Sphenoidotomy

Functional endoscopic surgery of the sphenoid sinus is less commonly performed than those previously mentioned. Treatment options for sphenoid sinus disease are varied. The natural ostium at the sphenoethmoidal recess may be widened via a transnasal approach without ethmoidectomy or the sphenoid sinus may be accessed through the posterior ethmoid air cells following

ethmoidectomy or sphenoid sinus marsupialization may be performed (Fig. 8). On preoperative or postoperative imaging for patients under consideration for revision endoscopic sinus surgery (RESS), it is critical to note a few anatomic variations in this region. Sphenoid sinus septa are variable in the number and site of insertion. If a sphenoid sinus septum inserts on the carotid canal or optic canal, it is important to know this preoperatively. Pneumatized anterior clinoid processes should be mentioned as dissection or instrumentation in this region could place the optic nerves or internal carotid arteries at risk of injury. Bony dehiscence or thinning of the optic or carotid canal walls should be noted. Additionally, the sphenoethmoidal air cell, also commonly known as the Onodi air cell, is an anatomic variant generally defined as the excessive pneumatization of the

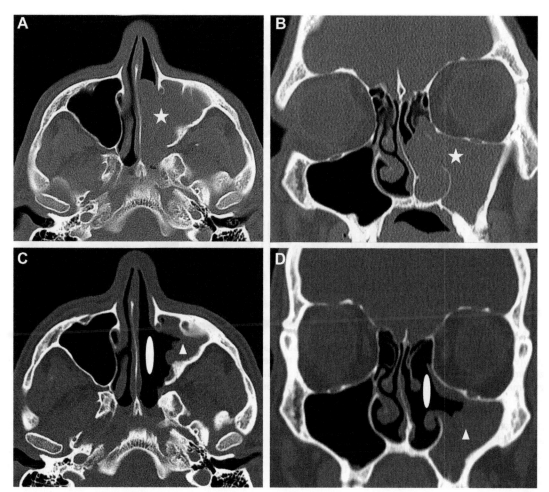

Fig. 4. Endoscopic tumor resection. Preoperative (*A, B*) axial and coronal CT shows a left-sided inverted papilloma, which was resected endoscopically. Postoperative (*C, D*) images show changes in tumor resection along with findings of left uncinectomy, partial left turbinectomies, ethmoidectomy, and left medial maxillary wall resection (*white oval, C, D*). Residual mucosal thickening is present in the left maxillary sinus (*white triangle, C, D*). Comparison with the preserved structures on the right helps illustrate the missing resected structures on the left.

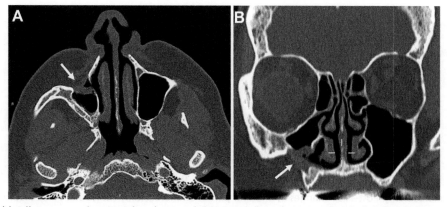

Fig. 5. Caldwell–Luc procedure. Axial and coronal CT images show large postsurgical defect (*white arrow A, B*) involving the anterolateral wall of the right maxillary sinus, consistent with history of Caldwell–Luc procedure.

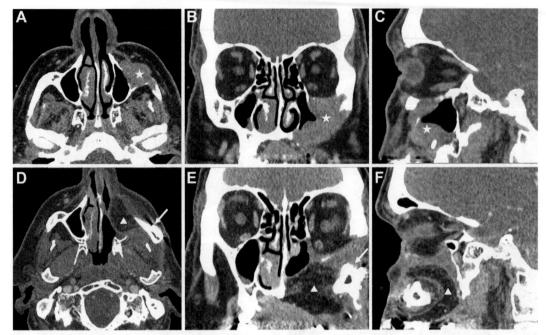

Fig. 6. Total maxillectomy. Pre (*A–C*) and post (*D–F*) surgical changes for the resection of a left maxillary sarcoma (*white star, A–C*), with left total maxillectomy, with the resection of hard palate, left orbital floor, and the left zygoma with free flap reconstruction of the left midface (*white triangle, D–F*), fibular graft for maxilla-zygomatic reconstruction (*white arrow, D*) and left infraorbital floor reconstruction using AlloDerm.

posterior-most ethmoid air cells superlateral to the sphenoid sinus. These air cells may lie in close proximity to the internal carotid artery or optic nerve or the air cells may extend into the anterior clinoid processes. Findings from endoscopic sphenoid sinus surgery are most often best appreciated in the sagittal and axial planes.[25]

Aside from functional sphenoid sinus surgery, sphenoidotomy is performed for transsphenoidal sellar approaches. Alteration of normal paranasal sinus anatomy whereas instruments are advanced toward the sella through the nasal cavity is minimized as much as possible, although as mentioned earlier various structures may need to be manipulated or resected to obtain adequate access.[26] Following the resection of a portion of the posterior nasal septum, a wide sphenoidotomy is performed. Sphenoid sinus septa are resected. Access to the sella is then obtained. Following the sellar phase of the procedure, skull base reconstruction must be performed. In some cases such as when a CSF leak was noted intraoperatively or a large dural defect is anticipated, a vascularized nasomucosal flap created from the

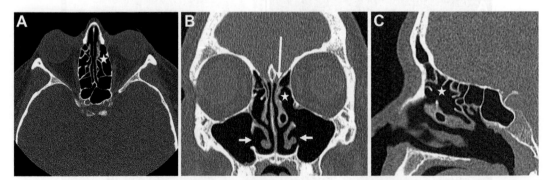

Fig. 7. Ethmoidectomy. Post–FESS changes in bilateral partial ethmoidectomy (*white star A–C*). Additional findings of bilateral uncinate resection and nasoantral defects (*short white arrows, B*) are also evident on the coronal images. Also, note the preservation of the vertical basal lamella of the middle turbinate (*long white arrow, B*).

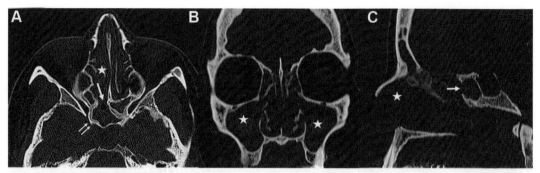

Fig. 8. Recurrent polyposis postsurgery. Recurrent pansinus polyposis (*star* in A–C) is seen in these images in this patient with extensive bilateral FESS surgery directed at both the anterior osteomeatal unit (including uncinectomy, antrostomy, and septoplasty) as well as the posterior osteomeatal unit (which includes posterior ethmoidectomy and right sphenoidotomy [*single white arrows* in A, C]). Note the diffuse neoosteogenesis surrounding the sphenoid sinus (*double arrows*, A).

previously described nasal septum resection or use of an autologous fat graft may be used.[26] (Fig. 9). Otherwise, the defect may be sealed with a combination of various synthetic materials such as gelfoam, fibrin glue, or synthetic grafts.[26]

FRONTAL SINUS SURGERY
Endoscopic Frontal Sinusotomy

Endoscopic frontal sinus surgery is divided into a 3-part Draf classification characterized by progressively more extensive procedures. The Draf type 1 procedure refers to the resection of the anterior ethmoid air cells and the uncinate process followed by a frontal sinusotomy.[27] (Fig. 10). A Draf type 2 procedure involves the resection of the frontal sinus floor from the nasal septum medially to the lamina papyracea laterally.[27] (Fig. 11). In the Draf type 3 or the modified Lothrop procedure, the frontal sinus septum, superior nasal septum, and the entire frontal sinus floor to the level of the orbit are resected[27](Fig. 12).

Various types of frontal sinus stents may also be used to maintain or restore patency of the frontal sinus outflow tract.[28]

The frontal sinus region may also be associated with many important anatomic variants including agger nasi cells, frontal cells, and supraorbital ethmoid cells. Residual frontal sinus region variants not identified preoperatively or intraoperatively can be a cause of recurrent frontal sinus disease following surgery. The frontal sinuses and frontal outflow tracts are generally best depicted on sagittal and coronal planes.

Osteoplastic Flap Frontal Sinus Obliteration

Osteoplastic flap frontal sinus obliteration, an external approach, was previously the gold standard for the treatment of chronic frontal sinusitis

and may still be performed for this indication in certain instances.[29] It is also used for the surgical treatment of frontal sinus pathology not amenable to endoscopic approach such as complex frontal sinus fractures and their complications, such as mucoceles. This procedure involves the resection of the frontal sinus mucosa and obliteration of the sinus with fat (usually abdominal) grafts.[29]

Postprocedural changes from frontal sinus obliteration with an osteoplastic flap demonstrate fat density or signal filling the frontal sinus and changes from prior osteotomy (Fig. 13).

ORBITAL DECOMPRESSION

Orbital decompression surgery is primarily used to treat thyroid eye disease, though it can be used to treat any cause of increased orbital pressure. The medial orbital wall, lateral orbital wall, and orbital floor may be resected to achieve decompression. Additionally, fat can be resected without the removal of bone using transcutaneous, transconjunctival, and transcaruncular approaches. Regarding surgical approaches that involve the sinonasal cavities, (eg, medial orbital wall and orbital floor approaches) these may be open, endoscopic, or via a Caldwell–Luc antrostomy. The orbital floor is rarely decompressed in isolation. Orbital floor decompression is usually combined with medial wall decompression as an inferomedial procedure. Endoscopic orbital decompression usually involves uncinectomy and ethmoidectomy to access the orbital floor and medial orbital wall, respectively. However, access is obtained, the orbital floor or medial orbital wall, and commonly both, are resected. Orbital fat can be resected along with bone resection if a greater reduction of proptosis is desired. On imaging, postsurgical changes from prior orbital

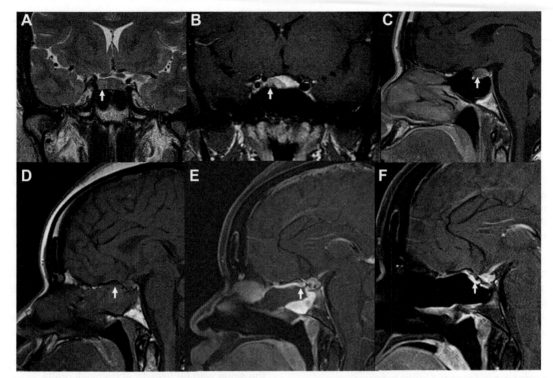

Fig. 9. Sphenoidotomy and nasoseptal flap. Preoperative coronal T2 (*A*), postcontrast coronal T1 (*B*), and sagittal T1 (*C*) show a pituitary microadenoma (*white arrow*). Immediate postoperative sagittal T1 pre (*D*) and postcontrast (*E*) shows the extensive changes in sphenoidotomy, packing materials, and nasoseptal flap reconstruction (*small white arrow*) of the anterior sellar floor. Later follow-up images (*F*) show the expected evolution of the findings with a resolution of the sinus mucosal thickening and thinning of the nasoseptal flap (small *white arrow*).

decompression include the absence of the lamina papyracea or orbital floor and projection of orbital contents into the ethmoid sinus region or maxillary sinus. Postsurgical changes from the various approaches to the orbital walls may also be noted.[30,31]

CRANIOFACIAL RESECTION

Patients with large sinonasal tumors that would otherwise be difficult to completely resect or with tumors involving the anterior skull base may undergo craniofacial resection. Traditionally this has been performed as an open surgery though in some cases, endoscopic approaches are now being used. In an open craniofacial resection, first, a bifrontal craniotomy is usually performed although other craniotomy variations may be used depending on the specific circumstances. Then a lateral rhinotomy or similar incision is performed, followed by an osteotomy to provide exposure to the sinonasal cavity. Depending on the sites of tumor involvement, partial or total maxillectomy, turbinectomy, ethmoidectomy, sphenoidotomy, nasal septal resection, frontal sinus cranialization,

or orbital exenteration can be performed to obtain adequate margins (**Fig. 14**). Intracranially, the frontal lobes may be retracted to expose the skull base and subsequent frontal lobe edema may be seen on postoperative imaging. If dura is found to be involved, dural dissection is performed, which increases the risk of CSF leak or subsequent intracranial infection. In the immediate postoperative period, pneumocephalus or intracranial hemorrhage may be seen. Following the resection of the tumor and any other associated structures, reconstruction is performed. Free flaps, local vascularized pedicle flaps (often using the inferior turbinate, middle turbinate, or nasal septum), synthetic material, and/or composite grafts may be used.[32–35]

POSTOPERATIVE COMPLICATIONS
Hemorrhage and Other Vascular Complications

As mentioned previously, the internal carotid arteries are at risk for injury during sinus surgery and several anatomic variants can increase this risk. Additional arterial structures which may be

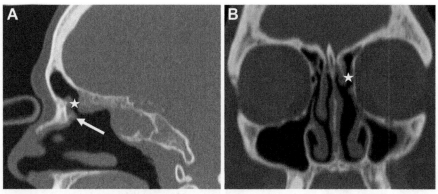

Fig. 10. Endoscopic frontal recess approach (Draf type 1 procedure). Parasagittal and coronal images show removal of anterosuperior ethmoidal and frontal recess air cells (*white star, A, B*) and the uncinate process on the left side with the preservation of the nasofrontal beak (*white arrow, A*).

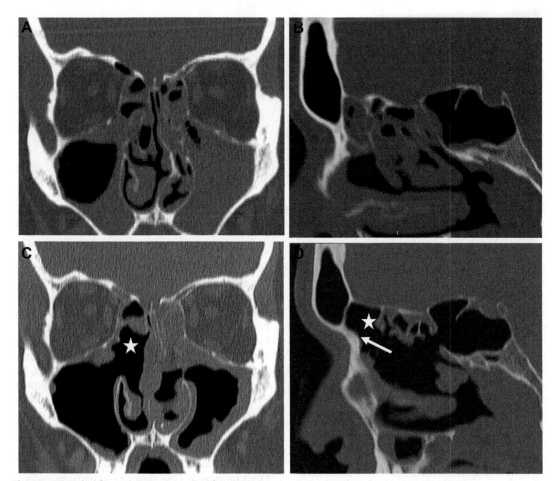

Fig. 11. Extended frontal sinusotomy (Draf type 2 procedure). Pre (*A, B*) and postoperative (*C, D*) images show the endoscopic approach resection of the floor of the frontal sinus extending from the lamina papyracea laterally to the nasal septum medially (*white star, C*). The parasagittal images on the right side show the typical postoperative changes in the enlargement of the frontal sinus drainage pathway, with the removal of the anterior ethmoid and frontal recess air cells (*white star, D*) as well as the loss of the nasofrontal beak (*white arrow, D*).

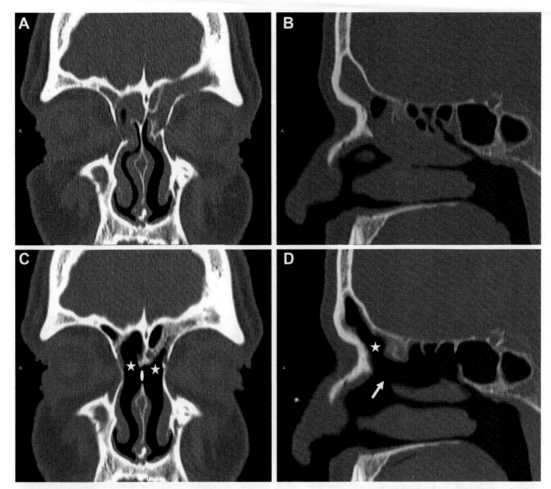

Fig. 12. Modified Lothrop procedure (Draf type 3). Pre (*A, B*) and postoperative (*C, D*) images show the findings of modified Lothrop procedure, which includes the clearance of bilateral frontal sinus drainage pathways (*white star, C, D*), with additional removal of the frontal sinus septum, superior nasal septum (*white oval, C*), parts of the middle turbinate anteriorly (*arrow, D*).

at risk for injury during sinonasal surgery include the anterior and posterior ethmoid arteries, the sphenopalatine arteries, and even the anterior cerebral arteries.[36,37] The internal carotid artery is most at risk for injury during procedures involving the posterior ethmoid air cells or the sphenoid sinuses.[38] Frontal sinus surgery, anterior ethmoid procedures, and procedures involving the anterior portions of the middle turbinates and anterior portions of the nasal septum place the anterior ethmoidal arteries or their branches at risk.[39] The sphenopalatine artery or its branches supply much blood supply to the posterior portion of the middle turbinates, nasal cavity including the nasal septum, and sphenoid sinuses.[40,41] The posterior ethmoidal artery supplies the posterior ethmoid air cells and part of the posterior nasal septum.[41] Arterial anatomy, as elsewhere in the body, is variable and CTA or catheter-based angiography may

be needed to delineate the specifically involved vascular structures.

Treatment of vascular complications varies by site of injury and severity of hemorrhage. Surgical packing or cautery with silver nitrate may be performed. Endovascular treatment with coils, covered stents, or balloon occlusion can be performed for heavy bleeding or refractory cases. Ultimately surgical cautery, ligation, or vascular bypass (in cases of internal carotid artery injury without reassuring findings on test balloon occlusion) in the operating room may be required.[41]

Cerebrospinal Fluid Leak and Skull Base Injury

Most iatrogenic CSF leaks or skull base defects are identified at the time of injury and successfully repaired intraoperatively.[12] For those cases not detected or repaired at the time of surgery, imaging in conjunction with the β2-transferrin test plays

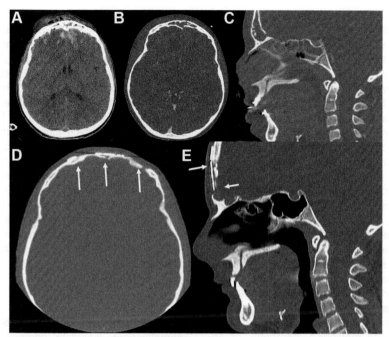

Fig. 13. Frontal sinus cranialization. Pretreatment axial (*A, B*) and sagittal (*C*) CT images show communited fractures involving the frontal calvarium with the involvement of both the inner and outer tables of the frontal sinuses and intracranial hemorrhage. Postprocedural changes in bifrontal craniotomy, followed by the cranialization of the frontal sinus along with repair using pericranial graft (*arrows* in *D, E*). Note the continuation of the intracranial compartment into the frontal sinus, with no inner table.

a vital role in diagnosis and localization. Complications resulting from the perforation of the skull base include intracranial hemorrhage, direct cerebral parenchymal injury, intracranial infection, or cephalocele. Most associated intracranial complications are best depicted on MRI.

On CT, findings suggestive of a leak include an osseous defect and adjacent paranasal sinus or nasal cavity opacification, or air-fluid level. CT performed before and following the administration of iodinated intrathecal contrast, or CT cisternography, may be performed.[42] CT cisternography

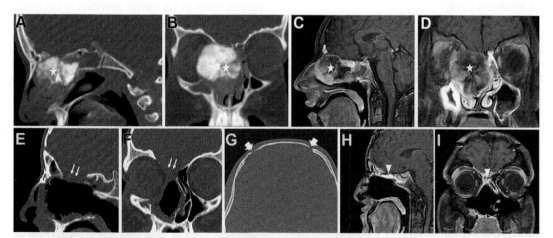

Fig. 14. Craniofacial resection. Presurgical CT (*A, B*) and MR (*C, D*) images show a large sinonasal osteosarcoma (*white star, A–D*) involving the upper sinonasal cavity with extension into the right orbit and the anterior skull base. Postsurgical CT (*E–G*) and MR (*H,I*) images show the findings of bifrontal craniotomy (*white arrowhead, G*) for craniofacial approach anterior skull base resection (*double white arrows E, F*) of the tumor with a reconstruction of the anterior skull base using vascularized pericranial flap (*white triangle, H, I*).

should be assessed both qualitatively and quantitatively. If a CSF leak is present, an increase in the attenuation of material within the sinonasal cavity following the administration of intrathecal contrast may be detected visually (**Fig. 15**). In more subtle cases, an increase in Hounsfield units within a region of interest by more than 50% on postintrathecal contrast images is considered positive for CSF leak.[42] In the immediate postoperative period, CT is the best choice for depicting suspected intracranial hemorrhage.

MRI may be performed particularly if there is a concern for cephalocele or intracranial complications. CT findings of osseous skull base defect and complete opacification of the adjacent sinuses/sinonasal cavity or especially the opacification of the adjacent sinus in a nondependent or lobular fashion should raise the concern for potential cephalocele and MRI should then be considered to exclude cephalocele.[42] MRI with and without intravenous contrast is also the study of choice to detect the intracranial complications of infection including meningitis, cerebritis, or abscess. Gliosis or encephalomalacia will also be best seen on MRI. MRI cisternography without contrast is characterized by the utilization of high-resolution three-dimensional heavily T2-weighted sequences and may be used to directly visualize CSF leaks, evidenced by a fluid-intensity column contiguous with both the intracranial and extracranial compartments.[42] MRI cisternography following the intrathecal administration of gadolinium may also be performed at some institutions.[43] Findings positive for CSF leak on intrathecal gadolinium-enhanced MRI cisternography are T1 hyperintense gadolinium material within the sinonasal cavity.[43]

Radionuclide cisternography is an additional technique that may be used to detect CSF leaks. Absorbent pledgets are first placed into the sinonasal cavity in various locations via endoscopy. Then a radiotracer, indium-111 (111In)-labeled diethylenetriamine-pentaacetic acid (DTPA) or technetium-99m (99mTc)-DTPA is administered intrathecally. Imaging with a gamma camera is then performed usually at 2 to 6 hours and 24 hours following radiotracer administration. Indium-111 imaging may be delayed up to 72 hours for slower leaks.[42] Activity in the region of the sinonasal cavity suggests a leak. Activity in the bowel can also suggest a leak which indicates that the patient has swallowed CSF following leakage in the sinonasal cavity.[12] Following nuclear medicine imaging, the absorbent pledgets are removed and the radiotracer activity of the pledgets is compared with serum radiotracer activity.[42,44] Ranges for a positive pledget-to-serum ratio vary by study and institution with the usual lower threshold considered to be a pledget-to-serum activity ratio of 1.5:1.[42,44]

Orbital Complications

Inadvertent penetration into the orbit can cause complications including hemorrhage, infection, extraocular muscle injury, and even permanent blindness. Imaging findings of orbital injury include medial or inferior orbital wall defect, hematoma, proptosis, orbital emphysema, fat stranding/edema, distortion of the extraocular muscles, distortion of the optic nerve, or distortion of the globe. Intraorbital infection can occur following orbital penetration and cellulitis or abscess may result.

The medial orbital wall is the most common site of penetration and various anatomic factors may predispose to orbital injury.[45] Preexisting lamina papyracea defects, usually secondary to prior trauma, result in the medial deviation of the medial orbital wall and adjacent intraorbital soft tissue. The medially deviated lamina papyracea can be mistaken for ethmoid septation and medially herniated soft tissues may be mistaken for hypertrophied sinonasal mucosa.[46] An additional anatomic

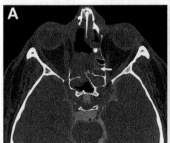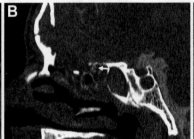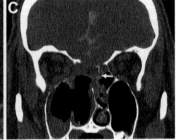

Fig. 15. CSF leak postsinonasal surgery. Axial (*A*), sagittal (*B*), and coronal (*C*) CT cisternogram images show a small amount of contrast pooling within the left posterior ethmoid cell (*white arrow*) status postresection of mass involving the sinonasal cavity and anterior skull base.

factor that may place a patient at risk for orbital complications is the lateralization of the uncinate process. Typically the medial orbital wall lies in the same vertical plane as the maxillary sinus ostium.[12] This can result from maxillary or ethmoid sinus underpneumatization or maxillary atelectasis.[47] When the normal anatomic relationship of the medial orbital wall and the maxillary sinus ostium are distorted, this predisposes to orbital penetration during FESS.[47]

Orbital hematomas can be venous or arterial. Although rare, arterial hemorrhage (secondary to injury of anterior ethmoidal artery) is a surgical emergency and is usually identified during or immediately following surgery within the recovery suite.[48] Venous hemorrhage is less rapid and therefore, likely to present later.[49] Regardless of the source, intraorbital hemorrhage can result in an orbital compartment syndrome and subsequent optic nerve ischemia.[49]

Extraocular muscle injury can occur. This most commonly involves the medial rectus.[45] Injuries range from muscle fiber disruption to complete laceration.[45] Even in the absence of direct muscular injury, scarring/fibrosis of the adjacent fat can result in restricted extraocular muscle movement or a change in the vector of muscle pull.[45] Additionally, muscles can become entrapped following iatrogenic bony orbital wall injury and subsequent herniation of soft tissue structures through the defect.

Nasolacrimal duct injury can result in epiphora or dacryocystitis. Most nasolacrimal duct injuries resolve without intervention.[12] Some cases may require stenting, dacryocystoplasty, or dacryocystorhinostomy.[3] Duct integrity can be assessed with CT or dacryocystography.

Lastly, direct optic nerve injury can occur. Several anatomic variants mentioned previously may be present in and around the sphenoid sinus which can predispose to optic nerve injury during procedures involving this region. These include an insertion of a sphenoid sinus septum onto the optic canal, pneumatized anterior clinoid processes, osseous thinning or dehiscence, or Onodi cells.[25]

Nasal Septum Perforation

Septoplasty can rarely result in nasal septal perforation.[50] As the nasal septal cartilage is relatively avascular, this is thought to occur due to the disruption of the nasal septum mucosa in corresponding areas on each side of the septum.[50] Most patients with nasal septal perforation are asymptomatic though symptomatic patients may report recurrent epistaxis, crusting, pain, or whistling.[50,51] If symptomatic, nasal septal perforation may be surgically treated with various types of tissue grafts or placement of a prosthesis.[52]

Empty Nose Syndrome

Empty nose syndrome (ENS) refers to a clinical entity most often following turbinate resection characterized by paradoxic nasal obstruction despite a patent nasal cavity on imaging, physical examination, and endoscopy.[53] (**Fig. 16**). Patients diagnosed with ENS may report symptoms of dyspnea, nasal crusting, dryness, and epistaxis.[53,54] Notably, ENS sufferers frequently report significant impacts on activities of daily living and many patients are diagnosed with depression and anxiety.[55] The pathogenesis of ENS is controversial but likely a multifactorial process related to the disruption of normal mucosal-assisted air humidification, postsurgical anatomic alterations leading to changes in airflow resistance, and disruption of neurosensory

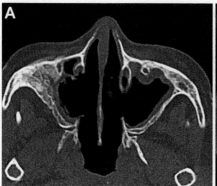 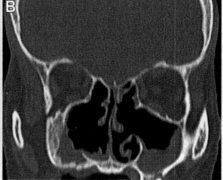

Fig. 16. Empty nose syndrome. Changes in bilateral FESS surgery are seen in this patient with a clinical diagnosis of Empty nose syndrome. There is near complete resection of bilateral superior, middle, and right inferior turbinates, with partial resection of the left inferior turbinate on axial (*A*) and coronal (*B*) CT images.

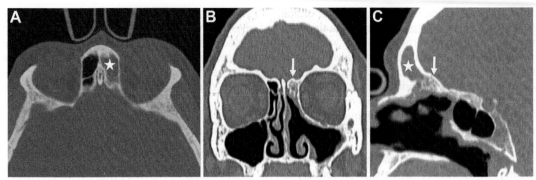

Fig. 17. Recurrent mucosal obstruction and neoosteogenesis. Axial, coronal, and sagittal CT images in this patient with prior frontal recess endoscopic surgery show recurrent obstruction with complete opacification of the left frontal sinus (*white star, A, C*). In addition, coronal and sagittal images also show thickening and sclerotic changes of residual ethmoid septa, suggestive for neoosteogenesis (*white arrow, B, C*).

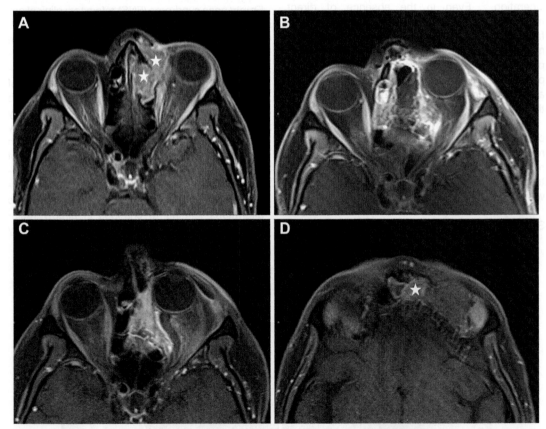

Fig. 18. Recurrent tumor. Preoperative (*A*) and immediate postoperative (*B*) images show endonasal approach resection of a sinonasal undifferentiated carcinoma (white star, A) involving the left anterior ethmoid, with extension into the left orbit and the left prenasal soft tissues. Follow-up imaging at 2 years shows expected postsurgical changes in the left ethmoid (*C*) with focal recurrence along the superior aspect of the postsurgical site, superomedial to the orbit (*white star, D*).

mechanisms.[53,56] Management of ENS is challenging.[57] Conservative treatment consists of topical corticosteroids, nasal lavage, and lubricants.[57] Surgical reconstruction of the turbinates with implantable biomaterials or autografts can also be performed.[57]

Recurrent Sinusitis

RESS is not uncommon and the need for RESS is affected by various factors such as the presence of polyps, asthma, aspirin-exacerbated respiratory disease, fungal sinusitis, and many others.[58] Initially, patients with symptoms of chronic sinusitis following FESS are managed medically with antibiotics and steroids.[59] If this fails, a CT scan is usually performed and revision surgery may be considered.[59] The most common anatomic findings identified in patients undergoing RESS are lateralized middle turbinate (due to postsurgical scarring/adhesions), recurrent polyps (see **Fig. 8**), residual ethmoid air cells, frontal recess scarring, residual agger nasi cells, and residual uncinate process.[23,59,60] Following FESS, it is common to see focal or diffuse sinus wall osseous thickening.[61,62] (**Fig. 17**). Although this finding, commonly referred to as osteitis or neoosteogenesis, can be seen in patients with chronic sinusitis who have not had surgery, it is more common in patients with a history of previous sinus surgery.[63] The pathogenesis of this finding is still inconclusive, though it has been associated with disease severity and an increased incidence of revision surgery.[63] When imaging patients being considered for revision surgery, it is important to identify any potential causes of sinonasal stenosis or obstruction, describe areas of sinonasal opacification, and to accurately detail any previously performed procedures and associated anatomic alterations to assist in preoperative planning for revision surgery.

Recurrent Malignancy

It can be difficult to discriminate recurrent disease from inflammation or granulation tissue. Both demonstrate variable patterns of enhancement, CT density, and MRI signal characteristics. Often, recurrence can only be reliably diagnosed with serial imaging or biopsy and careful evaluation of the baseline posttreatment imaging scan. Imaging findings that can suggest residual or recurrent tumor include new areas of nodular enhancement (**Fig. 18**), new bone erosion, and presence of restricted diffusion. If reconstruction techniques were used, close attention to the surgical flap margins is prudent.[64,65]

SUMMARY

Posttreatment imaging evaluation of sinuses encompasses a wide gamut of procedures, ranging from endoscopic procedures for sinonasal inflammatory diseases to markedly radical surgeries for malignant neoplasms (with or without reconstructions), as well as providing access for surgeries involving the anterior and central skull base. Advances in both techniques and devices have expanded the use of endoscopic approaches in managing both benign and malignant lesions, in addition to being the primary surgical method for treating all medically refractive sinonasal inflammatory disorders. Familiarity with the complex anatomy in the sinonasal region and knowledge of the various procedures is indispensable in interpreting these imaging studies.

CLINICS CARE POINTS

- Knowledge of various FESS surgical techniques and reconstructive methods, in addition to access to presurgical imaging and operative notes is essential in evaluating post treatment scans.

- A systematic approach is a prerequisite to evaluate all the various subsites and components within the paranasal sinuses, adjacent soft tissues and the skull base.

- Familiarity with various complications and recurrence patterns in surgeries for both benign and malignant sinonasal conditions is crucial in accurately interpreting post treatment scans.

DISCLOSURE

The authors have nothing to disclose.

REFERENCES

1. Rawal RB, Farzal Z, Federspiel JJ, et al. Endoscopic resection of sinonasal malignancy: a systematic review and meta-analysis. Otolaryngol–Head Neck Surg 2016;155(3):376–86.
2. Huang BY, Lloyd KM, DelGaudio JM, et al. Failed endoscopic sinus surgery: spectrum of ct findings in the frontal recess. RadioGraphics 2009;29(1):177–95.
3. Ginat DT. Posttreatment imaging of the paranasal sinuses following endoscopic sinus surgery. Neuroimaging Clin N Am 2015;25(4):653–65.

4. Workman AD, Palmer JN, Adappa ND. Posttreat-ment surveillance for sinonasal malignancy. Curr Opin Otolaryngol Head Neck Surg 2017;25(1): 86–92.

5. Hwang PH, McLaughlin RB, Lanza DC, et al. Endo-scopic septoplasty: indications, technique, and re-sults. Otolaryngol–head Neck Surg Off J Am Acad Otolaryngol-head Neck Surg 1999;120(5):678–82.

6. Schatz CJ, Ginat DT. Imaging features of rhino-plasty. Am J Neuroradiol 2014;35(2):216–22.

7. Dubin MR, Pletcher SD. Postoperative packing after septoplasty: is it necessary? Otolaryngol Clin North Am 2009;42(2):279–85, viii–ix.

8. Hosemann W, Schroeder HWS. Comprehensive re-view on rhino-neurosurgery [Internet]. GMS Curr Top Otorhinolaryngol Head Neck Surg 2015. Available at: https://www.ncbi.nlm.nih.gov/pmc/articles/PMC4702051/. Accessed April 30, 2021.

9. Chipp E, Prinsloo D, Rayatt S. Rhinectomy for the management of nasal malignancies. J Laryngol Otol 2011;125(10):1033–7.

10. Subramaniam T, Lennon P, O'Neill JP, et al. Total rhinectomy, a clinical review of nine cases. Ir J Med Sci 2016;185(3):757–60.

11. Levine H, Clemente M. Endoscopic and micro-scopic approaches. New York: Thieme; 2005.

12. Som P, Curtin H. Head and neck imaging. 5th edi-tion. Amsterdam: Elsevier; 2011. p. 3080.

13. Datta RK, Viswanatha B, Shree Harsha M. Caldwell luc surgery: revisited. Indian J Otolaryngol Head Neck Surg 2016;68(1):90–3.

14. Sireci F, Nicolotti M, Battaglia P, et al. Canine fossa puncture in endoscopic sinus surgery: report of two cases. Braz J Otorhinolaryngol 2017;83(5): 594–9.

15. Erbek SS, Koycu A, Buyuklu F. Endoscopic modified medial maxillectomy for treatment of inverted papil-loma originating from the maxillary sinus. J Craniofac Surg 2015;26(3):e244.

16. CARDELLI P, BIGELLI E, VERTUCCI V, et al. Palatal obturators in patients after maxillectomy. Oral Im-plantol 2015;7(3):86–92.

17. Kang Y-F, Liang J, He Z, et al. Orbital floor symmetry after maxillectomy and orbital floor reconstruction with individual titanium mesh using computer-assisted navigation. J Plast Reconstr Aesthet Surg 2020;73(2):337–43.

18. Park YY, Ahn HC, Lee JH, et al. Flap selection for reconstruction of wide palatal defect after cancer surgery. Arch Craniofac Surg 2019;20(1):17–23.

19. Sampathirao LMCSR, Thankappan K, Duraisamy S, et al. Orbital floor reconstruction with free flaps after maxillectomy. Craniomaxillofac Trauma Reconstr 2013;6(2):99–106.

20. Shukla A, Dudeja V. To study the effect of orbital sling on post operative vision in cases of maxil-lary carcinoma undergoing total maxillectomy. Indian J Otolaryngol Head Neck Surg 2014; 66(2):196–9.

21. Cordeiro PG, Chen CM. A 15-year review of midface reconstruction after total and subtotal maxillectomy: part II. Technical modifications to maximize aesthetic and functional outcomes. Plast Reconstr Surg 2012;129(1):139–47.

22. Cohen NA, Kennedy DW. Revision endoscopic sinus surgery. Otolaryngol Clin North Am 2006;39(3): 417–435, vii.

23. Musy PY, Kountakis SE. Anatomic findings in pa-tients undergoing revision endoscopic sinus sur-gery. Am J Otolaryngol 2004;25(6):418–22.

24. Ercan C, Imre A, Pinar E, et al. Comparison of submucosal resection and radiofrequency turbi-nate volume reduction for inferior turbinate hyper-trophy: evaluation by magnetic resonance imaging. Indian J Otolaryngol Head Neck Surg 2014;66(3):281–6.

25. Unal B, Bademci G, Bilgili YK, et al. Risky anatomic variations of sphenoid sinus for surgery. Surg Radiol Anat 2006;28(2):195–201.

26. Field M, Spector B, Lehman J. Evolution of endo-scopic endonasal surgery of the skull base and par-anasal sinuses. Atlas Oral Maxillofac Surg Clin North Am 2010;18(2):161–79.

27. Weber R, Draf W, Kratzsch B, et al. Modern con-cepts of frontal sinus surgery. Laryngoscope 2001; 111(1):137–46.

28. Khan MA, Alshareef WA, Marglani OA, et al. Outcome and complications of frontal sinus stenting: a case presentation and literature review. Case Rep Otolaryngol 2020 26;2020–e8885870.

29. Silverman JB, Gray ST, Busaba NY. Role of osteo-plastic frontal sinus obliteration in the era of endo-scopic sinus surgery. Int J Otolaryngol 2012. Available at: https://www.ncbi.nlm.nih.gov/pmc/articles/PMC3480005/. Accessed April 21, 2021.

30. Braun TL, Bhadkamkar MA, Jubbal KT, et al. Orbital decompression for thyroid eye disease. Semin Plast Surg 2017;31(1):40–5.

31. Rootman DB. Orbital decompression for thyroid eye disease. Surv Ophthalmol 2018;63(1):86–104.

32. Bhatki AM, Pant H, Snyderman CH, et al. The expanded endonasal approach for the treatment of anterior skull base tumors. Oper Tech Otolaryngol-head Neck Surg 2010;21(1):66–73.

33. Bhatki AM, Pant H, Snyderman CH, et al. Recon-struction of the cranial base after endonasal skull base surgery: local tissue flaps. Oper Tech Otolaryngol-head Neck Surg 2010;21(1):74–82.

34. Luu Q, Farwell DG. Microvascular free flap recon-struction of anterior skull base defects. Oper Tech Otolaryngol-head Neck Surg 2010;21(1):91–5.

35. Pereira L, Carron MA, Mathog RH. Traditional cranio-facial resection. Oper Tech Otolaryngol-head Neck Surg 2010;21(1):2–8.

36. Hudgins PA, Browning DG, Gallups J, et al. Endoscopic paranasal sinus surgery: radiographic evaluation of severe complications. AJNR Am J Neuroradiol 1992;13(4):1161–7.
37. Maniglia AJ. Fatal and other major complications of endoscopic sinus surgery. The Laryngoscope 1991; 101(4 Pt 1):349–54.
38. Weidenbecher M, Huk WJ, Iro H. Internal carotid artery injury during functional endoscopic sinus surgery and its management. Eur Arch Otorhinolaryngol 2005;262(8):640–5.
39. Lee WC, Ku PKM, van Hasselt CA. New guidelines for endoscopic localization of the anterior ethmoidal artery: a cadaveric study. The Laryngoscope 2000; 110(7):1173–8.
40. Georgakopoulos B, Le PH. Anatomy, head and neck, nasal concha [Internet]. In: StatPearls. Treasure Island (FL): StatPearls Publishing; 2021. Available at: http://www.ncbi.nlm.nih.gov/books/NBK546636/. Accessed April 21, 2021.
41. Halderman AA, Sindwani R, Woodard TD. Hemorrhagic complications of endoscopic sinus surgery. Otolaryngol Clin North Am 2015;48(5):783–93.
42. Lloyd KM, DelGaudio JM, Hudgins PA. Imaging of skull base cerebrospinal fluid leaks in adults. Radiology 2008;248(3):725–36.
43. Selcuk H, Albayram S, Ozer H, et al. Intrathecal gadolinium-enhanced mr cisternography in the evaluation of CSF leakage. Am J Neuroradiol 2010;31(1): 71–5.
44. Grantham VV, Blakley B, Winn J. Technical review and considerations for a cerebrospinal fluid leakage study. J Nucl Med Technol 2006;34(1):48–51.
45. Bhatti MT, Schmalfuss IM, Mancuso AA. Orbital complications of functional endoscopic sinus surgery: MR and CT findings. Clin Radiol 2005;60(8): 894–904.
46. O'Brien WT, Hamelin S, Weitzel EK. The preoperative sinus ct: avoiding a "CLOSE" call with surgical complications. Radiology 2016;281(1):10–21.
47. Meyers RM, Valvassori G. Interpretation of anatomic variations of computed tomography scans of the sinuses: a surgeon's perspective. The Laryngoscope 1998;108(3):422–5.
48. Khanna A, Sama A. Managing complications and revisions in sinus surgery. Curr Otorhinolaryngol Rep 2019;7(1):79–86.
49. Al-Mujaini A, Wali U, Alkhabori M. Functional endoscopic sinus surgery: indications and complications in the ophthalmic field. Oman Med J 2009;24(2): 70–80.
50. Bloom JD, Kaplan SE, Bleier BS, et al. Septoplasty complications: avoidance and management. Otolaryngol Clin North Am 2009;42(3):463–81.
51. Topal O, Celik SB, Erbek S, et al. Risk of nasal septal perforation following septoplasty in patients with allergic rhinitis. Eur Arch Oto-rhino-laryngol Off J Eur Fed Oto-rhino-laryngol Soc EUFOS Affil Ger Soc Oto-rhino-laryngol - Head Neck Surg 2011; 268(2):231–3.
52. Re M, Paolucci L, Romeo R, et al. Surgical treatment of nasal septal perforations. Our experience. Acta Otorhinolaryngol Ital 2006;26(2):102–9.
53. Kuan EC, Suh JD, Wang MB. Empty nose syndrome. Curr Allergy Asthma Rep 2015;15(1):493.
54. Moore EJ, Kern EB. Atrophic rhinitis: a review of 242 cases. Am J Rhinol 2001;15(6):355–61.
55. Manji J, Nayak JV, Thamboo A. The functional and psychological burden of empty nose syndrome. Int Forum Allergy Rhinol 2018;8(6):707–12.
56. Gill AS, Said M, Tollefson TT, et al. Update on empty nose syndrome: disease mechanisms, diagnostic tools, and treatment strategies. Curr Opin Otolaryngol Head Neck Surg 2019;27(4):237–42.
57. Leong SC. The clinical efficacy of surgical interventions for empty nose syndrome: A systematic review. The Laryngoscope 2015;125(7):1557–62.
58. Miglani A, Divekar RD, Azar A, et al. Revision endoscopic sinus surgery rates by chronic rhinosinusitis subtype. Int Forum Allergy Rhinol 2018 Sep;8(9): 1047–51.
59. Khalil HS, Eweiss AZ, Clifton N. Radiological findings in patients undergoing revision endoscopic sinus surgery: a retrospective case series study. BMC Ear Nose Throat Disord 2011;11:4.
60. Lazar RH, Younis RT, Long TE, et al. Revision functional endonasal sinus surgery. Ear Nose Throat J 1992;71(3):131–3.
61. Baban MIA, Mirza B, Castelnuovo P. Radiological and endoscopic findings in patients undergoing revision endoscopic sinus surgery. Surg Radiol Anat SRA 2020;42(9):1003–12.
62. Lee JT, Kennedy DW, Palmer JN, et al. The incidence of concurrent osteitis in patients with chronic rhinosinusitis: a clinicopathological study. Am J Rhinol 2006;20(3):278–82.
63. Snidvongs K, Sacks R, Harvey RJ. Osteitis in chronic rhinosinusitis. Curr Allergy Asthma Rep 2019;19(5):24.
64. Eggesbø HB. Imaging of sinonasal tumours. Cancer Imaging 2012;136–52.
65. Vandecaveye V, De Keyzer F, Nuyts S, et al. Detection of head and neck squamous cell carcinoma with diffusion weighted MRI after (chemo)radiotherapy: correlation between radiologic and histopathologic findings. Int J Radiat Oncol Biol Phys 2007;67(4): 960–71.

Surgical Free Flaps and Grafts in Head and Neck Reconstruction
Principles and Postoperative Imaging

Prashant Raghavan, MBBS[a],*, Kalpesh Vakharia, MD, MS[b],
Robert E. Morales, MD[c], Sugoto Mukherjee, MD[d]

KEYWORDS

- Head and neck reconstruction • Complications • Myocutaneous flaps • Posttreated neck
- Head and neck cancer

KEY POINTS

- Surgical management of advanced head and neck cancers requires complex reconstruction techniques after tumor extirpation to preserve preoperative function and cosmesis.
- A large variety of flaps and grafts, classified based on their blood supply, anatomic location in relation to the recipient site, and composition are used in such procedures.
- Knowledge of the anatomy of flaps and graft, their expected imaging appearance, the various complications (both early and delayed), and patterns of tumor recurrence after such procedures is essential in the interpretation of posttreatment surveillance imaging.

INTRODUCTION

The goals of surgical treatment of head and neck malignancy are tumor extirpation, restoration of deglutition, respiration, speech, and cosmesis. To this end, otolaryngologists have at their disposal a variety of reconstructive techniques that have been refined over the years. These techniques encompass a spectrum from simple skin grafts to complex free tissue transfer procedures. The radiologist is often presented with cross-sectional imaging studies in patients who have undergone such procedures whereby the altered anatomy makes image interpretation challenging. This review provides an overview of the more commonly used reconstructive techniques and the imaging findings of expected postoperative changes and the complications that may ensue from such procedures.

PRINCIPLES AND TERMINOLOGY

Mathes and Nahai proposed the concept of a "reconstructive ladder" in the 1970s. The ladder's rungs described steps of reconstructive techniques of increasing complexity from secondary intention healing, primary closure, delayed closure, simple skin grafts to local, distant, and free flaps (FF). The ladder underwent reassessment in the 1990s. A "reconstructive elevator"

[a] Neuroradiology, Department of Diagnostic Radiology and Nuclear Medicine, University of Maryland School of Medicine, 22 South Greene Street, Baltimore, MD 21201, USA; [b] Department of Otorhinolaryngology–Head and Neck Surgery, R Adams Cowley Shock Trauma Center, University of Maryland School of Medicine, 419 West Redwood Street, Suite 370, Baltimore, MD 21201, USA; [c] Neuroradiology, Diagnostic Neuroradiology Fellowship, Department of Diagnostic Radiology and Nuclear Medicine, University of Maryland School of Medicine, 22 South Greene Street, Baltimore, MD 21201, USA; [d] Department of Radiology and Medical Imaging, University of Virginia Health System, PO Box 800170, 1215 Lee Street, Charlottesville, VA 22908-1070, USA
* Corresponding author.
E-mail address: praghavan@umm.edu

Neuroimag Clin N Am 32 (2022) 75–91
https://doi.org/10.1016/j.nic.2021.09.002

was proposed by Gottlieb and colleagues, the principle of which is that the technique chosen must be that which achieves the best long term outcome, however complex it may be, tailored to the patient's needs and the nature of the clinical problem and that not every problem required a free flap.[1–3]

Although the terms "flap" and "graft" are sometimes used interchangeably, they represent distinct entities. A flap is tissue with intrinsic blood supply that is, not dependent on the recipient bed for perfusion whereas a graft must derive its blood supply from angiogenesis at the recipient bed. A flap's blood supply may be derived from intact donor vasculature or may require reestablishment using microvascular techniques.[4]

FLAP NOMENCLATURE

Flaps may be classified based on their constituent tissues, blood supply, proximity to the recipient site, or the method by which they are transferred (rotation, advancement, and so forth). Several classification schemes exist. **Fig. 1** provides a comprehensive overview of one such scheme (with permission from Wei FC and Mardini S. Flaps and Reconstructive Surgery. Elsevier).

Blood supply: Flaps may be "random" whereby they are supplied by unnamed vessels and derived from close proximity to the recipient site or "axial" whereby they are perfused by a named blood vessel. Random flaps are thin, comprised of skin and subcutaneous tissue, and perfused by unnamed subdermal vessels. Axial flaps are based on the "angiosome" concept of three-dimensional blocks of tissue comprised of skin and deeper structures supplied by specific source arteries.[5] The vascular supply of a "pedicled" axial flap remains connected anatomically to its parent vessel throughout transfer while that of a "free" flap requires disconnection and reattachment using microsurgical techniques. Examples of pedicled flaps include the pectoralis major, transverse rectus abdominis myocutaneous (TRAM), and latissimus dorsi flaps. A "perforator" flap, supplied by a transmuscular/fascial leash of blood vessel feeders is comprised only of skin and/or fascial tissue and is a less morbid alternative to a myocutaneous flap. It is technically more demanding, requiring a meticulous dissection of blood vessels through muscles, thereby potentially allowing the preservation of residual muscle function.[6,7]

Proximity: A "local" flap uses tissue that is anatomically contiguous with the recipient bed whereas a regional flap is derived from tissue that is in the vicinity but is not directly contiguous with the recipient site. "Regional" flaps, examples of which are nasoseptal and forehead flaps, used for skull base and nasal tip reconstruction respectively, derive their blood supply from the same anatomic area of the structure to be

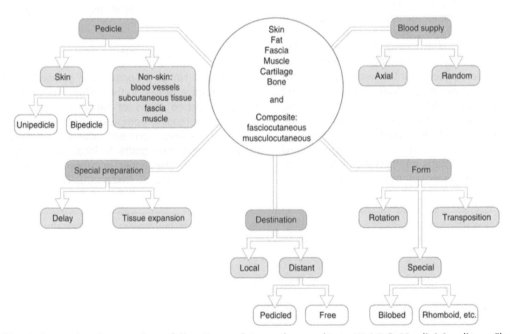

Fig. 1. Comprehensive overview of Flap Nomenclature schemes. (*From* Wei F-C, Mardini S, editors. Flaps and Reconstructive Surgery. Philadelphia: W B Saunders; 2009.)

reconstructed. These may be transferred from the donor site by releasing incisions or by tunneling beneath the skin to reconstruct the recipient bed. A "distant" flap is anatomically remote from the recipient bed and may be free or pedicled. The radial forearm free flap (RFFF), anterolateral thigh (ALT), fibula free flap (FFF), and the scapular free flap are among the more commonly used FF to reconstruct defects in head and neck.

Composition: Flaps may be comprised of skin, fascia, muscle, fat, bone, or a combination of these. The head and neck region can be divided into various subunits that comprise different types of tissue. When a defect of the head and neck is created after tumor extirpation or after traumatic injury, an understanding of the type of tissues that are missing in a particular subunit can help the reconstructive surgeon determine the ideal reconstructive tool to replace the lost tissue. For example, removal of a tumor involving the left body of the mandible and overlying gingiva and adjacent floor of mouth will result in a defect of bone and soft-tissue which must be reconstructed. Flaps in general but especially FF can be categorized as soft-tissue or bone flaps. The bone flaps usually have a soft-tissue component that can be used for reconstruction.

Soft-tissue flaps can be further characterized as skin flaps, fascial flaps, muscular flaps, musculocutaneous flaps, fasciocutaneous flaps, or visceral flaps depending on the soft-tissue components present within the flap. Each of these flaps has a distinct blood supply that supplies the associated soft-tissue. Depending on the type of flap it can either be transferred to the head and neck region in a pedicled fashion (whereby the blood vessels are left intact) or as a free flap with an associated microvascular anastomosis performed to reestablish the flaps blood supply. In addition to recognizing that type of tissue loss that needs to be reconstructed, an understanding of the volume, and surface area needed can assist in determining which flap is the ideal technique for any particular patient. Flaps that have a significant muscular component or often used to reconstruct defects of the head and neck, skull base, and aerodigestive tract. These flaps can be pedicled flaps or free. Commonly used flaps includes the pectoralis major, rectus abdominis, latissimus dorsi, sternomastoid, trapezius, and myocutaneous submental island flaps among others.[8,9] The pectoralis major flap, supplied by the pectoral branch of the thoracoacromial artery, can provide coverage over a large defect and is also useful for salvage or

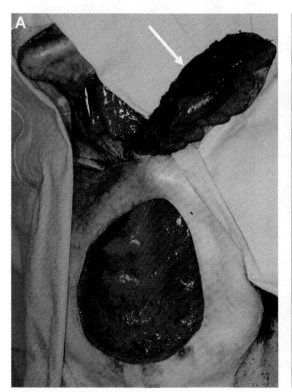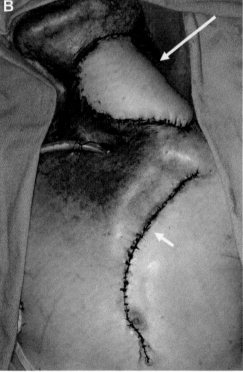

Fig. 2. Operative photo depicts rotation and tunneling of the myocutaneous pectoralis major pedicled flap (*arrow*) (*A*). The flap covers the large operative defect (*long arrow*) (*B*), and the donor site is closed primarily (*short arrow*) (*B*).

emergency reconstruction (Fig. 2). The latissimus dorsi flap, supplied by the thoracodorsal artery via the subscapular system, is a versatile flap with a large surface area and volume and a long pedicle that allows it to reach many regions in the head, neck, and scalp.[10] It can be transferred as either a pedicled flap or a free flap. The rectus abdominis flap, the use of which may be limited in obese patients, is supplied by the deep inferior epigastric artery and provides perhaps the largest skin coverage of any flap used in the head and neck. It can be used as a free flap to reconstruct defects in the scalp, face, skull base, and pharynx.[11] The forehead flap, known to Indian surgeons as early as 600 BCE, containing glabellar and frontalis muscle fibers and supplied by the supraorbital and supratrochlear vessels is a commonly used regional pedicled flap to repair nasal defects.[12]

The most common soft-tissue free flap used in head and neck reconstruction include the RFFF (Fig. 3) and the ALT free flap (Fig. 4). The RFFF obtains its blood supply from the radial artery and the associated venae comitantes along with the cephalic vein. This free flap is composed of skin and fascia and can be modified to incorporate tendon and bone. The RFFF may be rolled to create a tube for pharyngoesophageal reconstruction (Figs. 5 and 6). The RFFF may also be modified into an osteocutaneous flap to include the radius for maxillary or mandibular reconstruction (Fig. 7). Approximately 50% of the width of the radius bone can be harvested with an average length of 5 to 12 cm.[13] Benefits of the fasciocutaneous RFFF include thin, smooth, pliant skin, with potential for excellent sensory innervation and a long pedicle. Preoperative Allen's test to ensure adequate ulnar arterial perfusion of the hand is essential before harvesting the RFFF.[4,14] An alternative to the RFFF is the ulnar forearm FF which is a fasciocutaneous flap based on the ulnar artery and its venae comitantes.[15] Some authors arguing that the ulnar forearm free flap rarely results in flap loss, donor site morbidity, or hand ischemia, and

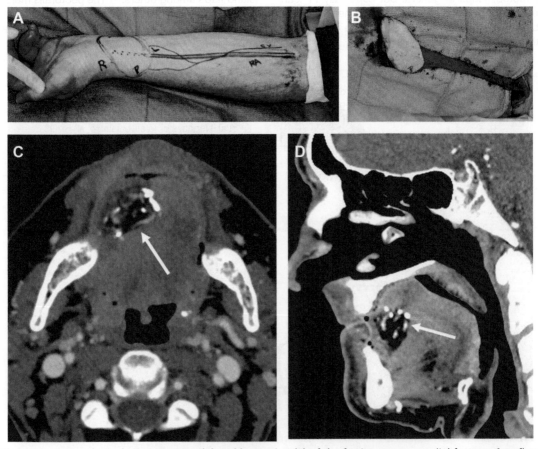

Fig. 3. Operative photo depicts mapping (A) and harvesting (B) of the fasciocutaneous radial forearm free flap. Axial (C) and sagittal (D) postcontrast CT reveal the flap reconstructing the tongue and floor of mouth defect (arrows).

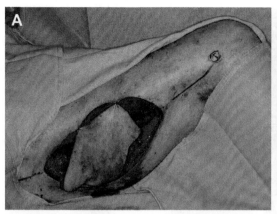
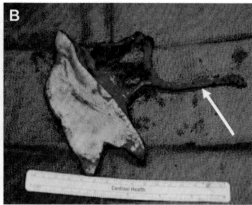

Fig. 4. Operative photos of an anterolateral thigh free flap (*A*, *B*) and its vascular supply (*arrow*) (*B*).

may be associated with less hair growth and better outcomes than the RFFF.[16] The ALT flap is based on the descending branch of the lateral femoral circumflex artery. It is a versatile flap in that it can be raised as a subcutaneous, musculocutaneous, fasciocutaneous, adipofascial, myofascial, or myocutaneous flap to reconstruct numerous head and neck defects such as those involving the scalp, skull base, pharynx, tracheal stoma, oral cavity, and oropharynx (**Fig. 8**).[17] A unique type of soft-tissue flaps are visceral flaps that are used in head and neck reconstruction. These include the free jejunal flap and tubed gastro-omental flap among others. Free jejunal flap transfers are the more frequently performed procedure due to low complication rates and low donor site morbidity. The low ischemic tolerance of the jejunum however may necessitate anastomosing more than one vascular pedicle to minimize postoperative thrombosis.[18,19]

The nasoseptal flap, the workhorse flap for anterior skull base defects, is discussed in a separate chapter in this issue.

Bone or osseous flaps used in the head and neck are usually derived from the fibula, radius, or scapula. Flaps for head and neck reconstruction, on rare occasion, are derived from the iliac crest, ribs, metatarsals, medial femoral condyle, and humerus.[20] The FFF has the ability to maintain mass over time (despite being subjected to postoperative radiation), it has a long pedicle length and it can provide a long segment of bone that can be cut contoured without impeding weight bearing thus make it the "work horse" flap for mandible reconstruction (**Fig. 9**)[21,22] The fibula flap has specific geometric attributes in terms of how the skin paddle and the bone and the pedicle relate to each other. Given this feature of the FFF the leg that is selected for the reconstruction of a specific defect is important. For example, consider a situation or if you have a left-sided mandibular body and associated adjacent floor of mouth defect with blood vessels available in either neck. In this situation, if you select the ipsilateral leg (left leg) and orient the skin paddle to preferentially sit in the oral cavity,

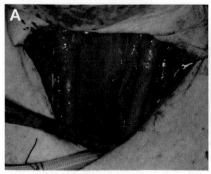
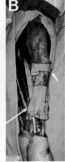
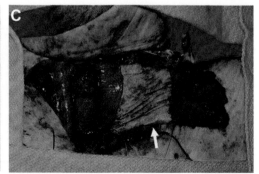

Fig. 5. Operative photo depicts the laryngectomy operative bed/defect (*A*). The radial forearm free flap is harvested. The component of the flap with skin (long *arrow*) (*B*) will be tubed to form the mucosal surface of the neopharynx. The smaller area with intact skin (short *arrow*) (*B, C*) will serve as the skin paddle which can be used to cover a defect and/or to monitor the flap's perfusion/viability.

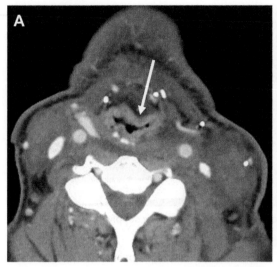
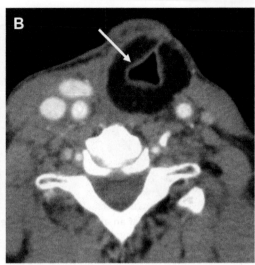

Fig. 6. Axial postcontrast CT reveals the fasciocutaneous radial forearm (*A*) and anterolateral thigh (*B*) free flaps with the skin surface of the flap tubed to form the lumen of the neopharynx (*arrows*). Note the more abundant subcutaneous fat in the anterolateral thigh free flap than the radial forearm free flap.

the pedicle will be oriented anteriorly, which will allow the surgeon to either anastomose either in the left neck or the right neck. If you select the contralateral (right) leg and orient the skin paddle to preferentially sit in the oral cavity, the pedicle will be oriented posteriorly, and the surgeon will be limited to anastomose in the ipsilateral (left) neck.

Scapular flaps may be obtained from the lateral scapular border or the tip; these flaps derive their blood supply from the circumflex or thoracodorsal branches of the subscapular artery, respectively. The scapular tip free flap (STFF) is used for shorter mandibular defects and offers the advantage of a long, reliable pedicle derived from the angular branch of the thoracodorsal artery. The FFFs and subscapular flaps provide complementary options for oromandibular reconstruction, with the former preferred for younger patients with extended

defects, multiple osteotomies, and limited soft-tissue requirements. The subscapular FFs are excellent options for elderly patients, those with peripheral vascular disease, and for short defects and those requiring large, complex soft-tissue reconstruction.[23–25]

A summary of the more commonly used flaps in head and neck reconstruction is presented in **Table 1** (with permission from McCarty JL, et al. Am J Neuroradiol. 2019 Jan;40(1):5–13).

PREOPERATIVE ASSESSMENT

The length and complexity of free tissue transfer procedures necessitate careful consideration of preoperative factors that may influence surgical

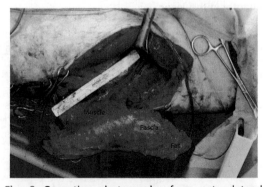

Fig. 8. Operative photograph of an anterolateral thigh free flap still attached in the left thigh. (AV – pedicle artery and vein, muscle – vastus lateralis muscle, fascia – fascia overlying the vastus lateralis muscle and tensor fascia lata, fat – subcutaneous fat, skin – skin paddle of the flap).

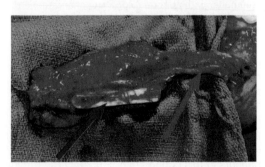

Fig. 7. - Operative photograph of an osteocutaneous radial forearm free flap depicts the radial bone that has been harvested (*black arrow*) with the pedicle (*red arrow*).

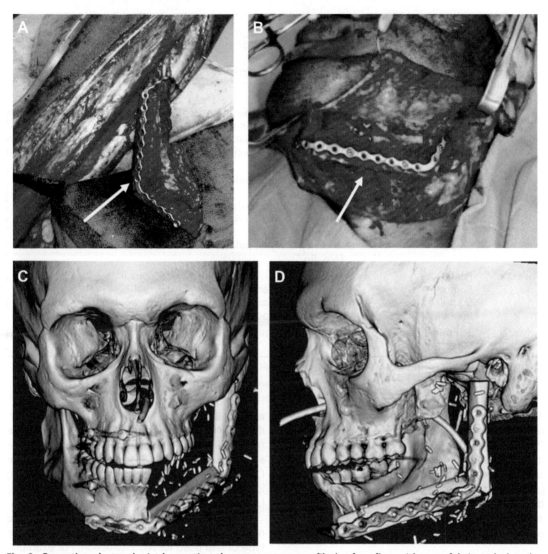

Fig. 9. Operative photos depict harvesting the osteocutaneous fibular free flap with a prefabricated plate (*arrow*) (*A*) and placement of the flap at the mandibulectomy site (*arrow*) (*B*). 3D reformatted CT images reveal the relationship of the flap and overlying hardware to the native mandible (*C*, *D*).

outcome. Although age and cardiovascular status are not directly associated with flap failure, factors that do increase the risk of its occurrence include malnutrition, diabetes mellitus, and preoperative radiation to the surgical bed. Smoking, although not directly linked to flap failure, may impair postoperative wound healing.[26]

The role of preoperative imaging in flap surgery is threefold. Imaging aids in assessing peripheral vascular disease (not uncommon comorbidity in patients with head and neck cancer), assessing flap perforator anatomy, and identifying congenital vascular anomalies that may impact/preclude graft harvest, thereby enabling shorter dissection and anesthesia times and minimizing complication

rates. No consensus exists in the choice of imaging modality and Doppler sonography, CT, and MR angiography may all be comparably effective in this regard. For flaps commonly used in head and neck reconstruction, preoperative imaging can be used to identify thoracodorsal perforators for latissimus dorsi flaps, lateral circumflex femoral perforators for ALT flaps, and peroneal perforators for fibular FF. Severe atherosclerotic disease (stenoses 50% in severity) in the aortoiliac system or distal lower extremity vessels may preclude surgery. Likewise, fibular FF harvest is contraindicated in the presence of variant arterial anatomy in the legs, seen in 5% to 7% of the population, whereby the peroneal artery provides the bulk of

Table 1
Surgical free flaps in head and neck reconstruction

category	Free Flap	Reconstructs	Donor Artery
Muscular	Rectus abdominis	Skull base, orbit	Deep inferior epigastric
	Latissimus dorsi	Skull base, scalp	Thoracodorsal
Fascial	Radial forearm	Oral cavity, tongue, palate, nose, face, scalp, lip, pharynx, larynx	Radial
	ulnar forearm	Oral cavity, tongue, palate, nose, face, scalp, lip, pharynx, larynx, cervical esophagus	Ulnar
	Lateral thigh	Oral cavity, tongue, palate, pharynx	Deep femoral
	Anterolateral thigh	oral cavity, tongue, palate, pharynx, larynx, cervical esophagus	Descending branch, lateral circumflex femoral
	Scapula	Oral cavity, tongue, palate, nose, face, lip	Subscapular
osseous	Fibula	Mandible	Peroneal
	Radius	Mandible & midface	Radial
	Scapula	Mandible & midface	Subscapular, thoracodorsal
	Iliac crest	Mandible & midface	Deep circumflex
visceral	Jejunum	Pharynx, esophagus	Superior mesenteric branches
	Omentum	Scalp	Gastroepiploic

From McCarty JL, Corey AS, El-Deiry MW, et al. Imaging of surgical free flaps in head and neck reconstruction. AJNR Am J Neuroradiol 2019 Jan;40(1):5–13.

arterial supply to the foot, either as a peroneal artery magna or when the peroneal artery is absent. Preoperative CTA may aid in the evaluation of the caliber of recipient vessels and select the optimal side for anastomosis. These include the facial, superior thyroid, and lingual arteries among branches of the external carotid system and the superficial cervical arteries and the internal and external jugular and facial veins.[26–32]

POSTOPERATIVE ASSESSMENT

Postoperative imaging following free flap reconstructions depends on the type of the reconstruction, the anatomic structures resected, and the presence of any complicating features or suspicion of tumor recurrence. Box 1 summarizes an approach to imaging interpretation. Although CT with contrast represents the workhorse in most institutions, MR imaging and PET (both PET-CT and PET-MRI) are essential complementary modalities in challenging cases. Lately, PET-CECT scans are increasingly being used as the imaging modality of choice in posttreated surveillance settings. Although there is a lack of consensus regarding the timing of surveillance scans, a consensus surveillance imaging algorithm as discussed in the ACR-NIRADS white paper suggests FDG-PET/CECT at 8 to 12 weeks after the completion of definitive therapy as a baseline, followed by

another CECT or FDG-PET/CECT 6 months later, if negative. If 2 consecutive FDG-PET/CECTs are negative, then surveillance imaging can be stopped. If only CECT is being done, another CECT neck is recommended at 6 months which is followed by a CECT neck and chest 12 months later if the second CECT is negative.[33]

The imaging appearance in the reconstructed neck is dictated by the resected tissue and the type of flap used for reconstruction. For example,

Box 1
Approach to interpretation of CT and MR studies after surgical reconstruction for head and neck cancer

- Review pretreatment imaging studies, and postoperative baseline studies if available and relevant clinical and operative notes

- Postsurgical changes may mimic tumor; be familiar with these

- Be familiar with complications, both early and late. Information from the clinical presentation can help direct attention to the presence of these.

- Evaluate for new mass-like or nodular enhancement not only within the operative bed, but also remote from the surgical site.

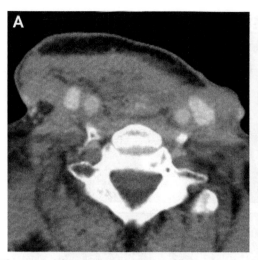 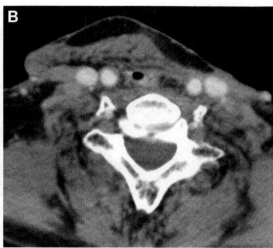

Fig. 10. Axial postcontrast CT in a patient with total laryngectomy and pectoralis major pedicled flap reconstruction, at baseline (A) and 4 years later (B), reveals atrophy of the flap. Notice the muscle typically atrophies and loses volume more prominently than the fat.

in muscular flaps such as the pectoralis major myofascial flap used to repair a defect in the oral cavity/oropharynx, imaging demonstrates a central fatty core and a surrounding superficial muscular tissue. However, in cases of extensive surgical defects such as in hypopharyngeal/laryngeal cancers, which require a total resection, a neopharynx is reconstructed in a tubed fashion from a myofascial flap, leading to a unique imaging appearance of the tissues (see Fig. 6), which are reversed with the skin/superficial fascial components on the inside recreating the inner pseudo mucosal layer of the neopharynx.[34] Muscular components of the flap appear similar to muscles elsewhere with a striated appearance. When imaged serially, FF show predictable changes on both CT and MR imaging, consisting of gradual atrophy of the muscular and fatty components, along with remodeling and varying degrees of scar formation (Fig. 10). MR examinations show the various components of the flap in a very elegant fashion,[35] with findings of T1 hypointensity, T2 hyperintensity with enhancement in the early periods which slowly transitions to a more heterogeneous pattern on both T1 and T2 sequences with fatty atrophy of the muscular component and shrinkage of the fatty portions of the flap. CECT studies are helpful in demonstrating the vascular anatomy of the flap and also can help in detecting osseous changes that may arise from nonunion, infection, or necrosis.

Fig. 11. Operative photograph of an anterolateral thigh free flap anastomosis. The ALT flap is at the top of the image (A – artery, V – vein, blue arrow – flower coupler venous anastomosis). Notice the implanted wire that emanates from the venous coupler (device that anastomoses 2 ends of a vein (see Fig. 16 for imaging appearance)) leaves the neck and is plugged into a box off the field, which monitors blood flow (bottom right of image).

Table 2
Immediate and delayed complications of flaps and grafts

Immediate/Early	Delayed/Late
• Thrombosis (arterial/venous)	• Infection/Abscess
• Bleeding/Hematoma	• Fistulas
• Infection/Abscess	• Osteonecrosis
• Seromas/Chyle leaks	• Hardware exposure/fractures and loosening
• Dehiscence	• Recurrent tumor

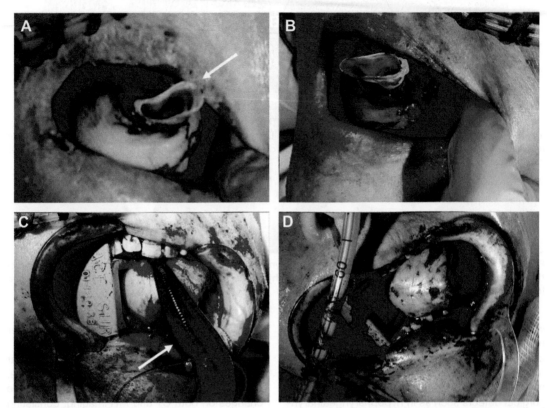

Fig. 12. Photographs depicting clinical example of venous congestion. (*A*) Postoperative day 1 shows a normal well perfused radial forearm free flap used for tongue reconstruction with a Penrose drain (*arrow*). (*B*) Postoperative day 4 when the patient has a neck hematoma resulting in venous compression and thrombosis of the vascular pedicle which leads to the venous congestion in the flap as evidenced by the dark, purple color of the flap. (*C*) The flap after the evacuation of the neck hematoma, reestablishment of the venous outflow, and application of leeches (*arrow*). (*D*) The salvaged radial forearm free flap after leech therapy.

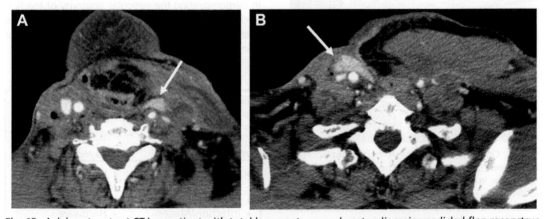

Fig. 13. Axial postcontrast CT in a patient with total laryngectomy and pectoralis major pedicled flap reconstruction, who presents with hemorrhage from a fistula. A hyperdense structure, that was questioned to represent possible extravasation of contrast (*arrow*) (*A*), is displaced thyroid tissue. Thyroid tissue is also identified on the contralateral side (*arrow*) (*B*). This can also be mistaken for residual/recurrent tumor.

COMPLICATIONS

The common complications following reconstructive flap surgery and an approach to their detection on imaging are summarized in **Box 1** and **Table 2** and include ischemia, necrosis, infection, osteonecrosis, and recurrent tumor. Complications are dependent on the type, complexity, and duration of the procedure, the stage of the tumor, whether additional nodal resections were performed, associated tracheostomy, patient factors such as age, anemia, malnutrition, and other comorbidities, along with continued tobacco and alcohol use.[36]

The immediate postoperative evaluation following flap reconstruction surgery is targeted toward assessing flap viability and ischemia (secondary to either arterial or venous thrombosis) leading to total or partial flap loss.[37] Frequent clinical monitoring represents the mainstay in this setting and includes evaluating flap color, capillary refill, pin-prick tests, and temperature assessments along with other adjunct techniques including bedside Doppler monitoring. When a flap has an external skin paddle, it is more amenable to monitor for flap perfusion through the above-mentioned techniques. When an entire flap is buried monitoring for flap perfusion becomes more challenging. However the development of implantable venous and arterial Doppler's allow clinicians to more intimately monitor blood flow to and from the flap at the level of the anastomosis thereby allowing clinicians to more easily monitor a buried flap (**Fig. 11**). A flap can have either arterial insufficiency or venous obstruction, both of which are surgical emergencies. In the setting of arterial insufficiency, there is not enough blood flowing through the artery in the flap. Such a flap would be pale, cold, lack tone, and capillary refill and would result in no blood or very slow blood return on pin-prick. However, a flap that has venous congestion occurs when there is an obstruction of venous outflow. A venous congested flap will be swollen, firm, look bruised, or purple and will have rapid dark blood return on pin-prick. Emergent thrombectomy and revision surgery may be required in cases of vascular compromise. In the setting of venous congestion applications of leeches can help salvage a compromised flap as demonstrated in (**Fig. 12**).

Cross-sectional imaging plays a major role in the delayed/later stages when evaluating for infections/abscesses, fistulas, dehiscence, and osteonecrosis. Radiologists should be aware of potential pitfalls with relation to pseudomasses secondary to missing contralateral structures

(such as salivary glands) or transplanted tissues (thyroid) (**Fig. 13**). The flap may itself appear mass-like and be mistaken for tumor and as discussed above, an awareness of the surgical procedure and its internal components will aid in differentiation from the latter. Vascular pedicle ossifications may present as a palpable abnormality, appear as linear/curvilinear densities and can be easily identified on CT.[38]

Infections/ abscess/Chyle leaks/seromas - These complications are not uncommon and are usually diagnosed and managed clinically. The imaging findings are nonspecific and can show the findings of a fluid collection with or without rim enhancement, soft-tissue edema, and thickening as well as the loss of tissue planes.[4] Reactive lymphadenitis can be seen, mimicking nodal recurrences. Rarely image guided drainages or aspirations are performed to allow for sampling and culture sensitivity.

Fistulas/dehiscence - Fistulas and dehiscences can happen secondary to infection, radiation, surgical factors, or due to tumor recurrences (**Figs. 14 and 15**). A significant association has been seen in patients who continue smoking/tobacco use. Fistulas and dehiscences can occur separately or together or may follow each other. It's not uncommon to have flap breakdowns overlying surgical hardware or overlying bones (following composite reactions and reconstructions). On imaging, direct evidence of flap breakdown, thinning, and exposure of surgical hardware and bones may be evident.[34] Particular attention should also be

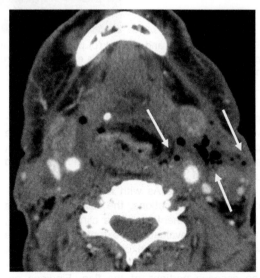

Fig. 14. Axial postcontrast CT reveals fistula formation from the neopharynx to the skin surface (*arrows*) in this patient who had a history of steroid therapy for COPD before total laryngectomy.

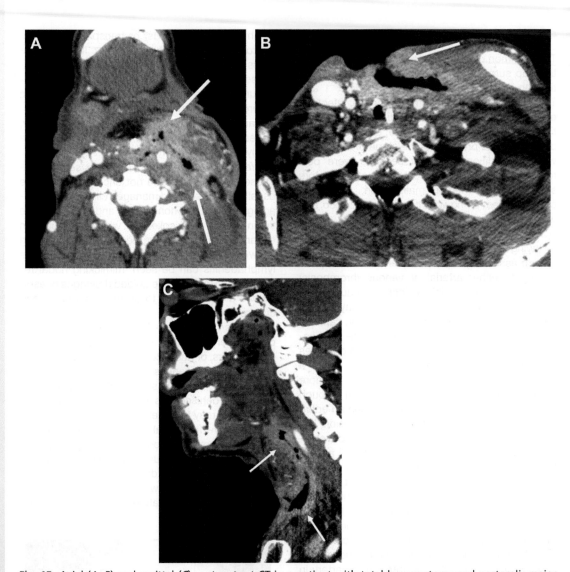

Fig. 15. Axial (A, B) and sagittal (C) postcontrast CT in a patient with total laryngectomy and pectoralis major pedicled flap reconstruction reveals extensive recurrent tumor along a large fistula between the neopharynx and skin surface/stoma (arrows).

paid to complications associated with metal hardware (both screws and plates), specifically in the mandible, evaluating for periprosthetic lucencies, screw loosening, hardware fractures, and diastasis.

Osteonecrosis - As with many of the above-described complications, the role of imaging is usually complementary to the clinical diagnosis, specifically to evaluate the extent of the osseous involvement and to exclude other etiologies. Osteonecrosis may affect the native mandible or the osseous portions of the flap. Findings on, CECT and MR imaging include osseous changes such as cortical irregularities, fragmentation, intra-osseous gas, periosteal reactions, and

pathologic fractures, and also, with coexistent infection, soft-tissue abnormalities which include sinuses/fistulae and abscesses (Fig. 16). Imaging findings are frequently complicated with an associated history of prior radiation (such as osteora-dionecrosis—which can also affect sites remote from the surgery) or bisphosphonate use (bisphosphonate-related osteonecrosis of the mandible).[39,40] Osteoradionecrosis is discussed in greater detail elsewhere in this issue.

Recurrences - Tumor recurrences represent the gravest complication and remain the primary focus of surveillance imaging especially in the delayed setting. Imaging for residual tumors in the immediate/early postsurgical setting is rare, the

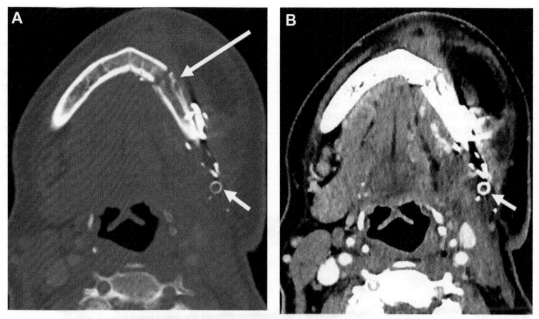

Fig. 16. Axial postcontrast CT reveals cortical irregularity and lytic destruction of the distal fibular free flap (*long arrow*) (*A*) without associated soft-tissue mass (*B*) in this patient with osteonecrosis of the graft. The circular surgical hardware is the venous coupler (*short arrows*) (*A*, *B*).

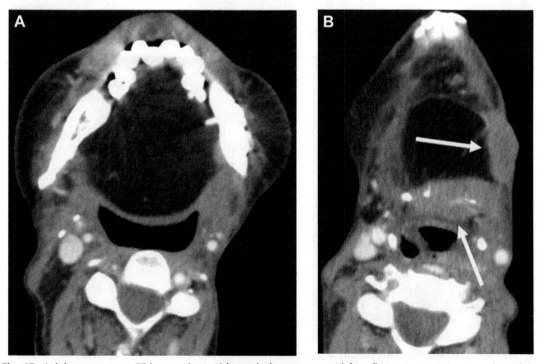

Fig. 17. Axial postcontrast CT in a patient with total glossectomy and free flap reconstruction reveals nodular enhancement (*A*) along the lateral and posterior margins of the flap representing tumor recurrence (*arrows*) (*B*).

evaluation for which is also complicated by the evolving postsurgical changes and presurgical radiation. CECT or combined FDG-PET/CECT is the usual imaging modality (for evaluating both the primary site and nodal recurrence) with MR imaging for evaluating skull base and intracranial involvement and perineural spread. Recurrences can be clinically silent and require careful evaluation of both the surgical site, margins of the surgical cavity and remotely elsewhere within the neck (including "nontraditional" sites such as in the retropharyngeal region or contralateral side both due to the resection of draining nodal stations and subsequently altered lymphatic drainage). The typical imaging pattern[34] is that of a new or increasing soft-tissue mass-like lesion or unusual thickening either at the interface of the surgical site/native tissue and the flap or within the surgical bed (**Figs. 17 and 18**). Rarely can they also be seen at the site of vascular anastomosis. When these recurrences are adjacent to the bone (eg, mandible), new osseous destruction can be seen with an adjacent soft-tissue mass and may require a high index of suspicion to accurately distinguish from changes secondary to chronic osteomyelitis or osteoradionecrosis (**Fig. 19**).

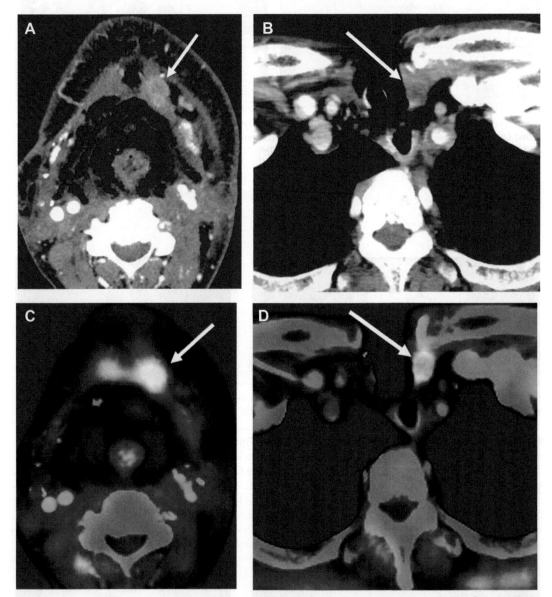

Fig. 18. Axial postcontrast CT in a patient with total laryngectomy and anterolateral thigh free flap reconstruction reveals nodular enhancement representing recurrent tumor at the anterior margin of the flap (*arrow*) (*A*) and along the left side of the stoma (*arrow*) (*B*). PET-CT reveals increased uptake of these lesions (*arrows*) (*C, D*).

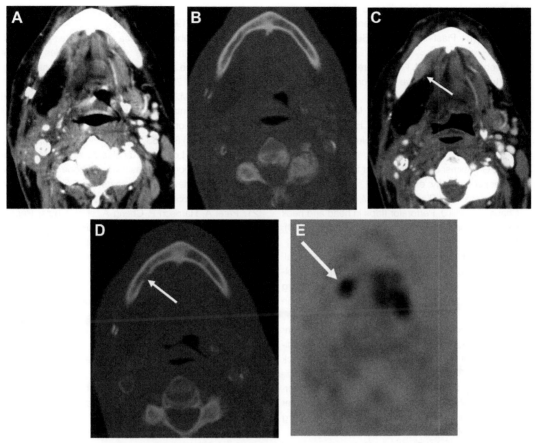

Fig. 19. Axial postcontrast CT at baseline in a patient with hemiglossectomy and radial forearm free flap reconstruction (*A, B*). On surveillance PET-CT imaging there is new nodularity along the anterior margin of the flap (*arrow*) (*C*) with adjacent osseous erosion (*arrow*) (*D*) and increased uptake on FDG-PET (*arrow*) (*E*). Although these imaging features are highly suggestive of tumor recurrence, on biopsy the lesion represented actinomycosis infection.

SUMMARY

Interpretation of imaging studies after reconstructive procedures in the head and neck is challenging. Knowledge of details of the surgical procedure performed the expected imaging features of flaps and grafts and a high index of suspicion for tumor recurrence are key while evaluating these studies.

CLINICS CARE POINTS

- A wide variety of reconstructive techniques are employed in head and neck cancer surgery.
- Awareness of surgical techniques employed in head and neck cancer surgery and reconstruction enables the radiologist to assess complications with confidence.

- Expected postoperative findings may be mistaken for tumor recurrence by the unwary radiologist. Conversely, complications may be missed under the assumption that findings represent expected sequela of surgery.

ACKNOWLEDGMENTS

The authors would like to acknowledge Brigitte Pocta, MLA for her assistance with the manuscript. The authors also acknowledge Scott Strome, MD and Joshua Lubek, MD, DDS, for the operative images.

DISCLOSURE

The authors have nothing to disclose.

REFERENCES

1. Wei F-C, Mardini S, editors. Flaps and reconstructive surgery. W B Saunders Co.; 2009.

2. Mathes SJ, Nahai F. Classification of the vascular anatomy of muscles: experimental and clinical correlation. Plast Reconstr Surg 1981;67(2): 177–87.

3. Gottlieb LJ, Krieger LM. From the reconstructive ladder to the reconstructive elevator. Plast Reconstr Surg 1994;93(7):1503–4.

4. McCarty JL, Corey AS, El-Deiry MW, et al. Imaging of Surgical Free Flaps in Head and Neck Reconstruction. AJNR Am J Neuroradiol 2019; 40(1):5–13.

5. Taylor GI, Palmer JH. The vascular territories (angiosomes) of the body: experimental study and clinical applications. Br J Plast Surg 1987;40(2):113–41.

6. Chana JS, Odili J. Perforator flaps in head and neck reconstruction. Semin Plast Surg 2010;24(3): 237–54.

7. Blondeel PN, Van Landuyt KHI, Monstrey SJM, et al. The "Gent" consensus on perforator flap terminology: preliminary definitions. Plast Reconstr Surg 2003;112(5):1378–83. quiz 1383, 1516; discussion 1384-1387.

8. Amin AA, Sakkary MA, Khalil AA, et al. The submental flap for oral cavity reconstruction: extended indications and technical refinements. Head Neck Oncol 2011;3:51.

9. Sebastian P, Cherian T, Ahamed MI, et al. The sternomastoid island myocutaneous flap for oral cancer reconstruction. Arch Otolaryngol Head Neck Surg 1994;120(6):629–32.

10. Har-El G, Bhaya M, Sundaram K. Latissimus dorsi myocutaneous flap for secondary head and neck reconstruction. Am J Otolaryngol 1999;20(5): 287–93.

11. Urken ML, Turk JB, Weinberg H, et al. The rectus abdominis free flap in head and neck reconstruction. Arch Otolaryngol Head Neck Surg 1991;117(9): 1031.

12. Ramsey ML, Brooks J, Zito PM. Forehead flaps. In: StatPearls. Treasure island (FL). StatPearls Publishing; 2021.

13. Shnayder Y, Tsue TT, Toby EB, et al. Safe osteocutaneous radial forearm flap harvest with prophylactic internal fixation. Craniomaxillofac Trauma Reconstr 2011;4(3):129–36.

14. Souter DS. In: Wei F-C, Mardini S, editors. Flaps and reconstructive surgery. W B Saunders Co.; 2009.

15. Huang J-J, Wu C-W, Lam WL, et al. Anatomical basis and clinical application of the ulnar forearm free flap for head and neck reconstruction. Laryngoscope 2012;122(12):2670–6.

16. Antony AK, Hootnick JL, Antony AK. Ulnar forearm free flaps in head and neck reconstruction: systematic review of the literature and a case report. Microsurgery 2014;34(1):68–75.

17. Park CW, Miles BA. The expanding role of the anterolateral thigh free flap in head and neck reconstruction. Curr Opin Otolaryngol Head Neck Surg 2011;19(4):263–8.

18. Kurita T, Kubo T, Tashima H, et al. Free jejunal flap transfer with multiple vascular pedicles for safe and reliable pharyngoesophageal reconstruction. Head Neck 2018;40(10):2210–8.

19. Genden EM, Kaufman MR, Katz B, et al. Tubed gastro-omental free flap for pharyngoesophageal reconstruction. Arch Otolaryngol Head Neck Surg 2001;127(7):847–53.

20. Brown JS, Lowe D, Kanatas A, et al. Mandibular reconstruction with vascularised bone flaps: a systematic review over 25 years. Br J Oral Maxillofac Surg 2017;55(2):113–26.

21. Patel A, Harrison P, Cheng A, et al. Fibular Reconstruction of the Maxilla and Mandible with Immediate Implant-Supported Prosthetic Rehabilitation: Jaw in a Day. Oral Maxillofac Surg Clin N Am 2019;31(3): 369–86.

22. Hidalgo DA, Pusic AL. Free-flap mandibular reconstruction: a 10-year follow-up study. Plast Reconstr Surg 2002;110(2):438–49. discussion 450-451.

23. Powell DK, Nwoke F, Urken ML, et al. Scapular free flap harvest site: recognising the spectrum of radiographic post-operative appearance. Br J Radiol 2013;86(1023):20120574.

24. Blumberg JM, Walker P, Johnson S, et al. Mandibular reconstruction with the scapula tip free flap. Head Neck 2019;41(7):2353–8.

25. Dowthwaite SA, Theurer J, Belzile M, et al. Comparison of fibular and scapular osseous free flaps for oromandibular reconstruction: a patient-centered approach to flap selection. JAMA Otolaryngol Head Neck Surg 2013;139(3):285–92.

26. Abouyared M, Katz AP, Ein L, et al. Controversies in free tissue transfer for head and neck cancer: a review of the literature. Head Neck 2019;41(9): 3457–63.

27. Kagen AC, Hossain R, Dayan E, et al. Modern perforator flap imaging with high-resolution blood pool MR angiography. Radiographics 2015;35(3): 901–15.

28. Syed F, Spector ME, Cornelius R, et al. Head and neck reconstructive surgery: what the radiologist needs to know. Eur Radiol 2016;26(10):3345–52.

29. Akashi M, Nomura T, Sakakibara S, et al. Preoperative MR angiography for free fibula osteocutaneous flap transfer. Microsurgery 2013;33(6): 454–9.

30. Carroll WR, Esclamado R. Preoperative vascular imaging for the fibular osteocutaneous flap. Arch Otolaryngol Head Neck Surg 1996;122(7): 708–12.

31. González Martínez J, Torres Pérez A, Gijón Vega M, et al. Preoperative vascular planning of free flaps: comparative study of computed tomographic angiography, color doppler ultrasonography, and hand-

held doppler. Plast Reconstr Surg 2020;146(2): 227–37.

32. Kelly AM, Cronin P, Hussain HK, et al. Preoperative MR angiography in free fibula flap transfer for head and neck cancer: clinical application and influence on surgical decision making. AJR Am J Roentgenol 2007;188(1):268–74.

33. Aiken AH, Rath TJ, Anzai Y, et al. ACR Neck Imaging Reporting and Data Systems (NI-RADS): a white paper of the ACR NI-RADS committee. J Am Coll Radiol JACR 2018;15(8):1097–108.

34. Wester DJ, Whiteman ML, Singer S, et al. Imaging of the postoperative neck with emphasis on surgical flaps and their complications. AJR Am J Roentgenol 1995;164(4):989–93.

35. Tomura N, Watanabe O, Hirano Y, et al. MR imaging of recurrent head and neck tumours following flap reconstructive surgery. Clin Radiol 2002;57(2):109–13.

36. Haughey BH, Wilson E, Kluwe L, et al. Free flap reconstruction of the head and neck: analysis of 241 cases. Otolaryngol–head Neck Surg 2001; 125(1):10–7.

37. Suh JD, Sercarz JA, Abemayor E, et al. Analysis of outcome and complications in 400 cases of microvascular head and neck reconstruction. Arch Otolaryngol Head Neck Surg 2004;130(8):962–6.

38. Glastonbury CM, van Zante A, Knott PD. Ossification of the vascular pedicle in microsurgical fibular free flap reconstruction of the head and neck. AJNR Am J Neuroradiol 2014;35(10):1965–9.

39. Ruggiero SL, Fantasia J, Carlson E. Bisphosphonate-related osteonecrosis of the jaw: background and guidelines for diagnosis, staging and management. Oral Surg Oral Med Oral Pathol Oral Radiol Endod 2006;102(4):433–41.

40. Chong J, Hinckley LK, Ginsberg LE. Masticator space abnormalities associated with mandibular osteoradionecrosis: MR and CT findings in five patients. AJNR Am J Neuroradiol 2000;21(1):175–8.

Imaging of Complications of Chemoradiation

Prashant Raghavan, MBBS[a],*, Matthew E. Witek, MD, MS[b], Robert E. Morales, MD[a]

KEYWORDS

- Radiation • Chemotherapy • Osteoradionecrosis • Radiation necrosis • Radiation vasculopathy
- Optic neuritis • Myelitis • Checkpoint inhibitor toxicity

KEY POINTS

- Complications from chemoradiation for head and neck malignancy may arise days to years after treatment.
- The radiologist's task while interpreting surveillance imaging studies is not only to detect tumor recurrence but also identify complications that may have arisen in regional osseous structures, soft tissues, vasculature and neuraxis.
- The imaging appearance of some of these may mimic that of tumor recurrence.
- Clinical and imaging features of some complications such as optic neuritis and myelitis may be nonspecific and a history of prior radiation is necessary for correct diagnosis.
- Checkpoint inhibitors are a class of novel immunotherapeutic agents that are associated with a variety of unique toxicities with imaging manifestations that radiologists must learn.

INTRODUCTION

The treatment of cancers of the head and neck, by the virtue of their proximity to and tendency to arise from and involve anatomic structures vital for deglutition, speech, and respiration, frequently results in adverse effects compromising one or more of these functions. Aggressive management of these tumors by combining radiation and chemotherapy, the latter whether administered as induction treatment or concurrently, has led to superior disease control, albeit with a higher toxicity cost.[1] Preservation of organ function and minimization of toxicity remain major goals in the use of chemoradiation in disease management.[2] Although a wide range of adverse phenomena may occur during or after the course of chemoradiation in patients with head and neck cancer, this review will focus on the imaging manifestations of those that affect the brain and the osseous and soft tissue structures of the head and neck.

CLINICAL CONSIDERATIONS

"Toxicity" may include any temporary or permanent change in normal tissues and/or related symptoms arising from cancer treatment[1] and may be local or systemic. Adverse events arising from chemoradiation may be "early" or "late" in nature. Traditional chemotherapeutic agents used in head and neck cancer are not only inherently associated with a wide range of toxic effects but also may exacerbate the adverse effects of radiation.[3] The emergence of immunotherapy with immune checkpoint inhibitors (ICI) has caused several widespread systemic immune-related adverse events that can cause significant morbidity and, rarely, mortality.[4] Early, acute adverse events are usually temporary and are defined based on observations from conventional fractionated radiation as those encountered within 90 days of commencement of treatment. Most late events arise in the first

[a] Neuroradiology, Department of Diagnostic Radiology and Nuclear Medicine, University of Maryland School of Medicine, 22 S Greene Street, Baltimore, MD 21201, USA; [b] Department of Radiation Oncology, University of Maryland School of Medicine, Maryland Proton Treatment Center, 22 S Greene Street, Baltimore, MD 21201, USA
* Corresponding author.
E-mail address: praghavan@umm.edu

Neuroimag Clin N Am 32 (2022) 93–109
https://doi.org/10.1016/j.nic.2021.08.012

3 years of treatment with rare long-term sequela noted thereafter[5] and may be permanent. The development of newer, more aggressive fractionation techniques and chemoradiation schedules has resulted in early toxicities manifesting beyond 90 days.[1] Early toxic events primarily affect oropharyngeal and laryngeal function; mucositis is the most commonly encountered intensity limiting adverse effect.[1,6] Xerostomia due to salivary gland injury is also common and may be minimized using highly conformal radiation techniques designed to spare salivary gland tissue[7]

Early adverse events from chemotherapy may include mucositis, exacerbation of radiation-induced dermatitis, hypersensitivity reactions, myositis, endocrinopathy, myelosuppression, neuropathy, and nephrotoxicity. Late complications after radiation include dental injury (exacerbated by impaired salivary function), osteoradionecrosis (ORN), radiation vasculopathy, radiation necrosis of brain tissue, optic neuritis, myelitis, thyroid dysfunction, and rarely second malignancies.

MUCOSITIS

Mucositis is a near universal, painful complication of cancer treatment. It is a biologically complex process believed to evolve through 5 cellular phases.[8] Its pathologic hallmark is ulceration arising from the loss of the basal epithelial/stem cell layer. Clinically evident mucositis is comprised of a confluence of such ulcers, covered by a pseudomembrane of inflammatory cells, cellular debris, fibrin, and exudate.[9,10] Mucositis becomes evident in the first few weeks after radiation but can persist for weeks to months thereafter.[11] Failure of healing may lead to permanent ulceration and mucosal necrosis. On computed tomography (CT) studies obtained shortly after treatment (Fig. 1), affected mucosa demonstrates a low density, edematous "boggy" appearance. Studies often demonstrate other changes in the superficial soft tissues of the neck including the reticulation of the subcutaneous and deep fat, often accompanied by the thickening of the skin, fascia and platysma, and retropharyngeal edema and effusion. Mucositis must be distinguished from frank mucosal and soft tissue necrosis (Fig. 2) that occurs in the first few years after radiotherapy. On CT and MR imaging, this presents as an irregular debris containing ulcer. Although lack of enhancement is a reassuring finding, this may be associated with enhancement that is indistinguishable from tumor recurrence. In the latter scenario, close observation and/or biopsy may be required for definitive diagnosis.[12,13]

SALIVARY GLAND INJURY

Xerostomia is a common, long term, dose-dependent complication of radiotherapy. Severe xerostomia may be avoided by minimizing dose and/or using highly conformal radiotherapy techniques to minimize parotid and submandibular gland exposure.[14] The salivary glands exhibit early and late changes after chemoradiation with dramatic reduction in salivary flow rates noted in the first 2 weeks after treatment and gradual glandular atrophy developing due to the loss of acinar cells approximately 6 weeks thereafter. Parotid glandular volume typically decreases soon after radiotherapy, with a degree of recovery occurring thereafter when parotid sparing radiation techniques are used.[15] On CT studies obtained soon after radiation, increased gland density may be apparent with correspondingly increased T2 signal on MRI due to edema (Fig. 3).[16–18] Increased vascular permeability and acinar loss in the parotid glands may underlie changes observed on dynamic contrast-enhanced perfusion MRI and intravoxel incoherent motion MR imaging parameters as soon as 2 weeks after radiotherapy.[19,20]

THYROID GLAND INJURY

Hypothyroidism, necessitating routine life-long screening with serum thyroid-stimulation hormone, develops in about one-third of patients undergoing external beam radiation for head and neck cancers, usually within the first 2 years after treatment and is more common in patients who also undergo surgery.[21] Checkpoint inhibitors may also cause autoimmune thyroid dysfunction.[22] Morphologic changes after external beam radiation, including gland shrinkage (and rarely, enlargement) and development of cystic and solid masses, are well-documented on cross-sectional and ultrasound studies.[23,24] In a CT study, 85% of patients demonstrated a decrease in thyroid gland width after radiation for laryngeal cancer, with change in gland size being no different in patients with hypothyroidism and those without. Pre-existing thyroglossal duct cysts may also enlarge after radiation (Fig. 4), usually evident on first post-treatment studies due to inflammation and must not be mistaken for metastatic nodal disease.[25] The evidence for a causal relationship between radiation exposure and the development of thyroid cancer, especially of the papillary type, is incontrovertible. Although screening of all individuals exposed to radiation by yearly physical examination is recommended, the use of ultrasound is controversial. The benefits of early tumor detection must be balanced against the risks of

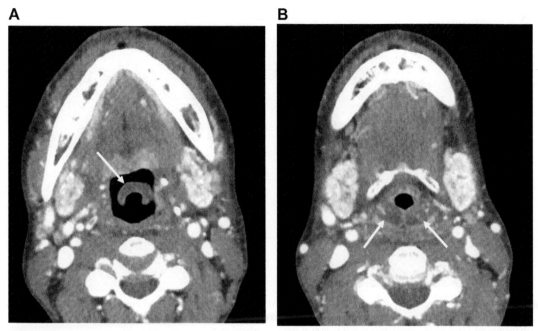

Fig. 1. Axial postcontrast CT after recent radiation therapy reveals the reticulation of the subcutaneous and deep fat planes. Mucosal/submucosal edema is typically evident involving the supraglottic larynx. The epiglottis (*arrow*) (*A*) and aryepiglottic folds (*arrows*) (*B*) are edematous with fullness and decreased attenuation.

unnecessary and expensive treatments and their attendant complications for tumors that may remain indolent and never become clinically apparent.[26] Surveillance ultrasound is offered widely to survivors of childhood cancer that have received radiation to the head and neck, given the greater likelihood of developing clinically relevant thyroid malignancies.[27]

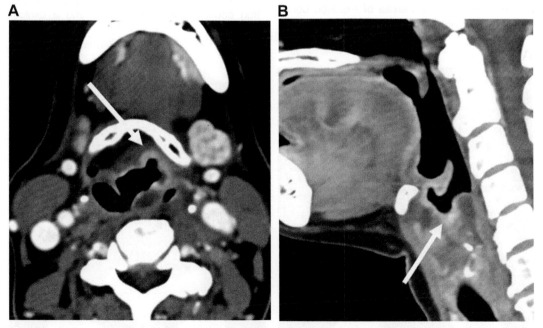

Fig. 2. Mucosal necrosis. Patient with supraglottic SCCA treated with radiation therapy 10 months prior. Biopsy revealed no recurrent tumor. Axial (*A*) and sagittal (*B*) postcontrast CT reveals thickened enhancing mucosa with overlying ulceration (*arrows*). (*Courtesy of* S Mukherjee, M.D., Charlottesville, VA).

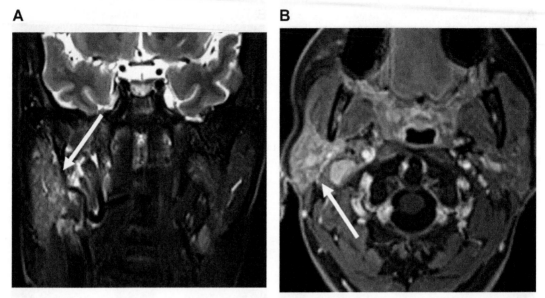

Fig. 3. Patient with adenoid cystic carcinoma of the right lip treated with resection and recent radiation therapy. Coronal T2WI with fat saturation (*A*) and postcontrast T1WI with fat saturation (*B*) reveals edema (*arrow*) (*A*) and enhancement (*arrow*) (*B*) involving the ipsilateral parotid gland in the treatment field.

OSTEORADIONECROSIS

ORN, although most commonly encountered in the mandible after radiation for oral cavity cancers, may affect any bony structure exposed to radiation in the head and neck. ORN may occur a few months to several years after radiation. The clinical presentation is variable and ranges from incidentally seen asymptomatic areas of exposed bone that may heal with conservative management to widespread bone loss necessitating extensive surgical reconstruction. ORN may present with pain, halitosis, dysgeusia, dysphagia, speech difficulty and with erythema, soft tissue swelling and abscess, and fistula formation when there is coexistent osteomyelitis.[28]

Its pathogenesis involves the development of hypoxia from radiation-induced vascular obliteration causing tissue breakdown and a clinically

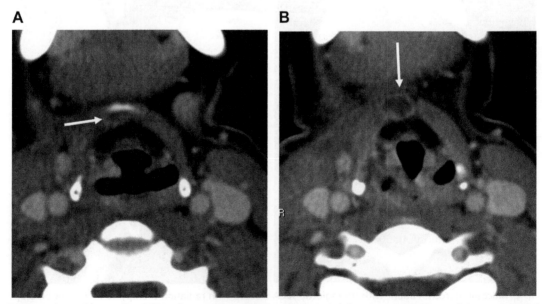

Fig. 4. Patient with tonsillar SCCA who received radiation therapy. Axial postcontrast CT reveals interval growth of a thyroglossal duct cyst between the pretreatment scan (*arrow*) (*A*) and the posttreatment scan (*arrow*) (*B*).

evident nonhealing wound, frequently containing exposed bone, with microorganisms playing only a contaminant role.[29] The risk of developing ORN is related to tumor T stage, proximity of tumor to bone, radiation dose and, perhaps, technique, trauma, dentition, nutritional status, alcohol abuse, smoking, underlying cardiovascular disease, and bisphosphonate use.[30]

Although studies indicate a decreasing prevalence of ORN attributed to newer radiation techniques, improved awareness and preventive care,[31] others contend that newer radiation modalities have not had a measurable impact on its occurrence; a meta-analysis[32] revealed similar prevalence rates of ORN between conventional radiotherapy (7.4%), intensity-modulated radiation therapy (IMRT) (5.1%), chemoradiation (6.8%), and brachytherapy (5.3%).

The CT findings (Fig. 5) of isolated ORN include bone erosion (frequently of the lingual mandibular cortex adjacent to the molar teeth being an early sign), loss of trabeculations, intraosseous gas, fragmentation, sclerosis, and fracture. On MRI, marrow edema (evident as low T1 and high T2 signal) is typical. The absence of associated soft tissue abnormality may enable differentiation of ORN from tumor recurrence, but is not always straightforward.[28,33] Coexistent osteomyelitis may result in adjacent soft tissue edema, periostitis, and formation of abscesses and sinus tracts. Imaging signs demonstrating signs of osteomyelitis in irradiated bone likely indicate underlying

ORN. Likewise, the presence of a solid or necrotic mass adjacent to affected bone may indicate tumor recurrence and must prompt biopsy. PET imaging is of limited value in differentiating ORN from recurrence with significant overlap in standardized uptake value (SUV) values being observed between the 2.[31] ORN of the cervical spine, a rare complication of radiation for nasopharyngeal, hypopharyngeal, and skull base cancers, may be difficult to differentiate from metastatic disease. However, contiguous, symmetric, upper cervical vertebral involvement, vertebral body collapse, and posterior pharyngeal wall soft tissue ulceration without paraspinal or epidural soft tissue components may help differentiate them.[34]

Radiation for nasopharyngeal, parotid, and external auditory canal malignancy rarely may result in temporal bone and skull base ORN (Fig. 6), with patients presenting with otalgia, hearing loss, and purulent otorrhea.[35] Imaging findings are similar to those encountered at other sites and include erosions of the bony external auditory canal in the early stages, mottled bone loss, mastoid and middle ear effusions, intraosseous gas, and destruction of the temporomandibular joint. In rare cases, soft tissue and intracranial abscesses and meningitis may occur due to superimposed infection.[36]

Laryngeal chondroradionecrosis (LCRN) (Fig. 7) presents with throat pain, hoarseness, dyspnea, and dysphagia and occurring soon after or several years after radiation. It is more likely to occur after

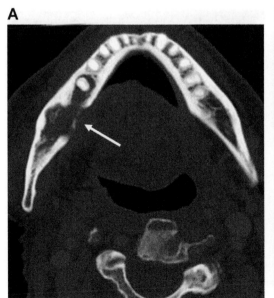 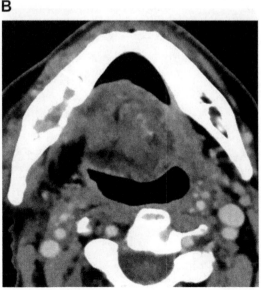

Fig. 5. Osteoradionecrosis of the mandible in a patient with oropharyngeal and oral cavity cancer who received chemoradiation after resection. Axial postcontrast CT reveals osseous erosion of the mandibular lingual cortex and fragmentation (*arrow*) (*A*) without evidence of associated soft tissue mass (*B*).

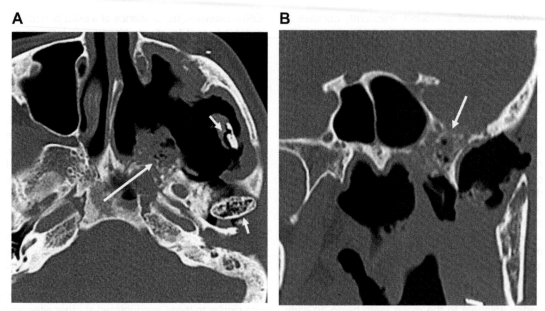

Fig. 6. Skull base osteoradionecrosis. Patient with adenoid cystic carcinoma of the maxillary sinus with orbital recurrence and history of partial maxillectomy, orbital exenteration, and chemoradiation. Axial (*A*) and coronal (*B*) CT reveals osseous erosion, fragmentation, intraosseous gas, and overlying mucosal ulceration involving the skull base (*long arrow*) (*A*) and (*arrow*) (*B*) and the mandible (*short arrows*) (*A*).

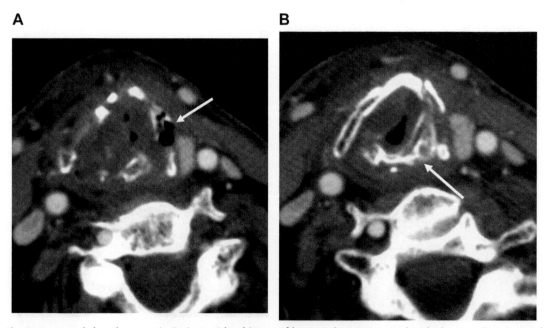

Fig. 7. Laryngeal chondronecrosis. Patient with a history of laryngeal cancer treated with chemoradiation. Axial postcontrast CT reveals fragmentation of and gas within the thyroid cartilage (*arrow*) (*A*) and deformity of the cricoid cartilage (*arrow*) (*B*).

the treatment of tumors that involve cartilage at presentation. The Chandler grading system classifies LCRN into 4 grades of progressively increasing severity with patients with grade IV disease (severe pain and odynophagia, weight loss and laryngeal obstruction causing severe respiratory distress) requiring laryngectomy. LCRN occurs due to radiation-induced end arteriolar obstruction in the perichondrium that nourishes cartilage. Findings on CT include cartilage fragmentation, collapse, and sloughing and gas bubbles within and around cartilage. PET imaging can show hypermetabolism, making distinction from tumor recurrence difficult.[37–39]

Mild/early-onset ORN is managed conservatively using a combination of debridement and antibiotics. Other approaches include the administration of hyperbaric oxygen after definitely ruling out tumor recurrence, although its efficacy remains controversial, and combination treatment pentoxifylline, vitamin E, and clodronate.[40,41] More severe ORN with large areas of bone exposure, discharging fistulae, or associated with fracture may require radical sequestrectomy or segmental mandibulectomy and free flap reconstruction.[42]

OPHTHALMOLOGICAL COMPLICATIONS

Radiation-induced optic neuropathy (RION) occurs due to ischemic necrosis of the anterior visual pathways. Vision loss usually occurs approximately 18 months (range 7–48 months) after treatment, is often profound, acute in onset and may be mono- or binocular, simultaneous, or sequential and is frequently irreversible.[43] Although the risk of RION increases with radiation dose, it may occur in patients at doses below "safe" radiation thresholds (<55 Gy; <8–10 Gy for stereotactic radiosurgery).[44] Increased T2 signal, subtle thickening, and enhancement of the prechiasmatic segment of the optic nerve(s) are typical findings on MRI (Fig. 8). It is important to note that these findings may be subtle, precede the development of visual loss and may persist for several months after treatment.[43] Management includes corticosteroids and hyperbaric oxygen, although no definitively effective therapeutic measures exist. Ocular complications may also include keratoconjunctivitis, xerophthalmia from lacrimal gland injury, nasolacrimal duct damage, injury to the iris and choroid, cataracts, and retinopathy.[45]

OTOTOXICITY

Radiation can affect all components of the auditory pathway. The median dose for the occurrence of ototoxicity after radiation for head and neck

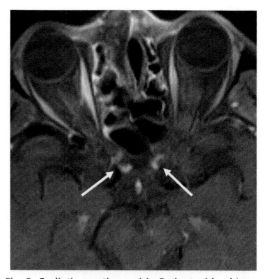

Fig. 8. Radiation optic neuritis. Patient with a history of sinonasal undifferentiated carcinoma who completed chemoradiation 6 months prior. Axial postcontrast T1WI with fat saturation reveals the enhancement of the prechiasmatic optic nerves bilaterally (*arrows*). (*Courtesy of* J Molitoris, M.D., Ph.D.,Baltimore, Maryland).

cancer is 60 to 66 Gy and above, although the threshold may be even lower (32–50 Gy).[46,47] Concurrent cisplatin administration significantly increases the risk of sensorineural hearing loss. The threshold cochlear dose for hearing loss with concurrent cisplatin-based chemotherapy may be as low as 10 Gy.[48] Rarely, enhancement of the labyrinthine structures may be evident after radiation on contrast-enhanced MRI (Fig. 9).

MYELITIS

Radiation myelopathy may occur a few months to several years after the treatment of head and neck cancer with radiation. The devastating nature of this entity compels the oncologist to prioritize excluding the spinal cord over tumor coverage during radiation planning and limiting total dose to the cord to less than 45 Gy in daily 1.8 to 2.0 Gy fractions.[49] The clinical and imaging manifestations of radiation myelopathy may be nonspecific, prompting consideration of other inflammatory, demyelinating, and autoimmune conditions unless a history of prior radiation is recognized. MRI abnormalities include long-segment cord T2 signal abnormality, cord expansion, and variable hemorrhage and enhancement with gadolinium contrast (Fig. 10). Khan and colleagues[50] suggest that predilection for this entity to affect the central gray matter to a greater degree than the white matter tracts in its periphery

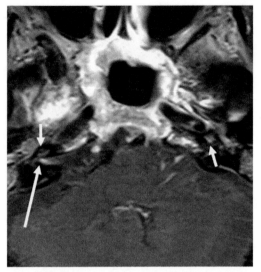

Fig. 9. Labyrinthine toxicity from radiation. Patient with a history of nasopharyngeal carcinoma treated with chemoradiation 2 years prior. Axial postcontrast T1WI with fat saturation reveals the enhancement of the bilateral cochlea (*short arrows*) and right internal auditory canal (*long arrow*).

perhaps implies ischemia and vasculitis as its underlying cause rather than demyelination. The presence of T1 hyperintense signal in the cervical vertebral bodies due to fatty marrow replacement in the radiation field is a useful clue to the diagnosis. Cord atrophy is frequently seen in survivors with a minority of patients demonstrating complete resolution of MRI changes.[50,51]

RADIATION NECROSIS IN THE BRAIN

The proximity of brain parenchyma to cancers of the craniofacial region and skull base make it susceptible to injury from radiation. This is especially true after radiation treatment for nasopharyngeal carcinoma (NPC). Although any part of the brain may be damaged by radiation, changes are most frequently seen in the temporal lobes. The incidence of temporal lobe necrosis is a function of radiation dose and technique and is influenced by a variety of genetic factors, underlying medical comorbidities and administration of chemotherapeutic agents such as the epidermal growth factor receptor inhibitor cetuximab.[52] The incidence of temporal lobe necrosis after radiation for NPC has declined in the era of IMRT with a 5-year actuarial incidence of 16% than 34.9% with conventional 2-dimensional radiotherapy.[53,54] Despite this, even with IMRT, particularly when NPC invades the skull base or the intracranial compartment, dosimetric "hot spots" maybe generated in the brain leading to necrosis.[53]

Radionecrosis may be detected incidentally on imaging studies in asymptomatic patients undergoing surveillance after treatment. It may also present with headache, seizures and deficits in memory, language, motor ability, and executive function.[55] Radiation injury is believed to occur in 3 temporal phases—an acute phase in the first few weeks after radiation mediated by vascular injury, that is, usually reversible; an early delayed phase, a few months after treatment, also reversible glial-cell related whereby demyelination of the affected white matter occurs; and a late delayed, irreversible phase about 6 months to several years after treatment characterized by inflammation and frank fibrinoid brain necrosis.[53,56] Management requires the use of corticosteroids and in lesions with mass effect, surgery, although the role of the latter is debatable. Other therapeutic approaches include anticoagulation, hyperbaric oxygen, and the use of more novel agents such as bevacizumab, ganglioside GM1, nerve growth factor, vitamin E, superoxide dismutase, and edavarone.[53]

In the early phase, MRI may demonstrate increased T2/FLAIR signal in the affected white matter without enhancement. In the early delayed phase, more extensive white matter involvement, mild swelling, and T2 hyperintensity and patchy areas of non–mass-like gray matter enhancement may appear. These changes may be unilateral or bilateral and also may be seen in the frontal lobes.[56,57] Structural changes in the temporal lobes also may be present even in the absence of obvious visual evidence of brain injury. Voxel based morphometric studies have revealed a decrease in gray matter volume in the bilateral superior temporal, left middle temporal, right fusiform, and right precentral gyri after radiation for NPC.[58] In the late stages, mass-like areas of necrosis with irregular peripheral, "feathery" enhancement surrounded by coalescent white matter signal abnormality are typical. Large lesions may exert considerable mass effect (**Fig. 11**). These findings should not be mistaken for locally recurrent or metastatic tumor. Although a history of radiation and their presence within or in close proximity to the radiation field may aid in this distinction, a definitive diagnosis may not always be possible. With the passage of time, areas of radiation necrosis may appear on imaging as foci of volume loss, encephalomalacia, and gliosis with dystrophic calcification.

On diffusion-weighted and diffusion tensor imaging, areas of necrosis tend to seem hypointense (higher ADC) than recurrent tumor, perhaps due to liquefaction and increased interstitial water.[59,60] Changes in MR spectroscopy (MRS), depending on the phase of the disease, that may support a

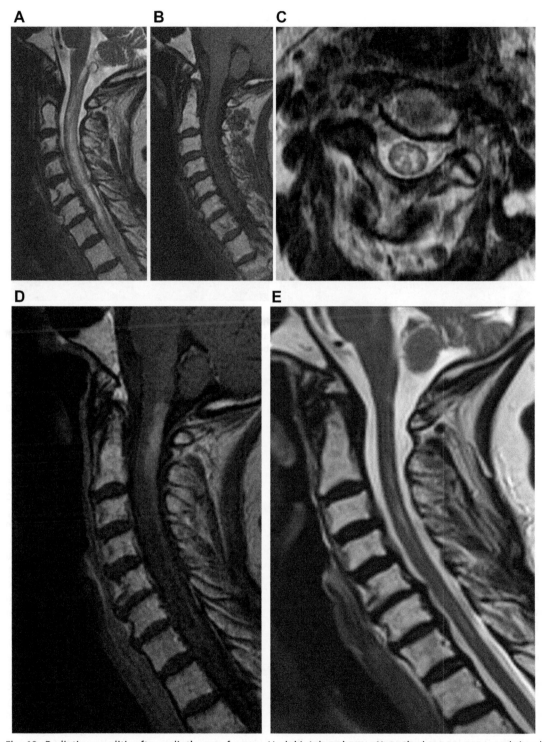

Fig. 10. Radiation myelitis after radiotherapy for non–Hodgkin's lymphoma. Note the long segment cord signal abnormality predominantly affecting the central cord (*A, C*) and patchy enhancement (*arrow, D*). The T1 hyperintense fatty marrow in the cervical vertebral bodies (*arrows, B*) is a clue to the diagnosis. Cord atrophy and decrease in edema are evident on the 6 month follow-up MR (*E*).

A

B

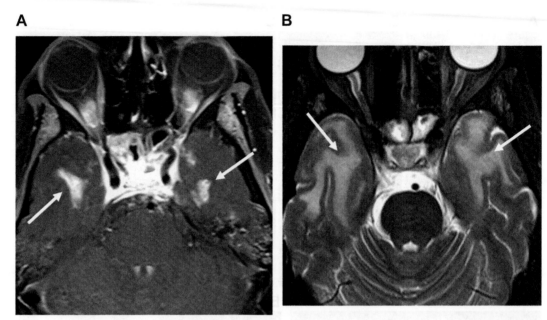

Fig. 11. Temporal lobe radiation necrosis. Patient with a history of nasopharyngeal carcinoma treated with chemoradiation 2 years prior. Axial postcontrast T1WI with fat saturation (A) and axial T2WI with fat saturation (B) reveals enhancing lesions within the bilateral temporal lobes (arrows) (A) with surrounding vasogenic edema (arrows) (B).

diagnosis of radiation necrosis include decrease in N-acetylaspartate, variable changes in choline and creatine levels and the presence of lactate and amino acid peaks. Although MRS offers a noninvasive way of characterizing these lesions at the metabolic level, no consensus exists regarding optimal technique, metabolite ratio calculation, accuracy and its value as a decision-making tool.[61] Dynamic susceptibility-weighted contrast-enhanced perfusion MRI parameters that maybe useful in distinguishing radiation necrosis from recurrent metastatic tumor include relative cerebral blood volume (rCBV), relative peak height (rPH), and percentage of signal-intensity recovery (PSR). In recurrent metastatic disease, rCBV, which correlates with microvascular density and rPH, which represents the maximal change in signal intensity during the transit of contrast, are significantly higher, whereas PSR which is believed to indicate capillary permeability, is lower.[62] Although early reports of the use of 2-[18F]fluoro-2-deoxy-D-glucose, (FDG)-PET imaging in distinguishing radiation necrosis from tumor were encouraging, the overlap in tracer uptake between the 2 can lead to diagnostic uncertainty. It is now recognized that radiation necrosis can be hypermetabolic and mimic tumor. Despite this, PET imaging, performed with either FDG or amino acid tracers, may still be superior to other imaging methods currently in practice.[63] Also, novel PET tracers and the use of hybrid PET-MRI systems

that enable accurate coregistration of simultaneously acquired PET and MR images may hold promise in differentiating the 2.[64]

VASCULOPATHY

Radiation may lead to a progressively occlusive cervical arteriopathy conferring a 2- to 9-fold increased the risk of stroke relative to comparable healthy individuals.[65] In the acute phase, radiation results in damage to adventitial vasa vasora, endothelial detachment, with splitting of the basement membrane and subintimal foam cell accumulation. These progress to medial atherosclerotic change and adventitial fibrosis that manifest as long segment stenoses several months to years after treatment.[65,66] Because the rate of significant carotid stenosis increases with time after radiation, the use of neck dissection and perhaps chemotherapy, screening using ultrasound is recommended for long-term survivors.[67] Angiographic findings of occlusive radiation vasculopathy include, in distinction to atherosclerotic stenoses in patients who have not undergone radiation, higher rates of contiguous involvement of the common and internal carotid arteries, greater involvement of the vertebral and external carotid arteries, and higher rates of bilaterality, tandem lesions, and completely occlusive and steno-occlusive lesions (Fig. 12). These patients also demonstrate more mature collateral pathways

A

B

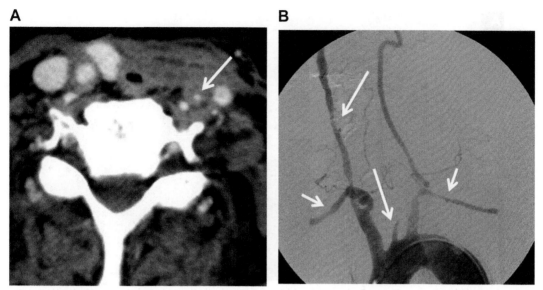

Fig. 12. Axial postcontrast CT (*A*) and angiogram (*B*), in 2 different patients, reveals radiation vasculopathy of the left common carotid artery (*arrow*) (*A*), bilateral common carotid arteries (*long arrows*) (*B*), and bilateral subclavian arteries (*short arrows*) (*B*). ([*B*] *Courtesy of* J Gomez, M.D., Jupiter, Florida).

than nonirradiated patients with a comparable level of vascular disease.[65] The best treatment strategy for clinically significant radiation induced carotid artery stenosis remains unclear. A recent meta-analysis[68] evaluating carotid endarterectomy (CEA) and stenting revealed similar risks of periprocedural stroke, myocardial infarction, and death with both procedures. Patients treated with CEA experience a higher risk of cranial nerve injury and a lower risk of long-term mortality.[68]

Carotid blowout syndrome (CBS) is a rare but devastating complication whereby hemorrhage occurs due to the loss of integrity of an arterial wall weakened by surgery and/or radiation. CBS is more likely to occur in patients who have undergone radical neck dissection and/or re-irradiation for salvage treatment. Hemorrhage can be precipitated by wound breakdown, infection, or formation of a pharyngocutaneous fistula.[69] CBS is more likely to occur with greater than 180° invasion of the circumference of the carotid wall by tumor. Strategies to prevent CBS include protecting the carotid arteries using distant well-vascularized myo- or fasciocutaneous flaps.[69] Several signs on CT angiography may point to impending or active CBS (**Fig. 13**). These include the exposure of an arterial structure, presence of pseudoaneurysms, and active contrast enhancement, with the presence of an exposed artery, a finding not identifiable on catheter angiography, being highly predictive of poor outcome.[70] Surgical ligation of the bleeding vessel may be difficult due to infection and/or scarring from radiation and is best used in unstable

patients with an open wound or fistula. Endovascular management strategies include embolization with particles, adhesives, or detachable balloon plugs, occlusion with Amplatzer vascular plugs and placement of covered stents.[69]

CHECKPOINT INHIBITOR TOXICITY

Checkpoint inhibitors are a group of immunomodulatory antibodies that have shown remarkable efficacy in treating a variety of malignancies. These include the programmed cell death receptor 1 (PD-1) antibodies such as nivolumab, cemiplimab, and pembrolizumab, used in the management of head and neck squamous cell carcinomas, programmed cell death ligand 1 (PD-L1) antibodies such as atezoliziumab and avelumab, used in melanoma and metastatic Merkel cell carcinoma, and ipilimumab, a cytotoxic T lymphocyte-associated antigen 4 (CTLA-4) antibody used to treat melanoma. Their use is associated with a wide variety of immune-related adverse events. Hypophysitis is a well-recognized complication not only associated with the use of ipilimumab, (incidence 3.2%), but also with nivolumab (0%,4%) and pembrolizumab (<0.1%) and is more likely to occur with a combination of ipilimumab plus nivolumab (6.4%).[22] Ipilimumab-induced hypophysitis occurs approximately 8 weeks after initiation and presents with clinical and laboratory evidence of hypopituitarism. Enlargement of the gland with geographic areas of hypoenhancement postulated to reflect fibrosis is typical on MRI (**Fig. 14**). These

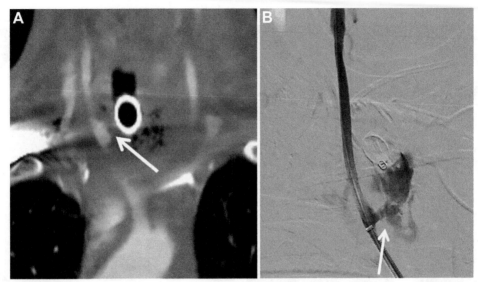

Fig. 13. Carotid blow out syndrome. Patient with a history of anaplastic thyroid carcinoma treated with resection and radiotherapy. Coronal postcontrast CT angiogram (*A*) reveals irregularity of the proximal right common carotid artery (*arrow*). Angiogram with selective catheterization of the right common carotid artery reveals the extravasation of contrast from the medial wall (*arrow*) (*B*). (*Courtesy of* J Gomez, M.D., Jupiter, Florida)

findings must not be mistaken for metastatic disease and a history of immunotherapy must always be sought in the setting of a patient with advanced malignancy. Pituitary enlargement has been noted to resolve within 40 days after steroid replacement. All patients with follow-up MR imaging performed within 40 days of diagnosis showed reversal of pituitary enlargement following the initiation of glucocorticoid treatment.[71,72] Leptomeningeal enhancement, not to be mistaken for metastatic disease, has also been reported in patients receiving ipilimumab.[73] Rarely encountered neurologic adverse events include peripheral neuropathy, Guillain–Barre syndrome, autoimmune encephalitis, aseptic meningitis, and posterior reversible encephalopathy syndrome.[74]

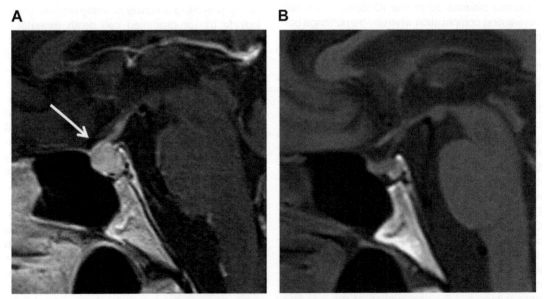

Fig. 14. Ipilimumab induced hypophysitis. Patient with a history of metastatic melanoma of the cheek treated with immunotherapy. Sagittal postcontrast T1WI (*A*) reveals diffuse enhancement and enlargement of the pituitary gland (*arrow*). Sagittal T1WI (*B*) 2 months prior reveals a normal pituitary gland.

RADIATION-INDUCED MALIGNANCY

Radiation-induced cancers are a rare complication after irradiation for head and neck malignancy, especially NPC. They occur several years after treatment (median 10–12 years) and carry a grim prognosis. Most of these are osteosarcomas (approximately 34%) and fibrosarcomas (approximately 19%) although several other types of malignant mesenchymal neoplasms and squamous cell carcinomas of the external auditory canal have been reported.[75,76] Their highly aggressive nature,[77] poor sensitivity to chemotherapy, and limited options for re-irradiation make surgery the only feasible treatment option in most cases.[75,76,78] These tumors are variable in their clinical and radiological presentation. On imaging, a heterogenous mass in the craniofacial region causing bone destruction must always prompt a diagnosis of a radiation-induced malignancy in a patient who has undergone therapeutic radiation in the past (**Fig. 15**). However, it may be difficult to distinguish these from recurrence of the treated tumor, metastases, or new lymphoma or melanoma. There are no histology specific imaging characteristics. Bone sarcomas may demonstrate a periosteal reaction and mineralization of the tumor matrix. The imaging features of radiation-induced osteosarcoma may differ from primary osteosarcoma in that the former may demonstrate greater heterogeneity of T2 signal and relatively lower FDG uptake on PET imaging.[12,79]

THE ONCOLOGIST'S PERSPECTIVE

Modern radiotherapy approaches to cancer management focus on optimizing tumor control and minimizing acute and late side effects through technologic advances in photon therapy planning, increasing the utilization of particle therapy, judiciously reducing radiotherapy doses and target volumes, and refining dose constraints of organs at risk.

IMRT uses multiple small radiation beams to enable a highly conformal dose distribution around the target volume while sparing surrounding healthy tissue. This is accomplished in part by the steep dose-gradient (ie, a rapid reduction from high to low dose) inherent to IMRT. Compared with 2D and 3D radiotherapy, IMRT has been associated with a reduction in dose to the parotid glands thereby reducing xerostomia. Other benefits of IMRT include reduced risk of temporal lobe necrosis in patients with nasopharynx cancer. In a prospective randomized trial, lateral temporal lobe necrosis was 21% with conventional radiotherapy than 13.1% with IMRT.[80] Further, randomized data demonstrated acute grade 3 mucositis rates of 14.5% with conventional radiotherapy than 6% with IMRT.[81] Similar to IMRT, intensity-modulated proton therapy (IMPT) is able to conform high doses of radiotherapy to the target. However, the unique dosimetric characteristics of protons in contradistinction to photons, enables physicians to reduce more intermediate, and low doses of radiation to nearby organs at risk than IMRT. In this context, IMPT has been associated with decreased mucositis, feeding tube dependency, xerostomia, dysgeusia, and mandibular ORN than IMRT.[82] Though encouraging, these data need to be confirmed in controlled randomized settings.

Beyond technologic advances, limited treatment volumes and refining organs at risk and their dose constraints have improved the therapeutic

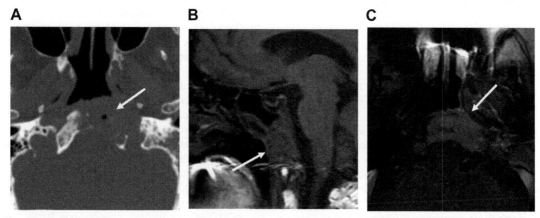

Fig. 15. Patient with a remote history of nasopharyngeal carcinoma treated with chemoradiation. Axial CT (*A*) reveals erosion of the clivus (*arrow*). Sagittal T1WI (*B*) reveals decreased signal throughout the marrow of the clivus (*arrow*). Axial postcontrast T1WI with fat saturation (*C*) reveals an enhancing mass within the clivus (*arrow*). Biopsy revealed undifferentiated sarcoma.

ratio of radiotherapy. For example, limiting contralateral irradiation for lateralized tumors spares contralateral organs at risk while maintaining excellent rates or regional control.[83] Similarly, eliminating low-risk elective nodal volumes was shown to reduce toxicity without sacrificing regional control.[84] Reducing margins around high-dose target volumes has been shown to maintain expected tumor control while reducing dose to organs at risk.[85–87] Finally, identifying structures and dose constraints for dysphagia and aspiration structures likely reduces the risk of long-term morbidity and mortality.[88] With pattern of failure analyses demonstrating a propensity for failing in high-dose target volumes, radiation oncologists have many tools at their disposal to limit dose to areas at low risk of containing disease to reduce acute and late side effects.

SUMMARY

Chemoradiation for head and neck cancers results in a variety of immediate and delayed complications that manifest on cross-sectional imaging studies. Awareness of the imaging appearances of these may aid the radiologist in distinguishing them from tumor recurrence. Delayed complications may present with nonspecific imaging findings and a history of radiation must be sought to arrive at the correct diagnosis.

ACKNOWLEDGMENTS

The authors would like to thank Brigitte Pocta, MLA for her assistance with the article.

DISCLOSURE

The authors have nothing to disclose.

REFERENCES

1. Trotti A. Toxicity antagonists in cancer therapy. Curr Opin Oncol 1997;9(6):569–78.
2. Seiwert TY, Salama JK, Vokes EE. The chemoradiation paradigm in head and neck cancer. Nat Clin Pract Oncol 2007;4(3):156–71.
3. Staar S, Rudat V, Stuetzer H, et al. Intensified hyperfractionated accelerated radiotherapy limits the additional benefit of simultaneous chemotherapy–results of a multicentric randomized German trial in advanced head-and-neck cancer. Int J Radiat Oncol Biol Phys 2001;50(5):1161–71.
4. Ferris RL, Blumenschein GJ, Fayette J, et al. Nivolumab for Recurrent Squamous-Cell Carcinoma of the Head and Neck. N Engl J Med 2016;375(19):1856–67.
5. Cox JD, Stetz J, Pajak TF. Toxicity criteria of the Radiation Therapy Oncology Group (RTOG) and the European Organization for Research and Treatment of Cancer (EORTC). Int J Radiat Oncol Biol Phys 1995;31(5):1341–6.
6. Givens DJ, Karnell LH, Gupta AK, et al. Adverse events associated with concurrent chemoradiation therapy in patients with head and neck cancer. Arch Otolaryngol Head Neck Surg 2009;135(12):1209–17.
7. Nutting CM, Morden JP, Harrington KJ, et al. Parotid-sparing intensity modulated versus conventional radiotherapy in head and neck cancer (PARSPORT): a phase 3 multicentre randomised controlled trial. Lancet Oncol 2011;12(2):127–36.
8. Sonis ST. The pathobiology of mucositis. Nat Rev Cancer 2004;4(4):277–84.
9. Sonis ST. Mucositis as a biological process: a new hypothesis for the development of chemotherapy-induced stomatotoxicity. Oral Oncol 1998;34(1):39–43.
10. Elting LS, Cooksley CD, Chambers MS, et al. Risk, outcomes, and costs of radiation-induced oral mucositis among patients with head-and-neck malignancies. Int J Radiat Oncol Biol Phys 2007;68(4):1110–20.
11. McCullough RW. Practice insights on patient care-management overview for chemoradiation toxic mucositis-guidelines, guideline-supported therapies and high potency polymerized cross-linked sucralfate (ProThelial). J Oncol Pharm Pract 2019;25(2):409–22.
12. Debnam JM, Garden AS, Ginsberg LE. Benign ulceration as a manifestation of soft tissue radiation necrosis: imaging findings. AJNR Am J Neuroradiol 2008;29(3):558–62.
13. Saito N, Nadgir RN, Nakahira M, et al. Posttreatment CT and MR imaging in head and neck cancer: what the radiologist needs to know. Radiographics 2012;32(5):1261–82 [discussion: 1282–4].
14. Deasy JO, Moiseenko V, Marks L, et al. Radiotherapy dose-volume effects on salivary gland function. Int J Radiat Oncol Biol Phys 2010;76(3 Suppl):S58–63.
15. Juan C-J, Cheng C-C, Chiu S-C, et al. Temporal Evolution of Parotid Volume and Parotid Apparent Diffusion Coefficient in Nasopharyngeal Carcinoma Patients Treated by Intensity-Modulated Radiotherapy Investigated by Magnetic Resonance Imaging: A Pilot Study. PLoS One 2015;10(8):e0137073.
16. Zhou N, Chu C, Dou X, et al. Early evaluation of radiation-induced parotid damage in patients with nasopharyngeal carcinoma by T2 mapping and mDIXON Quant imaging: initial findings. Radiat Oncol 2018;13(1):22.
17. Bronstein AD, Nyberg DA, Schwartz AN, et al. Increased salivary gland density on contrast-

enhanced CT after head and neck radiation. AJR Am J Roentgenol 1987;149(6):1259–63.

18. Wang Z-H, Yan C, Zhang Z-Y, et al. Radiation-induced volume changes in parotid and submandibular glands in patients with head and neck cancer receiving postoperative radiotherapy: a longitudinal study. Laryngoscope 2009;119(10):1966–74.

19. Zhou N, Chu C, Dou X, et al. Early evaluation of irradiated parotid glands with intravoxel incoherent motion MR imaging: correlation with dynamic contrast-enhanced MR imaging. BMC Cancer 2016;16(1):865.

20. Cheng C-C, Chiu S-C, Jen Y-M, et al. Parotid perfusion in nasopharyngeal carcinoma patients in early-to-intermediate stage after low-dose intensity-modulated radiotherapy: evaluated by fat-saturated dynamic contrast-enhanced magnetic resonance imaging. Magn Reson Imaging 2013;31(8):1278–84.

21. Tell R, Lundell G, Nilsson B, et al. Long-term incidence of hypothyroidism after radiotherapy in patients with head-and-neck cancer. Int J Radiat Oncol Biol Phys 2004;60(2):395–400.

22. Barroso-Sousa R, Barry WT, Garrido-Castro AC, et al. Incidence of Endocrine Dysfunction Following the Use of Different Immune Checkpoint Inhibitor Regimens: A Systematic Review and Meta-analysis. JAMA Oncol 2018;4(2):173–82.

23. Miller-Thomas MM, Kumar AJ, Sellin RV, et al. The shrinking thyroid: how does thyroid size change following radiation therapy for laryngeal cancer? AJNR Am J Neuroradiol 2009;30(3):613–6.

24. Soberman N, Leonidas JC, Cherrick I, et al. Sonographic abnormalities of the thyroid gland in long-term survivors of Hodgkin disease. Pediatr Radiol 1991;21(4):250–3.

25. Singh S, Rosenthal DI, Ginsberg LE. Enlargement and transformation of thyroglossal duct cysts in response to radiotherapy: imaging findings. AJNR Am J Neuroradiol 2009;30(4):800–2.

26. Schneider AB, Sarne DH. Long-term risks for thyroid cancer and other neoplasms after exposure to radiation. Nat Clin Pract Endocrinol Metab 2005;1(2):82–91.

27. Brignardello E, Felicetti F, Castiglione A, et al. Ultrasound surveillance for radiation-induced thyroid carcinoma in adult survivors of childhood cancer. Eur J Cancer 2016;55:74–80.

28. Hamilton JD, Lai SY, Ginsberg LE. Superimposed infection in mandibular osteoradionecrosis: diagnosis and outcomes. J Comput Assist Tomogr 2012;36(6):725–31.

29. Marx RE. Osteoradionecrosis: a new concept of its pathophysiology. J Oral Maxillofac Surg 1983;41(5):283–8.

30. Caparrotti F, Huang SH, Lu L, et al. Osteoradionecrosis of the mandible in patients with oropharyngeal carcinoma treated with intensity-modulated radiotherapy. Cancer 2017;123(19):3691–700.

31. Alhilali L, Reynolds AR, Fakhran S. Osteoradionecrosis after radiation therapy for head and neck cancer: differentiation from recurrent disease with CT and PET/CT imaging. AJNR Am J Neuroradiol 2014;35(7):1405–11.

32. Peterson DE, Doerr W, Hovan A, et al. Osteoradionecrosis in cancer patients: the evidence base for treatment-dependent frequency, current management strategies, and future studies. Support Care Cancer 2010;18(8):1089–98.

33. Glastonbury CM, Parker EE, Hoang JK. The postradiation neck: evaluating response to treatment and recognizing complications. AJR Am J Roentgenol 2010;195(2):W164–71.

34. Wu L-A, Liu H-M, Wang C-W, et al. Osteoradionecrosis of the upper cervical spine after radiation therapy for head and neck cancer: differentiation from recurrent or metastatic disease with MR imaging. Radiology 2012;264(1):136–45.

35. Yuhan BT, Nguyen BK, Svider PF, et al. Osteoradionecrosis of the Temporal Bone: An Evidence-Based Approach. Otol Neurotol 2018;39(9):1172–83.

36. Ahmed S, Gupta N, Hamilton JD, et al. CT findings in temporal bone osteoradionecrosis. J Comput Assist Tomogr 2014;38(5):662–6.

37. Chandler JR. Radiation fibrosis and necrosis of the larynx. Ann Otol Rhinol Laryngol 1979;88(4 Pt 1):509–14.

38. Gessert TG, Britt CJ, Maas AMW, et al. Chondroradionecrosis of the larynx: 24-year University of Wisconsin experience. Head Neck 2017;39(6):1189–94.

39. Hermans R, Pameijer FA, Mancuso AA, et al. CT findings in chondroradionecrosis of the larynx. AJNR Am J Neuroradiol 1998;19(4):711–8.

40. Annane D, Depondt J, Aubert P, et al. Hyperbaric oxygen therapy for radionecrosis of the jaw: a randomized, placebo-controlled, double-blind trial from the ORN96 study group. J Clin Oncol 2004;22(24):4893–900.

41. Delanian S, Chatel C, Porcher R, et al. Complete restoration of refractory mandibular osteoradionecrosis by prolonged treatment with a pentoxifylline-tocopherol-clodronate combination (PENTOCLO): a phase II trial. Int J Radiat Oncol Biol Phys 2011;80(3):832–9.

42. Hao SP, Chen HC, Wei FC, et al. Systematic management of osteoradionecrosis in the head and neck. Laryngoscope 1999;109(8):1324–7 [discussion: 1327–8].

43. Archer EL, Liao EA, Trobe JD. Radiation-Induced Optic Neuropathy: Clinical and Imaging Profile of Twelve Patients. J Neuro-ophthalmol 2019;39(2):170–80.

44. Doroslovački P, Tamhankar MA, Liu GT, et al. Factors Associated with Occurrence of Radiation-induced Optic Neuropathy at "Safe" Radiation Dosage. Semin Ophthalmol 2018;33(4):581–8.

45. Lin K-T, Lee S-Y, Liu S-C, et al. Risk of ocular complications following radiation therapy in patients with

nasopharyngeal carcinoma. Laryngoscope 2020; 130(5):1270–7.

46. Bhandare N, Antonelli PJ, Morris CG, et al. Ototoxicity after radiotherapy for head and neck tumors. Int J Radiat Oncol Biol Phys 2007;67(2): 469–79.

47. Pan C, Eisbruch A. Ototoxicity after radiotherapy of head-and-neck cancer: the perils of retrospective dose-response estimations: in regard to Bhandare et al. (Int J Radiat Oncol Biol Phys 2007;67:469-479). Int J Radiat Oncol Biol Phys 2007;68(5):1582 [author reply: 1582].

48. Hitchcock YJ, Tward JD, Szabo A, et al. Relative contributions of radiation and cisplatin-based chemotherapy to sensorineural hearing loss in head-and-neck cancer patients. Int J Radiat Oncol Biol Phys 2009;73(3):779–88.

49. Martel MK, Eisbruch A, Lawrence TS, et al. Spinal cord dose from standard head and neck irradiation: implications for three-dimensional treatment planning. Radiother Oncol 1998;47(2):185–9.

50. Khan M, Ambady P, Kimbrough D, et al. Radiation-Induced Myelitis: Initial and Follow-Up MRI and Clinical Features in Patients at a Single Tertiary Care Institution during 20 Years. AJNR Am J Neuroradiol 2018;39(8):1576–81.

51. Wang PY, Shen WC, Jan JS. MR imaging in radiation myelopathy. AJNR Am J Neuroradiol 1992;13(4): 1049–55 [discussion: 1056–8].

52. Niu X, Hu C, Kong L. Experience with combination of cetuximab plus intensity-modulated radiotherapy with or without chemotherapy for locoregionally advanced nasopharyngeal carcinoma. J Cancer Res Clin Oncol 2013;139(6):1063–71.

53. Zhou X, Liu P, Wang X. Temporal Lobe Necrosis Following Radiotherapy in Nasopharyngeal Carcinoma: New Insight Into the Management. Front Oncol 2020;10:593487.

54. Zhou G-Q, Yu X-L, Chen M, et al. Radiation-induced temporal lobe injury for nasopharyngeal carcinoma: a comparison of intensity-modulated radiotherapy and conventional two-dimensional radiotherapy. PLoS One 2013;8(7):e67488.

55. Cheung M, Chan AS, Law SC, et al. Cognitive function of patients with nasopharyngeal carcinoma with and without temporal lobe radionecrosis. Arch Neurol 2000;57(9):1347–52.

56. Landry D, Garsa AA, Glastonbury C. Imaging of Cerebral Radionecrosis: Collateral Damage from Head and Neck Radiation. Neurographics 2016;6(3): 151–8.

57. Chong VF, Fan YF, Mukherji SK. Radiation-induced temporal lobe changes: CT and MR imaging characteristics. AJR Am J Roentgenol 2000;175(2):431–6.

58. Lv X-F, Zheng X-L, Zhang W-D, et al. Radiation-induced changes in normal-appearing gray matter in patients with nasopharyngeal carcinoma: a

magnetic resonance imaging voxel-based morphometry study. Neuroradiology 2014;56(5): 423–30.

59. Asao C, Korogi Y, Kitajima M, et al. Diffusion-weighted imaging of radiation-induced brain injury for differentiation from tumor recurrence. AJNR Am J Neuroradiol 2005;26(6):1455–60.

60. Xu J-L, Li Y-L, Lian J-M, et al. Distinction between postoperative recurrent glioma and radiation injury using MR diffusion tensor imaging. Neuroradiology 2010;52(12):1193–9.

61. Sundgren PC. MR spectroscopy in radiation injury. AJNR Am J Neuroradiol 2009;30(8):1469–76.

62. Barajas RF, Chang JS, Sneed PK, et al. Distinguishing recurrent intra-axial metastatic tumor from radiation necrosis following gamma knife radiosurgery using dynamic susceptibility-weighted contrast-enhanced perfusion MR imaging. AJNR Am J Neuroradiol 2009;30(2):367–72.

63. Li H, Deng L, Bai HX, et al. Diagnostic Accuracy of Amino Acid and FDG-PET in Differentiating Brain Metastasis Recurrence from Radionecrosis after Radiotherapy: A Systematic Review and Meta-Analysis. AJNR Am J Neuroradiol 2018;39(2): 280–8.

64. Overcast WB, Davis KM, Ho CY, et al. Advanced imaging techniques for neuro-oncologic tumor diagnosis, with an emphasis on PET-MRI imaging of malignant brain tumors. Curr Oncol Rep 2021; 23(3):34.

65. Zou WXY, Leung TW, Yu SCH, et al. Angiographic features, collaterals, and infarct topography of symptomatic occlusive radiation vasculopathy: a case-referent study. Stroke 2013;44(2):401–6.

66. Murros KE, Toole JF. The effect of radiation on carotid arteries. A review article. Arch Neurol 1989; 46(4):449–55.

67. Brown PD, Foote RL, McLaughlin MP, et al. A historical prospective cohort study of carotid artery stenosis after radiotherapy for head and neck malignancies. Int J Radiat Oncol Biol Phys 2005; 63(5):1361–7.

68. Giannopoulos S, Texakalidis P, Jonnalagadda AK, et al. Revascularization of radiation-induced carotid artery stenosis with carotid endarterectomy vs. carotid artery stenting: A systematic review and meta-analysis. Cardiovasc Revasc Med Mol Interv 2018;19(5 Pt B):638–44.

69. Suárez C, Fernández-Alvarez V, Hamoir M, et al. Carotid blowout syndrome: modern trends in management. Cancer Manag Res 2018;10:5617–28.

70. Lee C-W, Yang C-Y, Chen Y-F, et al. CT angiography findings in carotid blowout syndrome and its role as a predictor of 1-year survival. AJNR Am J Neuroradiol 2014;35(3):562–7.

71. Wang H, Mustafa A, Liu S, et al. Immune Checkpoint Inhibitor Toxicity in Head and Neck Cancer: From

Identification to Management. Front Pharmacol 2019;10:1254.

72. Kurokawa R, Ota Y, Gonoi W, et al. MRI Findings of Immune Checkpoint Inhibitor-Induced Hypophysitis: Possible Association with Fibrosis. AJNR Am J Neuroradiol 2020;41(9):1683–9.

73. Ali S, Lee S-K. Ipilimumab Therapy for Melanoma: A Mimic of Leptomeningeal Metastases. AJNR Am J Neuroradiol 2015;36(12):E69–70.

74. Spain L, Wong R. The neurotoxic effects of immune checkpoint inhibitor therapy for melanoma. Melanoma Manag 2019;6(2):MMT16.

75. Wei Z, Xie Y, Xu J, et al. Radiation-induced sarcoma of head and neck: 50 years of experience at a single institution in an endemic area of nasopharyngeal carcinoma in China. Med Oncol 2012;29(2):670–6.

76. Zhang X, Bai S, Li H, et al. CT and MRI findings of radiation-induced external auditory canal carcinoma in patients with nasopharyngeal carcinoma after radiotherapy. Br J Radiol 2015;88(1050):20140791.

77. Tucker MA, D'Angio GJ, Boice JDJ, et al. Bone sarcomas linked to radiotherapy and chemotherapy in children. N Engl J Med 1987;317(10):588–93.

78. Giannini L, Incandela F, Fiore M, et al. Radiation-Induced Sarcoma of the Head and Neck: A Review of the Literature. Front Oncol 2018;8:449.

79. Sheppard DG, Libshitz HI. Post-radiation sarcomas: a review of the clinical and imaging features in 63 cases. Clin Radiol 2001;56(1):22–9.

80. Peng G, Wang T, Yang K-Y, et al. A prospective, randomized study comparing outcomes and toxicities of intensity-modulated radiotherapy vs. conventional two-dimensional radiotherapy for the treatment of nasopharyngeal carcinoma. Radiother Oncol 2012; 104(3):286–93.

81. Gupta T, Agarwal J, Jain S, et al. Three-dimensional conformal radiotherapy (3D-CRT) versus intensity modulated radiation therapy (IMRT) in squamous cell carcinoma of the head and neck: a randomized controlled trial. Radiother Oncol 2012;104(3):343–8.

82. Meijer TWH, Scandurra D, Langendijk JA. Reduced radiation-induced toxicity by using proton therapy for the treatment of oropharyngeal cancer. Br J Radiol 2020;93(1107):20190955.

83. Huang SH, Waldron J, Bratman SV, et al. Re-evaluation of Ipsilateral Radiation for T1-T2N0-N2b Tonsil Carcinoma at the Princess Margaret Hospital in the Human Papillomavirus Era, 25 Years Later. Int J Radiat Oncol Biol Phys 2017;98(1):159–69.

84. Sher DJ, Pham N-L, Shah JL, et al. Prospective Phase 2 Study of Radiation Therapy Dose and Volume De-escalation for Elective Neck Treatment of Oropharyngeal and Laryngeal Cancer. Int J Radiat Oncol Biol Phys 2021;109(4):932–40.

85. Burr AR, Harari PM, Haasl AM, et al. Clinical outcomes for larynx patients with cancer treated with refinement of high-dose radiation treatment volumes. Head Neck 2020;42(8):1874–81.

86. Burr AR, Harari PM, Ko HC, et al. Reducing radiotherapy target volume expansion for patients with HPV-associated oropharyngeal cancer. Oral Oncol 2019;92:52–6.

87. Zukauskaite R, Hansen CR, Grau C, et al. Local recurrences after curative IMRT for HNSCC: Effect of different GTV to high-dose CTV margins. Radiother Oncol 2018;126(1):48–55.

88. Eisbruch A, Schwartz M, Rasch C, et al. Dysphagia and aspiration after chemoradiotherapy for head-and-neck cancer: which anatomic structures are affected and can they be spared by IMRT? Int J Radiat Oncol Biol Phys 2004;60(5):1425–39.

PET/CT and PET/MR Imaging of the Post-treatment Head and Neck
Traps and Tips

Gloria J. Guzmán Pérez-Carrillo, MD, MSc, MPH[a],*, Jana Ivanidze, MD, PhD[b,c]

KEYWORDS

- PET/MR Imaging • PET/CT • FDG • DOTATATE • PSMA • FMISO • Post-treatment change • Head and neck cancer

KEY POINTS

- PET/CT can result in false-positive and false-negative results; it is imperative to understand normal variants of FDG uptake in the head and neck.
- Intimate understanding of surgical procedures and expected imaging changes is key to avoid misdiagnosis.
- Although 18F-FDG, which visualizes glucose metabolism, is helpful in the staging and treatment response assessment of head and neck cancer, more recently developed PET radiotracers targeting specific surface markers, such as 68Ga-DOTATATE for somatostatin receptor–positive neoplasms including paraganglioma, meningioma, and esthesioneuroblastoma, are promising for applications of diagnostic problem solving and may be a helpful adjunct in the differential diagnosis of head and neck neoplasms, and improve the sensitivity and specificity for the detection of certain pathologies.

INTRODUCTION

Head and neck tumors represent 3% of all malignant tumors in the United States.[1] In the United States, there were an estimated 53,000 new cases and 10,860 estimated deaths in 2019, with approximately 1.2% of men and women being diagnosed with this disease.[2] 2-Deoxy-2-(fluorine-18) fluoro-D-glucose (18F-FDG) uptake on PET with computed tomography (CT) is effective for monitoring head and neck cancer. However, variable physiologic FDG uptake and asymmetric FDG distribution in the neck can make image interpretation difficult. This is particularly evident in the post-treatment head and neck region, where alteration of expected anatomy makes diagnosis of recurrence or differentiating between recurrence and post-treatment change particularly challenging.[3]

Thus, having an extensive understanding of the normal variants of FDG uptake, the causes of false-positive (FP) and postnegative results, surgical procedures, and expected imaging changes and imaging protocols and reporting methods are key in avoiding diagnostic pitfalls.

Accurate localization of head and neck cancer primary neoplasms and nodal metastases is critical, particularly in the setting of locoregional

[a] Neuroradiology Section, Mallinckrodt Institute of Radiology, Washington University School of Medicine, 510 South Kingshighway, Campus Box 8131, St Louis, MO 63110, USA; [b] Division of Molecular Imaging & Therapeutics, Department of Radiology, Weill Cornell Medicine, 525 East 68th Street, Starr Building, 2nd Floor, New York, NY 10065, USA; [c] Division of Neuroradiology, Department of Radiology, Weill Cornell Medicine, 525 East 68th Street, Starr Building, 2nd Floor, New York, NY 10065, USA
* Corresponding author.
E-mail address: guzman.gloria@wustl.edu

Neuroimag Clin N Am 32 (2022) 111–132
https://doi.org/10.1016/j.nic.2021.09.003

advanced disease and in the setting of recurrence. 18F-FDG-PET/CT allows for accurate visualization of lesions with increased metabolism and has been shown to have high diagnostic accuracy in newly diagnosed and recurrent head and neck cancer, and in the context of treatment response assessment. The specificity, sensitivity, positive predictive value (PPV), and negative predictive value (NPV) of PET/CT in the evaluation of the post-treatment neck has been extensively described in the literature.[4,5] A meta-analysis by Gupta and colleagues[5] encompassing 51 studies and 2335 subjects determined that, for post-treatment FDG-PET/CT for the primary site, the sensitivity was 79.9%, specificity was 87.5%, PPV was 58.6%, and NPV was 95.1%.

PET/MR imaging has been available in the research setting for the past decade, and in recent years has found its way into clinical practice. PET/MR imaging has the advantage of decreased radiation dose given that MR is used for attenuation correction, obviating the need to acquire a CT; this advantage is of limited importance in the oncologic patient population often undergoing radiation therapy. Another key advantage is the increased soft tissue contrast allowing improved diagnostic performance compared with MR imaging alone or PET/CT alone (diagnostic accuracy of 0.926 vs 0.836 and 0.847; $P<.05$, respectively).[6] A potential drawback of PET/MR imaging is the decreased detection rate of lung nodules, particularly when they are not FDG-avid. PET requires accurate quantification of radiotracer distribution, which in turn requires accurate attenuation correction. PET/CT accomplishes attenuation correction based on electron density as assessed with low-dose CT, allowing for a linear attenuation coefficient to be assigned based on Hounsfield units. However, MR imaging–based attenuation correction is more complex given that MR imaging signal intensity is dependent on proton density and relaxation times, and does not directly translate to electron density.[7] The two main approaches to address the MR imaging–based attenuattion correction (AC) challenge are segmentation-based methods, which classify tissues based on MR imaging signal intensity into different tissue compartments (eg, air, fat, soft tissue, lung) that are then assigned a predefined linear attenuation coefficient; and atlas-based methods, which rely on a reference database of matching MR and CT images.[8] Additionally, there are reconstruction-based methods with simultaneous reconstruction of attenuation and activity data, based on the so-called maximum likelihood estimation of attenuation and activity algorithm, which relies on deriving the patient's body contours from non-AC images.[9]

However, the maximum likelihood estimation of attenuation and activity based approach is limited in that it relies on nonspecific accumulation of radiotracer in the skin, which is the case for FDG but not necessarily for many other radiotracers.[8] The question of synergy arising from concurrent FDG-PET and MR imaging evaluation remains to be fully answered; however, PET/MR imaging represents a promising approach in the diagnosis and follow-up of head and neck cancer.

UTILITY OF PET/COMPUTED TOMOGRAPHY IN DIAGNOSIS OF RECURRENT TUMOR IN THE POST-TREATMENT NECK

PET/CT performed in the early period after chemoradiation can help differentiate residual tumor from treatment-related changes.[10,11] It can help identify locoregional primary or nodal recurrence, new distal nodal, or distal organ metastatic disease,[11,12] and also assess response to treatment (Figs. 1 and 2).

ANATOMIC AND PHYSIOLOGIC ENTITIES IN THE HEAD AND NECK THAT RESULT IN FALSE-POSITIVE AND FALSE-NEGATIVE FINDINGS ON 18F-FDG-PET

Although PET has a high NPV, it also suffers from several FPs that result in low PPV. This is caused in part by numerous normal anatomic structures demonstrating physiologically increased 18F-FDG uptake. The tonsillar pillars, parotid glands, minor salivary glands in the soft and hard palate, the sublingual and the submandibular glands and nasopharyngeal lymphoid tissues known as Waldeyer ring (Fig. 3) can all demonstrate elevated 18F-FDG avidity.[13,14] Such lymphoid and glandular tissue can also be asymmetric and be mistaken for abnormality (Fig. 4).[14]

PEARL: To differentiate tumor from normal metabolic activity in cases of asymmetric 18F-FDG avidity, tonsillar maximum standardized uptake value (SUV) ratios may enable such distinction, with an SUV ratio greater than 1.6 conveying 62% sensitivity and 100% specificity.[15]

Brown adipose tissue (BAT), also known as brown fat, can also demonstrate normal increased FDG uptake because of its high metabolic activity,[16] and must not be confused with lymphadenopathy.[17]

PEARL: BAT is most commonly seen in those with BAT activation on prior studies, lower body mass index, female gender, lower temperatures, late morning scans, and with lower blood glucose.[17]

Skeletal muscle can also demonstrate intense metabolic activity because of shivering or tension

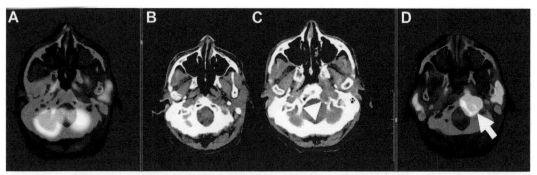

Fig. 1. A 73-year-old man with history of T2N2b left pyriform squamous cell carcinoma (SCC) status post incomplete conformal radiation treatment and salvage surgery a few months after had normal skull base findings and no abnormal 18F-FDG uptake on initial PET/CT follow-up after salvage surgery axial fused PET/CT (*A*) and noncontrast axial CT (*B*). Two months later, the patient presents with new decreased left soft palate mobility and abnormal left-sided tongue movements. The patient went on to have a second repeat PET/CT that showed a destructive osseous lesion centered at the petroclival junction and left hypoglossal canal in noncontrast axial CT (*C, arrowhead*) that demonstrates abnormal elevated 18F-FDG uptake on axial fused PET/CT (*D, arrow*), compatible with new regional metastatic disease.

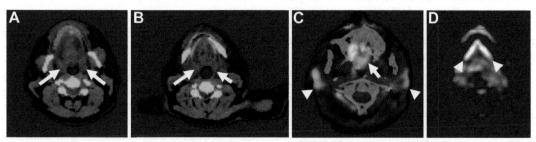

Fig. 2. A 57-year-old man with T2N0 supraglottic larynx SCCa treated with 70-Gy radiation therapy. 18F-FDG uptake is seen circumferentially in the supraglottic larynx (*A*) with a partially necrotic nodule seen on the right paraepiglottic fat, indicated with white arrow in (*B*). 18F-FDG uptake resolved 4 months after completion of radiation treatment, compatible with complete metabolic response (*C*).

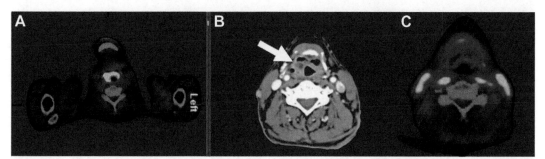

Fig. 3. (*A, B*) Axial fused PET/CT demonstrates elevated 18F-FDG uptake in tonsillar pillars (*arrows*). (*C*) Axial fused PET/CT demonstrates elevated 18F-FDG uptake in the bilateral parotid glands (*arrowheads*) and the minor salivary glands of the hard palate (*arrow*). (*D*) Axial PET demonstrates normal sublingual activity (*arrowheads*). All of these represent normal variants of metabolic activity.

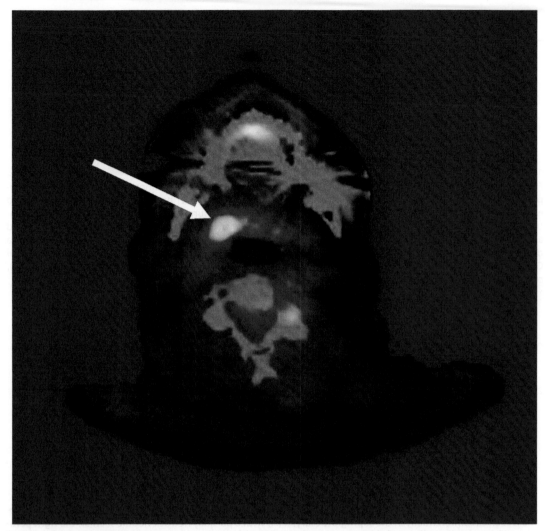

Fig. 4. Axial fused PET/CT demonstrates asymmetric FDG uptake in a normal left tonsillar pillar (*arrow*).

(Fig. 5). Note than in thin patients with minimal fat planes, intense muscle activity can obscure nodal disease (Fig. 6).[18] An addition, artifacts of attenuation correction, such as calcium and surgical clips, can result in artefactually increased 18F-FDG uptake (Fig. 7).[14] Symmetric vocal cord activity can be seen, especially if the patient is talking or vocalizing during the scan (Fig. 8).[18]

Finally, in about 90% of cases with metastatic cervical lymphadenopathy with primary tumors of "unknown" origin, a small primary in the oropharynx may be obscured by lingual or palatine tonsillar physiologic lymphoid 18F-FDG uptake,[19] which can result in a false-negative (FN) result.

PEARL: Narrow the window significantly to increase tissue contrast.

SPECIAL CONSIDERATIONS IN IMAGING PROTOCOLS AND REPORTING SYSTEMS
PET/Computed Tomography to Follow Quantitative Imaging Biomarkers Alliance Parameters

In order to standardize parameters to improve SUV comparisons across time and equipment, and to allow for big-data analysis, it is highly desirable that all PET/CT units follow the Radiological Society of North America's Quantitative Imaging Biomarkers Alliance (QIBA) parameters. QIBA, formed in 2007, aims to advance quantitative imaging through a collaboration among clinicians, medical physicists, researchers, health care professionals, and industry. QIBA parameters have a rigorous system of implementation, with FDG-

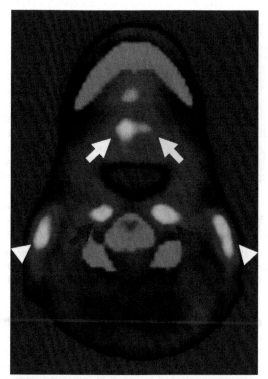

Fig. 5. Axial fused PET/CT shows normal intense 18F-FDG uptake in muscle, either caused by tension or shivering from cold. Here we see intense activity in the bilateral sternocleidomastoid muscles (*white arrowheads*), bilateral longus colli muscles (*black arrows*), and the bilateral genioglossus muscles (*white arrows*).

PET/CT as an imaging biomarker for tumor response currently in the most advanced stage of development (stage 3). QIBA Radiological Society of North America profiles for FDG-PET/CT are found in http://qibawiki.rsna.org/images/1/1f/QIBA_FDG-PET_Profile_v113.pdf.[20] This profile provides not only indications for image acquisition, but also the preimaging and postimaging stages, region of interest placement, and calculations.

PEARL: Update your protocols to follow QIBA parameters, which will standardize your data and allow easier data aggregation for research purposes.

Time of Flight PET/Computed Tomography and Digital PET Technique for Improved Lesion Visualization

Although currently standard of care, it is important to be familiar with time-of-flight (TOF) PET/CT and the effect it has of increasing the SUV value of lymph nodes.[21] This knowledge is especially critical if one interprets studies at an institution that has PET/CT units with and without TOF capability.

PITFALL: While comparing a prior study performed without TOF with a current study performed with TOF, one might incorrectly diagnose increased metabolic activity.

Likewise, using digital PET allows for smaller image resolution of 1 to 2 mm and enhanced definition of SUV, thus improving visualization and

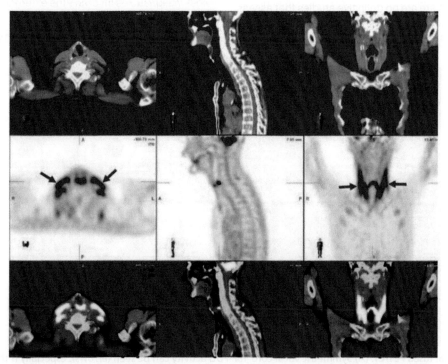

Fig. 6. Prominent normal muscle activity (*arrows*) obscuring abnormal nodal 18F-FDG uptake. This is especially problematic in patients with thin fat planes. (*From* Yao, M. (2012). PET Imaging of the Head and Neck, An Issue of PET Clinics. Elsevier Health Sciences; with permission).

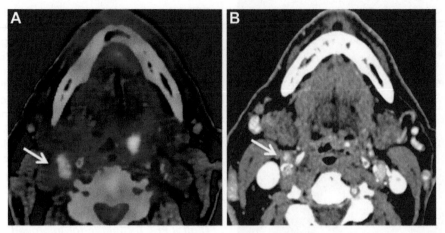

Fig. 7. Increased 18F-FDG activity (*A, arrow*) caused by attenuation correction in a calcified carotid atheromatous plaque (*B, arrow*). (*From* Purohit, B. S., Ailianou, A., Dulguerov, N., Becker, C. D., Ratib, O., & Becker, M. (2014). FDG-PET/CT pitfalls in oncological head and neck imaging. *Insights into imaging*, 5(5), 585-602; with permission).

diagnosis of small nodal or tumoral disease (**Fig. 9**).[22] This occurs because of improvements in solid state (digital) photodetectors, which allows better detection of the two coincident photons generated by positron annihilation, permitting improved localization of the event.[23]

Contrast-Enhanced PET/Computed Tomography and Value of Performing Dedicated Neck PET/Computed Tomography

Although there are no definitive studies that assess the question of whether there is improvement in diagnostic accuracy with the use of contrast-

enhanced CT, contrast is useful in evaluating extracapsular spread of nodal disease and necrosis, which affect management.[24] Dedicated PET/CT acquisition in the head and neck region has been demonstrated to result in improved spatial resolution and increased accuracy of SUV, compared with assessment of the head and neck region based on whole-body PET/CT images alone (**Fig. 10**).[18]

Neck Imaging Reporting and Data System

In 2016, the Neck Imaging Reporting and Data System (NI-RADS) was established with the

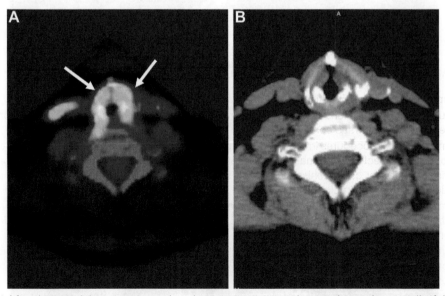

Fig. 8. Axial fused PET/CT. (*A*) Symmetric vocal cord 18F-FDG activity can be seen (*arrows*), especially if the patient is talking or vocalizing during the scan. Accompanying noncontrast axial CT (*B*) shows no underlying lesion.

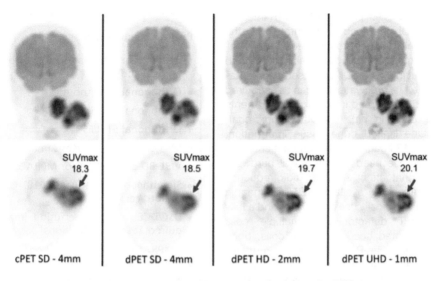

| SUVmax 18.3 | SUVmax 18.5 | SUVmax 19.7 | SUVmax 20.1 |
| cPET SD - 4mm | dPET SD - 4mm | dPET HD - 2mm | dPET UHD - 1mm |

Fig. 9. Improved visualization and SUV detection of conventional analog photomultiplier tube-based PET (cPET) versus digital PET (dPET) using different reconstruction matrix (in standard definition [SD], high definition [HD], and ultrahigh definition [UHD]) and different voxel volume sizes (4 mm, 2 mm, and 1 mm). (*From* Wright CL, Washington IR, Bhatt AD, Knopp MV. Emerging Opportunities for Digital PET/CT to Advance Locoregional Therapy in Head and Neck Cancer. *Semin Radiat Oncol.* 2019;29(2):93-101; with permission).

purpose of "standardizing assessment and reporting in surveillance imaging for patients with head and neck squamous cell carcinomas and their subsequent management."[25] The categories have been published by the American College of Radiology.[26,27] The role of PET/CT in NI-RADS is to help stratify the imaging results in combination with anatomic imaging findings. Normal 18F-FDG uptake corresponds to NI-RADS 1, mild 18F-FDG uptake is categorized as NI-RADS 2,

suspicious high 18F-FDG uptake is NI-RADS 3, and SUV uptake representing definite tumor recurrence is considered NI-RADS 4. The NI-RADS system is evaluated in detail elsewhere in this issue.

PET/MR Imaging Protocol Considerations

MR imaging–based attenuation correction is primarily accomplished on the basis of segmentation-based or atlas-based methods as

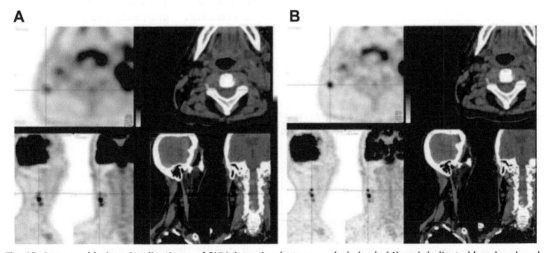

Fig. 10. Improved lesion visualization and SUV detection between whole body (*A*) and dedicated head and neck PET/CT (*B*). (*From* Yao, M. (2012). PET Imaging of the Head and Neck, An Issue of PET Clinics. Elsevier Health Sciences; with permission).

described previously.[8] For body PET/MR imaging applications, Dixon-based segmentation is the most commonly used approach, because of relatively fast acquisition and processing times and good reproducibility. For Dixon-based segmentation, separate fat- and water-images are acquired coronally and segmented into four compartments (soft tissue, fat, lung, air).[8,28] Methodologic challenges include limited bone tissue information, truncation of MR imaging data along patients' extremities, and the need for additional hardware components that affect AC (eg, radiofrequency coils).[29] Commercially available PET/MR imaging scanners today typically use a 3.0-T MR and a fully integrated PET detector with multiple coils including dedicated head and neck coils, body coils, and spine coils. Patient preparation, radiotracer dose, and uptake period are identical to established PET/CT protocols as detailed previously. Following acquisition of an MR-scout image, whole-body PET is acquired from the vertex to the mid-thigh, with 3 minutes of acquisition time per bed position and simultaneous MR imaging acquisition. Attenuation correction in the body is typically performed based on attenuation maps generated from the two-point Dixon sequence. Dedicated head-and-neck PET with concurrent diagnostic MR imaging is typically additionally acquired with a longer acquisition time of up to 10 minutes; although protocols vary from institution to institution, basic sequences acquired during PET/MR imaging studies are included in **Box 1**.

ADVANCED MR IMAGING IN THE CONTEXT OF PET/MR IMAGING IN HEAD AND NECK CANCER
Diffusion-Weighted Imaging

Diffusion-weighted imaging (DWI) reflects the random, microscopic translational motion of water molecules. Certain malignant neoplasms including head and neck cancer typically demonstrate high cellularity resulting in high nuclear-to-cytoplasmic ratio, and thereby reduced diffusion with low apparent diffusion coefficient (ADC) values compared with benign lesions caused by increased cellularity.[30] Diffusion imaging is a complementary sequence in MR imaging in head and neck cancer and improves diagnostic accuracy. It is important to note that certain benign entities also demonstrate reduced diffusion, including abscess, epidermoid cyst, and cholesteatoma.

Artifacts to be aware of include geometric distortion, susceptibility, and incomplete fat saturation. Additionally, motion artifacts related to respiratory motion, swallowing, and eye movements

---

Box 1
PET/MR imaging sequences

- Imaging for attenuation correction (eg, two-point Dixon)
- Orthogonal T1 without FS
- Orthogonal T2 without FS
- Orthogonal STIR/FS T2
- DWI or diffusion kurtosis imaging
- VIBE 3D or SPACE 3D or MPRAGE[a]
- Simultaneous or sequential 18F-FDG or other radiotracer
- DSC/DCE or other perfusion imaging is acquired at some institutions

[a] If MPRAGE is acquired, orthogonal FS TSE T1-weighted views may also be required.

---

are a concern for MR imaging acquisition in general but particularly for DWI.

Conventional DWI involves a single-pulsed echo planar sequence acquired in one gradient direction. Although it has advantages of a short acquisition time and ability to perform at low field strength, it is not suitable for head and neck imaging.[31] The shortcomings of conventional DWI can be overcome using trace imaging with ADC mapping, acquiring in at least three diffusion-sensitized directions and mathematically combined into a single trace sequence, with resulting decreased directional dependence within the voxels. The ADC map is important to differentiate between true reduced diffusion and T2 effects, similar to its applications in the brain for ischemic stroke and brain tumor evaluation.[30] In general, malignant head and neck neoplasms tend to have reduced diffusion with low ADC values (**Fig. 11**); however, exceptions exist including benign lesions with low ADC values (abscess, Warthin tumor, nerve sheath tumors, meningioma, cholesteatoma) and malignant neoplasms with lack of reduced diffusion (chordoma, chondrosarcoma). Overall, DWI MR imaging has shown utility as an adjunct tool in the evaluation of head and neck cancer.

Diffusion tensor imaging allows to measure the direction of diffusivity in addition to its magnitude. Parameters generated from diffusion tensor imaging, fractional anisotropy, and mean diffusivity reflect the shape and size of diffusion ellipsoids, respectively, and have been shown to correlate with cellular density, increasing the diagnostic confidence when used in conjunction with ADC.[32] Diffusion kurtosis imaging provides a

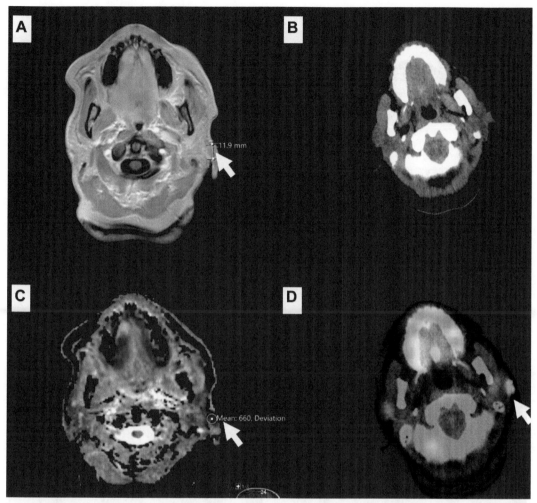

Fig. 11. Advantages of MR imaging DWI-based evaluation of lymphoma in the head and neck. Postgadolinium T1-weighted axial image demonstrates a minimally hypoenhancing lesion in the left parotid gland (*A, arrow*), which was not apparent on CT (*B*). The lesion demonstrates low ADC values on MR imaging DWI (*C, arrow*). FDG-PET demonstrated a corresponding focus of increased FDG avidity (*D, arrow*). Biopsy demonstrated lymphoma.

measure of deviation from Gaussian distribution in the degree of diffusion displacement in a given tissue. It requires acquisition with high b-values (>2000 s/mm^2).

Intravoxel incoherent motion uses a series of b-values ranging from 0 to 1000 s/mm^2 and takes advantage of differential signal loss seen at lower b-values to estimate tissue perfusion. Although intravoxel incoherent motion remains investigative at this time, there is increasing evidence for its utility in prediction of response to chemotherapy.[33,34]

MR Spectroscopy

MR spectroscopy evaluates tissue metabolite concentrations by measuring the signal of MR spectrum with different frequencies within a specific voxel set in the target tissue. Limitations include low signal-to-noise ratio and prolonged acquisition time. In the head and neck, single voxel technique is more commonly used compared with multivoxel technique. Volume of interest selection in the head and neck is challenging because of small target lesion size and complex anatomy. Squamous cell carcinoma of the head and neck has been shown to have distinct MR spectroscopy spectra compared with surrounding normal soft tissues, specifically demonstrating increased choline/creatine ratio, with the caveat that benign neoplasms, such as paragangliomas and schwannomas, can also demonstrate this finding.[35]

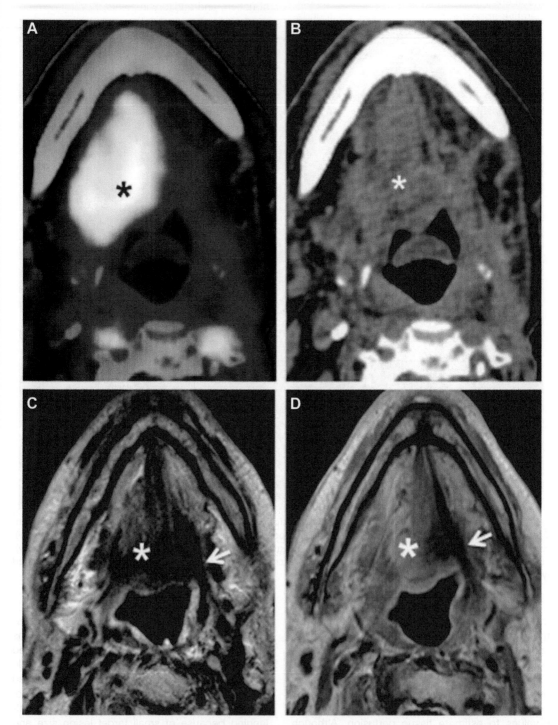

Fig. 12. Abnormal elevated 18F-FDG is seen at the right tongue (*asterisk*), caused by compensatory activity and hypertrophy secondary to postsurgical atrophy of the left tongue, as indicated by white arrow (*A*), with no corresponding lesion seen on axial noncontrast CT (*B*), axial T2-weighted (*C*), or contrast-enhanced T2-weighted (*D*) images. (*From* Purohit, B. S., Ailianou, A., Dulguerov, N., Becker, C. D., Ratib, O., & Becker, M. (2014). FDG-PET/CT pitfalls in oncological head and neck imaging. *Insights into imaging*, 5(5), 585-602; with permission).

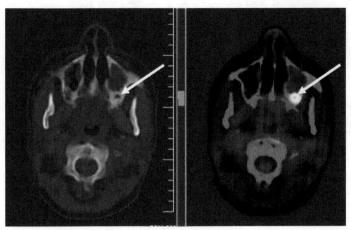

Fig. 13. A 61-year-old woman with past history of gingival hyperplasia and oral cavity dysplasia who presents in follow-up for right T2N0 p16-base of tongue SCC carcinoma in situ of the soft palate status post 70-Gy radiation treatment. Post-treatment increased abnormal metabolic activity in the left maxilla is related to dental abscess (*arrow*) and not recurrence associated with the soft palate lesion.

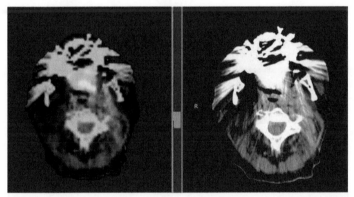

Fig. 14. A 71-year-old man with SCC of the base of tongue, status post nine cycles of treatment with pembroli-zumab and known residual lesion on physical examination. Note how extensive streak artifact precludes evalu-ation of the base of tongue.

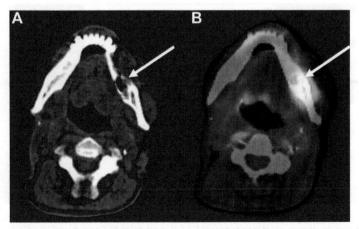

Fig. 15. Osteoradionecrosis seen as fragmentation and erosion of the left mandible on axial imaging (*A*, *B*, *arrows*) demonstrated elevated 18F-FDG activity.

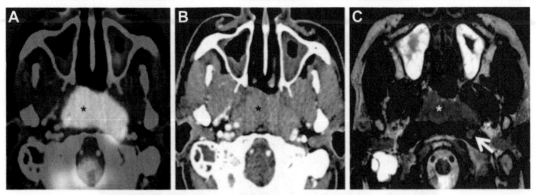

Fig. 16. Elevated 18F-FDG activity of large nasopharyngeal mass (*asterisk*) in axial PET/CT (*A*), axial contrast-enhanced CT (*B*), and axial contrast-enhanced T1-weighted (*C*) obscures a left retropharyngeal lymph node (*C, arrow*). (*From* Purohit, B. S., Ailianou, A., Dulguerov, N., Becker, C. D., Ratib, O., & Becker, M. (2014). FDG-PET/CT pitfalls in oncological head and neck imaging. *Insights into imaging*, 5(5), 585-602; with permission).

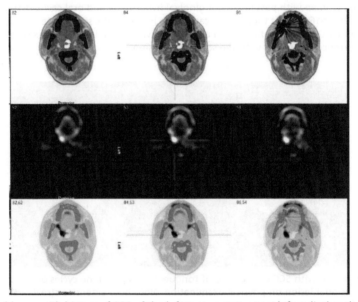

Fig. 17. A 53-year-old man with history of SCC of the left tongue status post left radical neck dissection and tonsillectomy presents with elevated 18F-FDG activity on the right tongue base (*cross-reference lines*) caused by normal tissue remnant as compared with the left.

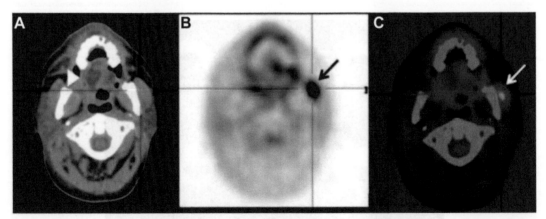

Fig. 18. Altered mechanics postsurgery can result in asymmetric metabolic activity of muscles of mastication. Localization to masseter muscle in axial noncontrast CT (*A*), and axial PET and fused PET/CT (*B, C*), the latter localizing the 18F-FDG activity to the left masseter muscle after right jaw surgery. (*From* Purandare, N. C., Puranik, A. D., Shah, S., Agrawal, A., & Rangarajan, V. (2014). Post-treatment appearances, pitfalls, and patterns of failure in head and neck cancer on FDG PET/CT imaging. Indian journal of nuclear medicine: IJNM: the official journal of the Society of Nuclear Medicine, India, 29(3), 151; with permission).

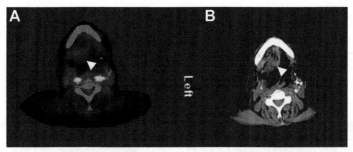

Fig. 19. A 68-year-old woman with T4N2c transglottic SCC status post near-total glossectomy presents for follow-up PET/CT. Axial fused PET/CT (*A*) and axial noncontrast CT (*B*) show the flap reconstruction demonstrating mild increased 18F-FDG activity (*arrowhead*).

POSTSURGICAL IMAGING FDG-PET/computed TOMOGRAPHY FINDINGS

Although PET/CT is the workhorse of post-treatment evaluation, it has diagnostic multiple pitfalls. First of all, it requires waiting 2 to 3 months to avoid FP results.[10,27,36] PET/CT studies performed 3 months after completion of treatment have moderately higher diagnostic accuracy on meta-regression analysis as compared with those performed before that time frame.[5]

Although PET/CT in the postoperative setting has been reported to have high NPV, it has a high rate of FPs that can result in incorrect diagnosis of recurrent tumor.[37] An intimate understanding of expected appearance of multiple surgical procedures is key to decrease the number of FP results during standard of care PET/CT imaging. These surgical procedures are evaluated in detail elsewhere in this issue. Next is a pictorial case-based review of some of these pitfalls.

Case 1: Denervation Change

PITFALL: Post-treatment denervation and atrophy can result in pseudomass on the contralateral side, which can give a FP result (**Fig. 12**).[14]

Case 2: Post-Treatment Ulceration/Abscess

PITFALL: Ulceration/abscess: Post-treatment ulceration and abscess (**Fig. 13**) can result in FP elevated 18F-FDG activity.[13,36]

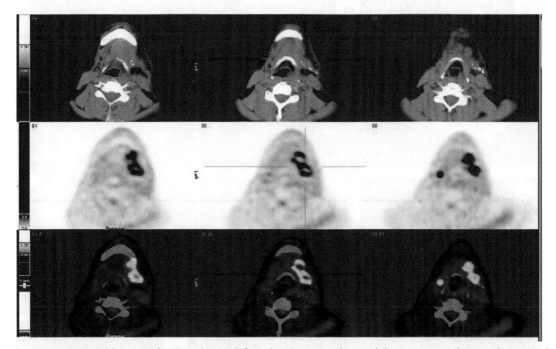

Fig. 20. A 45-year-old man with original T3N0 left oral cavity tumor has nodular recurrence deep to the surgical flap (*cross-reference lines*) demonstrating abnormal elevated 1 8F-FDG activity, compatible with recurrence.

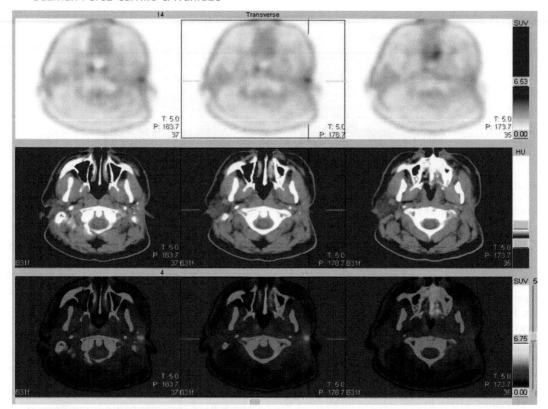

Fig. 21. A 45-year-old man with left T2N0 left pleomorphic adenoma has nodular tissue at treatment bed (*cross-reference lines*) demonstrating elevated 18F-FDG activity, originally diagnosed as recurrence. Subsequent MR imaging showed elevated ADC mean and biopsy showed no evidence of recurrence, thus the original diagnosis was an FP.

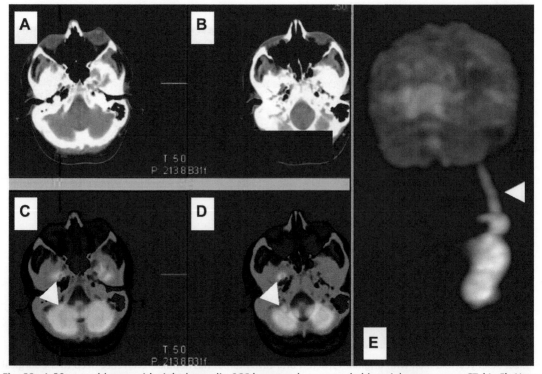

Fig. 22. A 38-year-old man with right lower lip SCC has grossly unremarkable axial noncontrast CT (*A, B*). However, axial fused 18F-FDG-PET/CT images demonstrated abnormal elevated 18F-FDG activity in the right foramen ovale (*C, D, arrowheads*), and seen as well on maximum-intensity projection PET image (*E, arrowhead*).

Case 3: Streak Artifact From Metallic Implants

PITFALL: Extensive streaking caused by metallic artifact, which results in FN results from obscuration of an underlying lesion (**Fig. 14**).[14]

Case 4: Osteoradionecrosis/Osteomyelitis

PITFALL: Post-treatment osteonecrosis/osteomyelitis can have elevated 18F-FDG activity and be misdiagnosed as recurrent tumor, a FP result (**Fig. 15**).[13]

Case 5: Nasopharyngeal Activity

PITFALL: Retropharyngeal lymph nodes affect the TNM staging and thus treatment. Especially in large nasopharyngeal masses with significant activity, these can be missed (**Fig. 16**).[13] This is also a blind spot for the surgeon, and they need to be aware of this finding ahead of time.

PEARL: Always make searching for retropharyngeal lymph nodes part of your search pattern, even if the PET is negative.

Case 6: Surgical Distortion

PITFALL: Normal FDG uptake in remnants of normal anatomy within distorted anatomy caused by surgical changes can be mistaken as recurrent tumor, a FP result (**Fig. 17**).[13,14]

Case 7: Altered Mechanics

PITFALL: Altered mechanics postsurgery can result in asymmetric metabolic activity of muscles of mastication caused by overcompensation (**Fig. 18**).[13]

Case 8: Surgical Flaps

PITFALL: Surgical flaps can have elevated 18F-FDG activity, which can be mistaken for recurrent tumor (**Fig. 19**).[38]

PEARL: Nodular more intense regions of FDG uptake deep to the flap are more consistent with tumor recurrence (**Fig. 20**).

Case 9: Post-treatment Inflammatory Changes

PITFALL: Inflammatory changes post-treatment can result in FP results (**Fig. 21**).[13,14]

Case 10: Perineural Spread of Disease

PEARL: Perineural spread of disease can be a blind spot on CT (**Fig. 22**), and thus careful search pattern on PET facilitates identification of this entity.[39]

FDG-PET/MR IMAGING APPLICATIONS

PET/MR allows for the combination of improved anatomic resolution and accurate localization of avid lesions in a synergistic manner. Technical aspects of MR imaging in head and neck cancer are discussed previously. There are notable clinically significant advantages of MR imaging relative to CT that PET/MR imaging can take advantage of. Thus, the presence of extracapsular spread, an important prognostic factor in head and neck cancer, can be diagnosed with MR imaging with

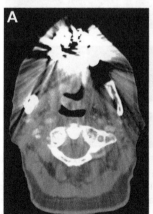
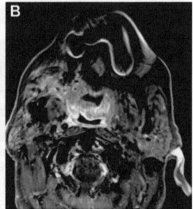
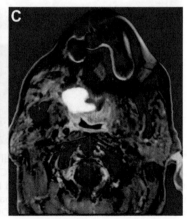

Fig. 23. Axial contrast-enhanced CT (*A*) shows streak artifact from dental amalgam limiting evaluation of the oropharynx, although there is subtle fullness of the right palatine fossa. Axial T1-weighted postcontrast fat-saturated image (*B*) obtained during FDG-PET/MR imaging acquisition shows reduction in metal artifact from dental amalgam compared with CT, allowing the asymmetric soft tissue thickening of the right palatine tonsil to be better appreciated. Fused axial FDG-PET/MR imaging with T1-weighted postcontrast fat-saturated image (*C*) shows marked FDG avidity in the area of masslike thickening of the right palatine tonsil, compatible with recurrent squamous cell carcinoma. (*From* Ryan JL, Aaron VD, Sims JB. PET/MR imaging vs PET/CT in Head and Neck Imaging: When, Why, and How? Semin Ultrasound CT MR. 2019;40(5):376-390; with permission).

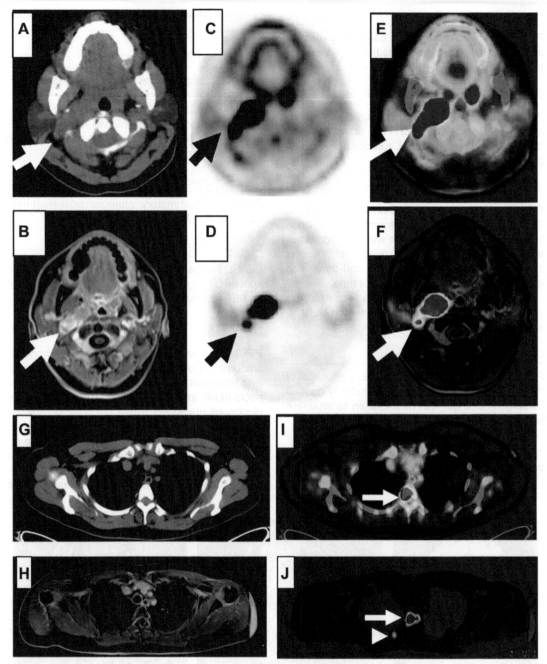

Fig. 24. Axial noncontrast CT (*A*), axial T1-weighted postcontrast (*B*), axial 18F-FDG-PET (*C*), axial 68Ga-DOTA-TATE-PET (*D*), axial fused 18F-FDG-PET/CT (*E*), and axial fused 68Ga-DOTATATE-PET/MR imaging (*F*). Axial noncontrast CT at the T4 level (*G*), axial fused FDG-PET/CT at the same level (*I*), axial T1-weighted postcontrast (*H*) and axial fused 68Ga-DOTATATE-PET/MR imaging (*J*) at the same level. The tumor located in the right parapharyngeal space (*arrows*) demonstrates intense FDG avidity (*C, E*) and DOTATATE avidity (*D, F*), less well delineated on axial CT noncontrast images (*A*) and axial T1-weighted postcontrast images (*B*). DOTATATE-PET in conjunction with MR imaging better resolved the two adjacent discrete lesions (*F*). In the T4 vertebral body, both FDG- and DOTATATE-PET demonstrate a circumscribed intensely avid metastasis (*arrow* in *I* and *J*); however, the increased target-to-background ratio on DOTATATE-PET allows visualization of additional small lesions, such as in the right posterior fourth rib (*arrowhead* in *J*).

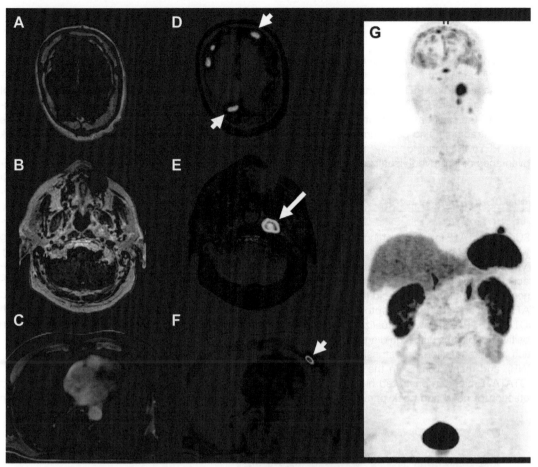

Fig. 25. Anatomic MR imaging axial T1-weighted postcontrast (*A–C*), axial fused 68Ga-DOTATATE PET/MR imaging (*D–F*), and whole-body 68Ga-DOTATATE PET maximum intensity projection image (*G*) in a patient with metastatic ENB. White arrowheads in (*D*) demonstrate dural based foci of circumscribed moderate avidity, compatible with metastases, less clearly delineated as subtle nodularity on postcontrast T1 imaging (*A*). A nodal metastasis is also visualized in the left parapharyngeal space (*E*), again less well delineated on MR imaging alone (*B*). Whole-body 68Ga-DOTATATE PET/MR additionally demonstrated a distant rib metastasis (*F*).

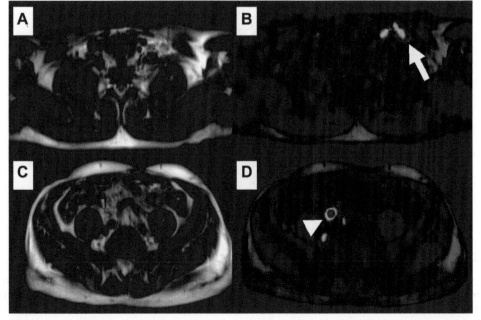

Fig. 26. Axial T1-weighted (*A, C*), axial fused 68Ga-PSMA (*B, D*). *Arrow* in *B* demonstrates prostate metastatic lesions in the left supraclavicular region that were not well seen on anatomic images in *A*. More tumor burden on the right iliac chain demonstrates similar 68Ga-PSMA uptake (*arrowhead* in *D*).

higher sensitivity compared with CT.[40] In patients with significant dental artifact, CT is of limited diagnostic utility, and PET/MR imaging thus holds an advantage over PET/CT (Fig. 23).[41] In cases of invasion of the skull base or orbits and in assessment of intracranial and perineural spread of disease, PET/MR imaging may provide distinct advantages of improved visualization.[42,43]

Non-FDG-PET Radiotracers

68Ga-DOTATATE

68Ga-DOTATATE is a radioconjugate consisting of the somatostatin analogue tyrosine-3-octreotate (Tyr3-octreotate or TATE) labeled with the PET tracer Gallium (68Ga) via the macrocyclic chelating agent dodecanetetraacetic acid (DOTA).[44] DOTATATE binds somatostatin receptor (SSTR) 2a, and DOTATATE PET allows visualization of SSTR-positive neoplasms with high diagnostic accuracy, such as paragangliomas, esthesioneuroblastoma (ENB), and meningiomas. In the head and neck, DOTATATE has demonstrated high sensitivity for detection of head and neck paragangliomas and

has proven to be particularly useful in the identification of additional lesions not identified with CT or MR imaging alone, in the confirmation of recurrent disease, and in the delineation of contiguous DOTATATE avidity throughout the entire course of large but poorly defined head and neck paragangliomas (Fig. 24).

ENB is a rare sinonasal neuroectodermal malignancy with favorable 5-year survival; however, it has a propensity for delayed locoregional recurrence. Current treatment options include resection, adjuvant radiotherapy, and/or chemotherapy; however, because of its rarity and location, determining the optimal treatment for ENB has been challenging. Because ENB expresses high levels of SSTR2A, imaging with DOTATATE PET/CT and PET/MR imaging has been found to have clinical utility, and peptide receptor radionuclide therapy (PRRT) with Lu177-DOTATATE is a promising treatment option in patients with metastatic ENB (Fig. 25).

68Ga-PSMA

68Ga-PSMA PET/MR imaging has demonstrated high diagnostic accuracy and prognostic value in

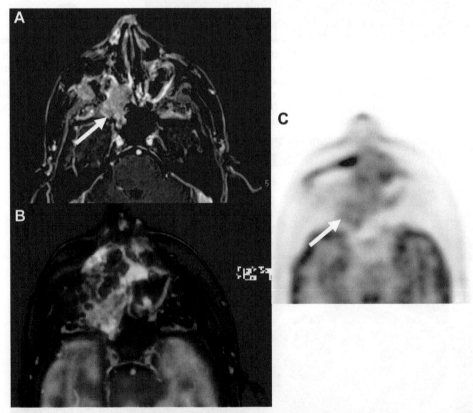

Fig. 27. Axial T1-weighted RPRT postcontrast (A), axial fused 18F-FDG-PET/MR imaging (B), and axial 18F-FDG PET (C). Arrow demonstrates mass-like enhancement centered at the right pterygopalatine fossa (A). Although anatomically this would be concerning for tumor recurrence, the lesion demonstrates no increased FDG activity (B, C).

prostate cancer and is on track to be Food and Drug Administration approved for clinical use in the near future. Although cervical nodal metastases in prostate cancer are uncommon, they do occur, and whole-body PET/MR imaging performed for clinical follow-up purposes allows identification of such metastases with higher sensitivity and specificity compared with CT or MR imaging alone (**Fig. 26**).

18F-Fluoromisonidazole

Hypoxia is an established poor prognostic factor in various solid tumors. In head and neck cancer, a meta-analysis demonstrated that assessment of hypoxia for targeting of radiotherapy improves.[45] 18F-Fluoromisonidazole allows hypoxia imaging with high reproducibility. Dynamic fluoromisonidazole PET allows pharmacokinetic modeling that produces a biomarker reflecting hypoxia more

directly and additionally providing information on perfusion, and allowing a more comprehensive assessment of radiation treatment response.[46]

Case Study Presentation

Case 1: post-treatment fibrosis
PITFALL: Post-treatment change of fibrosis can be masslike and demonstrate enhancement. PET/MR imaging might provide better anatomic delineation of the post-treatment change and physiologic information to help differentiate it from tumor recurrence (**Fig. 27**).

Case 2: perineural spread of disease
PEARL: The MR imaging portion of PET/MR imaging better delineates perineural spread of disease, which could be missed or mischaracterized on PET/CT (**Fig. 28**).

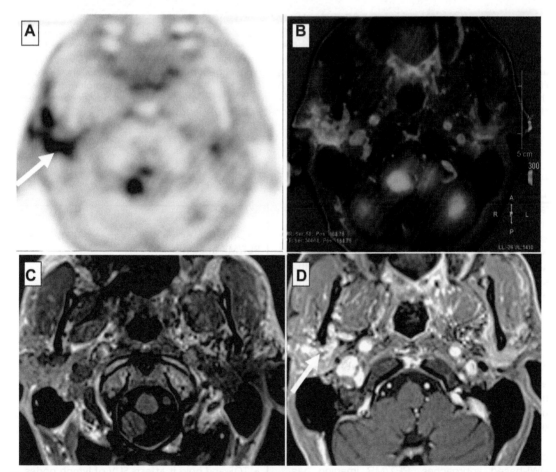

Fig. 28. Axial 18F-FDG-PET (*A*), axial fused 18F-FDG-PET/MR imaging (*B*), axial T1-weighted precontrast (*C*), and axial T1-weighted postcontrast (*D*). Although demonstrating increased FDG activity (*A*, *arrow*), the anatomic region of involvement (ie, the perineural spread) is best delineated in the MR image. The *arrow* demonstrates cordlike enhancement of the right auriculotemporal nerve (*D*), compatible with perineural spread of disease. The perineural spread was missed on original PET-CT study. (*Case courtesy of* Prashant Raghavan).

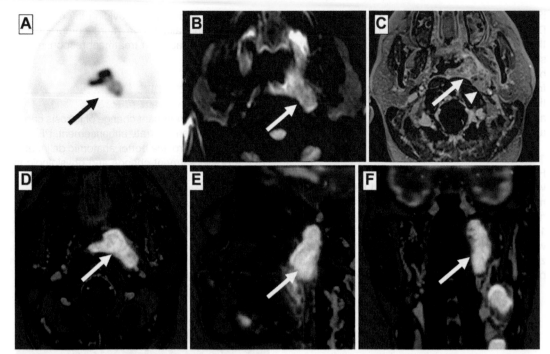

Fig. 29. Axial 18F-FDG-PET (*A*), axial DWI (*B*), axial T1-weighted postcontrast (*C*), and fused 18F-FDG-PET/MR imaging in axial (*D*), sagittal (*E*), and coronal (*F*). Left nasopharyngeal mass demonstrates abnormal increased 18F-FDG activity (*arrow* in *A*), and restricted diffusion (*B*). Anatomic MR image (*C*) allows the radiologist to realize there are two distinct masses, a nasopharyngeal mass (*arrow*), and a retropharyngeal lymph node (*arrowhead*). Notice how the lesions blend into each other on the fused PET/CT (*D–F, arrows*).

Case 3: nasopharyngeal activity
PITFALL: Retropharyngeal lymph nodes affect the TNM staging and thus treatment. Especially in large nasopharyngeal masses with significant activity, these can be missed.[13] MR imaging offers superior soft tissue differentiation as compared with CT[42] and can more easily delineate distinct lesions (**Fig. 29**). This area is also a blind spot for the surgeon, and they need to be aware of this finding ahead of time.

SUMMARY

Although PET/CT is a very sensitive tool in the evaluation of recurrence of the post-treatment neck, the radiologist must be aware of pitfalls and limitations of PET/CT to avoid FP and FN diagnosis.

PET/MR imaging allows advanced MR imaging evaluation of head and neck neoplasms including DWI-based approaches. PET/MR imaging has promising applications, both with FDG and with emerging radiotracers targeting other biologic mechanisms, such as DOTATATE, PSMA, and fluoromisonidazole.

CLINICS CARE POINTS

Potential traps in post-treatment PET/CT and PET/MR imaging

- Post-treatment inflammatory changes
- Denervation or atrophy of the treated side, with resulting hypertrophy of normal tissue on the contralateral side
- Post-treatment complication of ulceration or abscess
- Streak artifact from metallic structures, such as clips or fixation devices
- Obscuration of retropharyngeal lymph nodes
- Remnants of normal tissue in the surgical bed
- Altered motion mechanics postsurgery
- Reconstruction flaps
- TOF and how it affects SUV of lymph nodes

Pearls in post-treatment PET/CT and PET/MR imaging

- BAT activation increased in certain cases

- SUVmax ratio to evaluate asymmetric tonsillar activity
- QIBA protocols to optimize and standardize imaging
- Use narrow windows or use dual-energy CT to increase tissue contrast
- Evaluate perineural spread of disease on maximum intensity projection PET

DISCLOSURE

G.J. Guzmán Pérez-Carrillo: Consultant for Medtronic. J. Ivanidze: Principal investigator, investigator-initiated clinical trial research grant funded by Novartis Pharmaceuticals, NCT04081701, DOTATATE PET/MRI in SSTR2-positive CNS neoplasms (DOMINO-START).

REFERENCES

1. Jemal A, Siegel R, Xu J, et al. Cancer statistics, 2010. CA Cancer J Clin 2010;60(5):277–300.
2. National Cancer Institute. Head and Neck Cancer – Health Professional Version. Available at: https://www. cancer.gov/types/head-and-neck/hp. Accessed November 19, 2020.
3. Fukui MB, Blodgett TM, Snyderman CH, et al. Combined PET-CT in the head and neck: part 2. Diagnostic uses and pitfalls of oncologic imaging. Radiographics 2005;25(4):913–30.
4. Taghipour M, Sheikhbahaei S, Wray R, et al. FDG PET/CT in patients with head and neck squamous cell carcinoma after primary surgical resection with or without chemoradiation therapy. AJR Am J Roentgenol 2016;206(5):1093–100.
5. Gupta T, Master Z, Kannan S, et al. Diagnostic performance of post-treatment FDG PET or FDG PET/CT imaging in head and neck cancer: a systematic review and meta-analysis. Eur J Nucl Med Mol Imaging 2011;38(11):2083–95.
6. Park J, Pak K, Yun TJ, et al. Diagnostic accuracy and confidence of [18F] FDG PET/MRI in comparison with PET or MRI alone in head and neck cancer. Sci Rep 2020;10(1):9490.
7. Liu G, Cao T, Hu L, et al. Validation of MR-based attenuation correction of a newly released whole-body simultaneous PET/MR system. Biomed Res Int 2019;2019:8213215.
8. Rausch I, Quick HH, Cal-Gonzalez J, et al. Technical and instrumentational foundations of PET/MRI. Eur J Radiol 2017;94:A3–13.
9. Nuyts J, Dupont P, Stroobants S, et al. Simultaneous maximum a posteriori reconstruction of attenuation and activity distributions from emission sinograms. IEEE Trans Med Imaging 1999;18(5): 393–403.
10. Sheikhbahaei S, Marcus C, Subramaniam RM. 18F FDG PET/CT and head and neck cancer: patient management and outcomes. PET Clin 2015;10(2): 125–45.
11. Subramaniam RM, Truong M, Peller P, et al. Fluorodeoxyglucose-positron-emission tomography imaging of head and neck squamous cell cancer. AJNR Am J Neuroradiol 2010;31(4):598–604.
12. Tantiwongkosi B, Yu F, Kanard A, et al. Role of (18)F-FDG PET/CT in pre and post treatment evaluation in head and neck carcinoma. World J Radiol 2014; 6(5):177–91.
13. Purandare NC, Puranik AD, Shah S, et al. Post-treatment appearances, pitfalls, and patterns of failure in head and neck cancer on FDG PET/CT imaging. Indian J Nucl Med 2014;29(3):151–7.
14. Purohit BS, Ailianou A, Dulguerov N, et al. FDG-PET/CT pitfalls in oncological head and neck imaging. Insights Imaging 2014;5(5):585–602.
15. Pencharz D, Dunn J, Connor S, et al. Palatine tonsil SUVmax on FDG PET-CT as a discriminator between benign and malignant tonsils in patients with and without head and neck squamous cell carcinoma of unknown primary. Clin Radiol 2019;74(2):165 e117–23.
16. Steinberg JD, Vogel W, Vegt E. Factors influencing brown fat activation in FDG PET/CT: a retrospective analysis of 15,000+ cases. Br J Radiol 2017; 90(1075):20170093.
17. Ogawa Y, Abe K, Sakoda A, et al. FDG-PET and CT findings of activated brown adipose tissue in a patient with paraganglioma. Eur J Radiol Open 2018; 5:126–30.
18. Yao M. PET imaging of the head and neck, an issue of PET Clinics, vol. 7–4. Philadelphia: Elsevier Health Sciences; 2012.
19. Maghami E, Ismaila N, Alvarez A, et al. Diagnosis and management of squamous cell carcinoma of unknown primary in the head and neck: ASCO guideline. J Clin Oncol 2020;38(22):2570–96.
20. QIBA Profile. FDG-PET/CT as an imaging biomarker measuring response to cancer therapy. Radiological Society of North America (RSNA); 2016. Available at: http://qibawiki.rsna.org/images/1/1f/QIBA_FDG-PET_Profile_v113.pdf. Accessed November 19, 2020.
21. Akamatsu G, Mitsumoto K, Taniguchi T, et al. Influences of point-spread function and time-of-flight reconstructions on standardized uptake value of lymph node metastases in FDG-PET. Eur J Radiol 2014;83(1):226–30.
22. Wright CL, Washington IR, Bhatt AD, et al. Emerging opportunities for digital PET/CT to advance locoregional therapy in head and neck cancer. Semin Radiat Oncol 2019;29(2):93–101.

23. Van den Wyngaert T, De Schepper S, Carp L. Quality assessment in FDG-PET/CT imaging of head-and-neck cancer: one home run is better than two doubles. Front Oncol 2020;10:1458.

24. Antoch G, Freudenberg LS, Beyer T, et al. To enhance or not to enhance? 18F-FDG and CT contrast agents in dual-modality 18F-FDG PET/CT. J Nucl Med 2004;45(Suppl 1):56S–65S.

25. Juliano AF, Aiken AH. NI-RADS for head and neck cancer surveillance imaging: what, why, and how. Cancer Cytopathol 2020;128(3):166–70.

26. Aiken AH, Rath TJ, Anzai Y, et al. ACR neck imaging reporting and data systems (NI-RADS): a white paper of the ACR NI-RADS committee. J Am Coll Radiol 2018;15(8):1097–108.

27. Colevas AD, Yom SS, Pfister DG, et al. NCCN Guidelines insights: head and neck cancers, version 1.2018. J Natl Compr Canc Netw 2018;16(5):479–90.

28. Beyer T, Lassen ML, Boellaard R, et al. Investigating the state-of-the-art in whole-body MR-based attenuation correction: an intra-individual, inter-system, inventory study on three clinical PET/MR systems. MAGMA 2016;29(1):75–87.

29. Boellaard R, Quick HH. Current image acquisition options in PET/MR. Semin Nucl Med 2015;45(3):192–200.

30. Srinivasan A, Dvorak R, Perni K, et al. Differentiation of benign and malignant pathology in the head and neck using 3T apparent diffusion coefficient values: early experience. AJNR Am J Neuroradiol 2008;29(1):40–4.

31. Hagmann P, Jonasson L, Maeder P, et al. Understanding diffusion MR imaging techniques: from scalar diffusion-weighted imaging to diffusion tensor imaging and beyond. Radiographics 2006;26(Suppl 1):S205–23.

32. Abdel Razek AAK. Diffusion tensor imaging in differentiation of residual head and neck squamous cell carcinoma from post-radiation changes. Magn Reson Imaging 2018;54:84–9.

33. Guo W, Luo D, Lin M, et al. Pretreatment intra-voxel incoherent motion diffusion-weighted imaging (IVIM-DWI) in predicting induction chemotherapy response in locally advanced hypopharyngeal carcinoma. Medicine (Baltimore) 2016;95(10):e3039.

34. Paudyal R, Oh JH, Riaz N, et al. Intravoxel incoherent motion diffusion-weighted MRI during chemoradiation therapy to characterize and monitor treatment response in human papillomavirus head and neck squamous cell carcinoma. J Magn Reson Imaging 2017;45(4):1013–23.

35. King AD, Yeung DK, Ahuja AT, et al. Salivary gland tumors at in vivo proton MR spectroscopy. Radiology 2005;237(2):563–9.

36. Schoder H, Fury M, Lee N, et al. PET monitoring of therapy response in head and neck squamous cell carcinoma. J Nucl Med 2009;50(Suppl 1):74S–88S.

37. Cheung MK, Ong SY, Goyal U, et al. False positive positron emission tomography/computed tomography scans in treated head and neck cancers. Cureus 2017;9(4):e1146.

38. Escott EJ. Role of positron emission tomography/computed tomography (PET/CT) in head and neck cancer. Radiol Clin North Am 2013;51(5):881–93.

39. Larson CR, Wiggins RH. FDG-PET imaging of salivary gland tumors. Semin Ultrasound CT MR 2019;40(5):391–9.

40. Su Z, Duan Z, Pan W, et al. Predicting extracapsular spread of head and neck cancers using different imaging techniques: a systematic review and meta-analysis. Int J Oral Maxillofac Surg 2016;45(4):413–21.

41. Ryan JL, Aaron VD, Sims JB. PET/MRI vs PET/CT in head and neck imaging: when, why, and how? Semin Ultrasound CT MR 2019;40(5):376–90.

42. Xiao Y, Chen Y, Shi Y, et al. The value of fluorine-18 fluorodeoxyglucose PET/MRI in the diagnosis of head and neck carcinoma: a meta-analysis. Nucl Med Commun 2015;36(4):312–8.

43. Schaarschmidt BM, Heusch P, Buchbender C, et al. Locoregional tumour evaluation of squamous cell carcinoma in the head and neck area: a comparison between MRI, PET/CT and integrated PET/MRI. Eur J Nucl Med Mol Imaging 2016;43(1):92–102.

44. Ivanidze J, Roytman M, Sasson A, et al. Molecular imaging and therapy of somatostatin receptor positive tumors. Clin Imaging 2019;56:146–54.

45. Horsman MR, Mortensen LS, Petersen JB, et al. Imaging hypoxia to improve radiotherapy outcome. Nat Rev Clin Oncol 2012;9(12):674–87.

46. Grkovski M, Lee NY, Schoder H, et al. Monitoring early response to chemoradiotherapy with (18)F-FMISO dynamic PET in head and neck cancer. Eur J Nucl Med Mol Imaging 2017;44(10):1682–91.

Advanced CT and MR Imaging of the Posttreatment Head and Neck

Remy Lobo, MD[a], Sevcan Turk, MD[a], J. Rajiv Bapuraj, MD[b],
Ashok Srinivasan, MD[b],*

KEYWORDS

- Head and neck cancer - Imaging surveillance - MRI - CT - Diffusion imaging - Perfusion imaging
- Dual-energy CT

KEY POINTS

- Posttreatment morphologic alterations cause a significant change in the morphology and function of head and neck structures.
- Advanced magnetic resonance imaging (MRI) and computed tomography (CT) techniques have increased the accuracy in the detection of residual and recurrent lesions.
- Advanced techniques need to be tailored for the locoregional assessment of the head and neck.
- A summary review of these techniques is presented with highlights of the recent studies on the advances in imaging techniques in evaluating posttreatment sequela.

INTRODUCTION

Anatomic localization and preoperative functional assessment are the 2 important foundations for successful outcomes in the treatment of head and neck cancers. Given the complexity of the soft tissues including the vascular, neural, and lymphoid structures, the aim of the successful management of these cancers involves the transspatial excision of one or more groups of these structures followed by a combination of radiotherapy, chemotherapy, or both.[1] Excision of the soft tissue structures often entails reconstruction using transposed, interposed material, or free flaps. Each of the other above-mentioned therapeutic interventions causes profound changes in the anatomy of the region. These morphologic alterations can obscure tumor recurrence. Advanced computed tomography (CT) and magnetic resonance imaging (MRI) techniques have, therefore, been developed to assess for posttreatment sequela and to assess for residual and recurrent disease (Tables 1 and 2). Advances in both CT and MRI techniques form the basis of the initial assessment of the patients undergoing treatment for head and neck malignancies.

ANATOMIC CONSIDERATIONS

Squamous cell carcinomas are the most common malignancies encountered in the head and neck. Management of these cancers in the nasopharynx, oropharynx, hypopharynx, and larynx is often multimodality-based. Lesions in the sinonasal region and the oral cavities are primarily surgically excised and treated by adjuvant radiation or chemotherapy.[2] Additionally, surgical treatment involves the removal of draining lymph nodes. Nodal metastases occur along the expected regional drainage pathways and a thorough knowledge of these locations is helpful in managing these patients.[3]Nodal anatomy and the lymphatic pathways are nearly always distorted following surgery and radiotherapy, and this may result in

[a] Neuroradiology Division, Radiology, Michigan Medicine, 1500 E Medical Center Drive, Ann Arbor, MI 48109, USA; [b] Neuroradiology Division, Radiology, Michigan Medicine, 1500 E Medical Center Drive, B2A209, Ann Arbor, MI 48109, USA
* Corresponding author.
E-mail address: ashoks@med.umich.edu

neuroimaging.theclinics.com

Table 1
Sample scan parameters for CT perfusion from the authors' institution

Scan Type	Helical Noncontrast CT
Gantry Rotation Time/Length	0.8s Full
Detector Coverage	40 mm
Slice Thickness	2.5 mm
Interval	2.5 mm
Speed	20.62
Pitch	0.516:1
KVP	120
mA	80
DVOV	18

Scan Type	Cine – CT Perfusion
HiRes Mode	Off
Gantry Rot Time/Length	1.0s Full
Detector Coverage	40 mm
Slice Thickness	5 mm
# of Images/Rotation	8i
Cine Time b/w Images	1.0s
Scan Duration	50s
Interval	0
KVP/mA	120/65
DFOV	25
Delay	5s

Perfusion is conducted with 50 mL of Isovue 300 (iopamidol, Bracco) injected at 4 mL/s with 20 mL of normal saline 4 mL/s to follow. A routine postcontrast neck is acquired after the perfusion study with an additional 75 mL injected at 2 mL/s because we use a split bolus technique at our institution.
Abbreviation: CT, Computed tomography.

challenges in locating metastases that may not correspond to the lymphatic drainage territories of the resected tumor.[4]

CT and MRI remain the mainstay in the primary diagnosis of head and neck cancers. Multidetector CT and MRI with conventional sequences have been used for the initial preoperative staging of both the primary tumor and the nodal anatomy. Modification to the conventional techniques for the regional assessment of malignancies has been described.[4–6]

Surgical interventions can be broadly classified into neck dissection for lymph nodes, reconstructions of the postsurgical defects using, or a combination of both procedures. Surgical procedures can be followed by radiation treatment or radiation treatment may be the sole method of treatment, as in the case of early laryngeal carcinomas.

There are many types of neck dissection including radical, modified radical, selective, and extended radical neck dissections that involve either the removal or sparing of multiple normal adjacent structures such as the ipsilateral sternocleidomastoid muscle, spinal accessory nerve, and internal jugular vein.[7] A detailed description of these types is beyond the scope of this article and has been dealt with in another article in this issue.

Radiation therapy induces significant morphologic and histopathological alterations of the cutaneous, subcutaneous, muscular, and glandular structures of the neck, which ranges from early edematous changes and later fibrotic sequelae giving the neck the characteristic woody feel on palpation.[8] Changes following radiation therapy are most pronounced during the first few months after the end of radiation treatment and are visualized on both CT and MRI. They include the reticulation of the subcutaneous fat and deep fat planes, with the thickened appearance of the skin and platysma muscle. Enhancement and thickening of the pharyngeal walls and edema in the retropharyngeal space together with increased enhancement of the major salivary glands can also be observed. Later sequela includes atrophy of the salivary glands (postirradiation sialadenitis) and atrophy of the lymphatic tissues.[9] Surgical reconstruction of the postsurgical defects involves the placement of flaps composed of skin, subcutaneous fat, fascia, with or without muscle; and usually a vascular pedicle.[10] Detailed descriptions of the complications of chemoradiation and the imaging appearances of different types of flaps and their contents are presented in a different article in this issue.

PATHOLOGY AND ADVANCED IMAGING TECHNIQUES
Magnetic Resonance Diffusion

MR diffusion sequences have been designed to measure the Brownian motion of water molecules in tissues exposed to strong uniform magnetic fields. The random motion of water molecules in tissues is impeded when they encounter cell membranes, cellular organelles, and nerve fibers. Similarly, increased cellularity and cytotoxic edema associated with tumors hinder the motion of water molecules. Quantification of diffusion is performed by inbuilt software algorithms and the resulting value is termed as apparent diffusion coefficient (ADC), which is expressed in millimeters squared per second. Values for solid tumors in the head and neck vary depending on the cell type.

Table 2
Sample DCE perfusion MRI technique from the authors' institution

Vendor Neutral Parameter	Sample 3T Value
Coil	At least 16 channel
Parallel Imaging	On
Sequence	3D T1 weighted
TR/TE	4.91/1.91
Flip Angle	12 degrees
Slice Thickness	4.0 mm
Slices Per Slab	36
Field of View	230 mm
Temporal Resolution	8.85s
Number of Sections/Scan	40
Total Scan Time	6:07 min

We use 20 mL of MultiHance (gadobenate dimeglumine, Bracco) injected at 4 mL/s followed by 20 mL of saline at 4 mL/s.

Abbreviations: DCE, dynamic contrast-enhanced; MRI, magnetic resonance imaging.

Malignant lesions have a lower value than benign tumors and lymphomas have a lower value than carcinomas.[11] ADCs values for lymphomas are reported to be between 0.5 and 0.9 $\times$ 10^{-3} mm^2/s, for thyroid cancers they are higher at 1.3 to 3 x10^{-3} mm^2/s, and for squamous cell carcinomas they have an intermediate value of 0.6 to 1.5 $\times$ 10^{-3} mm^2/s with a mean of 0.9 to 1.2 $\times$ 10^{-3} mm^2/s. Poorly differentiated squamous cell carcinomas have lower values than well-differentiated carcinomas.[12] Lower ADC values have been attributed to hypercellularity, hyperchromatism, and a higher nuclear-to-cytoplasm ratio. The limitation of routine use of ADC values lies with the images being often motion degraded by breathing and swallowing, and due to single-shot EPI sequences which are frequently used for the acquisition of these sequences. A workaround for greater fidelity of the calculation of ADC values is to use multiexponential models with several B-values, with higher b values of 800–1000 s/mm^2 being more suitable for the accurate assessment of these parameters.[12]

Detection of larger metastatic lymphadenopathy is more easily accomplished by conventional CT or MRI; however, diffusion imaging can help in determining metastatic lymphadenopathy in subcentimeter nodes (less than 10 mm in diameter). This may have important implications while evaluating the postirradiated neck whereby small metastatic nodes may be impalpable. For the detection of impalpable metastatic nodes, a study has revealed an ADC threshold of 1.0 $\times$ 10^{-3} mm^2/s

leading to a high sensitivity of 92.3% and a specificity of 83.9% as a discriminator of benign and metastatic nodes.[13]

Differentiation of recurrent and residual tumors from posttreatment sequelae can be made with reasonable accuracy by diffusion imaging. Morphologic distortions following surgery and radiation therapy with and without chemotherapy may result in extensive fibrosis and scarring on follow-up. Biopsies in these treated areas for the suspicion of tumor recurrence often result in equivocal results.[14] Repeat surgical intervention may induce further radiation necrosis. Continued surveillance is, therefore, key in the assessment of recurrence which most frequently occurs at the site of the primary lesion. Diffusion-weighted imaging was noted to help in the differentiation of chronic postradiation sequelae and recurrence based on the ADC measurements in this situation. Changes in the ADC values were seen early and late in the posttreatment course with a high sensitivity of 94.6% and specificity of 95.9%.[15] Recurrent lesions characteristically appear as low-intensity areas on ADC maps than posttreatment scarring which tends to show higher signal intensities.[16] The predictive value of ADC maps in the postoperative assessment for head and neck squamous cell carcinoma recurrence was studied by Brenet and colleagues.[17] The authors compared ADC values in patients up to 8 days before the commencement of chemotherapy and 3 months after the completion of chemotherapy. In a univariate analysis, the initial ADC values were significantly lower in patients presenting with residual tumors (0.56 $\pm$ 0.11 vs 0.79 $\pm$ 0.13; P<.001). In disease-free individuals followed-up for additional 12 months after chemotherapy, the only factor which was significantly correlated with disease recurrence was the relative change in the ADC values.[17] Studies by Kim and colleagues,[18] however, showed that ADC values initially were lower (1.04 $\pm$ 0.19 $\times$ 10^{-3} mm^2/s) in patients who responded favorably to chemoradiation than in partial responders (1.35 $\pm$ 0.30 $\times$ 10^{-3} mm^2/s). They also found a significant increase in the ADC values in tumors which showed complete response as early as 1 week after the commencement of the treatment. In another study by Vandecaveye and colleagues,[19] the authors compared the ADC values before and after the treatment, and concluded that the change in ADC values before and after treatment.

(Δ ADC) for recurrent tumors was significantly lower than those who showed complete remission for the primary lesion (−2.3% $\pm$ 0.3% than 80% $\pm$ 41%; P = .0001). These studies underline the importance of DWI in both the diagnosis, treatment, and follow-up of head and neck cancers. Moreover, the importance of this technique is further enhanced with assessment with conventional MRI sequences, as was shown by Tshering Vogel and colleagues[20] (Fig. 1).

Perfusion Magnetic Resonance Imaging

Perfusion MRI is less frequently performed for the assessment of head and neck malignancies. The technique is based on the concept of interrogating a steady state of delivery of blood in normal tissues that can be disturbed by either increase or decrease in the vascular supply to the bed of tissues by using exogenous paramagnetic gadolinium chelates or by endogenous magnetically labeled arterial blood water acting as a diffusible tracer. The former technique is the basis for dynamic contrast-enhanced (DCE) perfusion studies and the latter technique forms the basis of arterial spin labeling (ASL) perfusion sequence.

DCE perfusion MRI permits the semiquantitative estimation of the vascularity of tissues depending on the flow intensity curves generated and measured after the bolus administration of contrast (see Table 2). Parameters such as maximum contrast index (CI), time to reach maximum CI, maximum slope, washout slope, and area under the curve (AUC) at a specific time can be measured. Pharmacokinetic modeling enables the measurement of parameters for the transfer of the contrast between the intravascular space to the extracellular extravascular space.[21] Three of the most useful DCE parameters are Vp, Ve, and Ktrans. Vp is the volume of blood plasma, Ve is the volume of the extravascular extracellular space, and Ktrans is the rate of transfer from the blood plasma into the extravascular extracellular space. Ktrans essentially measures how leaky a system is, considering the flow, surface area, and permeability. Ktrans correlates with the wash in phase (the slope of signal gain) as gadolinium enters the tissue slab. An additional useful parameter is Kep, sometimes considered the opposite of Ktrans. Kep is the backflow leakage of material from the extravascular extracellular space into the blood plasma.

Application of DCE perfusion MRI in head and neck malignancies has been explored for the assessment of the prediction of tumor response (Fig. 2), differentiating residual or recurrent cancers from posttreatment changes (Figs. 3 and 4), and from differentiating squamous cell carcinomas from other head and neck malignancies which could influence treatment strategies.

The pathophysiological basis for DCE perfusion studies is based on the concept of tissue hypoxia resulting from impaired perfusion resulting in suboptimal response to chemotherapy. Tissue hypoxia is thought to result in disordered angiogenesis due to the upregulation of vascular endothelial growth factor (VEGF) pathways, resulting in the development of abnormal, tortuous, and leaky vessels. This abnormal vasculature, in turn, prevents the optimal delivery of chemotherapeutic agents to the tumor bed. Newbold and colleagues showed that increasing perfusion parameters such as K(trans) and V(e) were associated with decreased tissue hypoxia.[22] K(trans) values were the strongest predictors for progression-free survival and overall survival in Stage 4 patients in a series of 74 patients with head and neck squamous cell carcinomas (HNSCC) as pretreatment prognostic markers[23] (see Fig. 4). Baer and colleagues used parametric response analyses for the evaluation of volume transfer constant and AUC at 60 seconds as predictors of survival in a cohort of 10 patients with locoregional HNSCC undergoing chemotherapy. They found that the volume transfer constant was more sensitive ($P = .002$) than AUC60 ($P = .2$) in determining overall survival in their cohort of patients. They concluded that with appropriate validation their method could be useful in the prediction of survival in patients with HNSCC.[24] Furthermore, Bernstein and colleagues[25] could differentiate responders and nonresponders to induction chemotherapy based on the measurements of baseline tumor plasma flow (F(P)). The tumor plasma flow was significantly greater in responders than nonresponders in the primary tumor (53.2 vs 23.9 mL/100 mL/min; $P = .27$) echoing the fact that the increased vascularity would be key in reducing hypoxia, which in turn diminishes the efficacy of chemotherapy. In a similar vein, Ng and colleagues[26] concluded that higher Ktrans values predicted a better 2-year local control rate of the primary tumor. Agrawal and colleagues[27] also showed higher blood flow (BF) and higher blood volumes (BVs) in responders than in nonresponders (Figs. 5 and 6).

The second aspect of perfusion imaging in the evaluation of head and neck cancers concerns the detection of residual and recurrent tumors in the background of treatment-related changes. Ishiyama and colleagues[28] investigated the utility of measuring BV and the permeability surface area (PS) in postradiation benign changes and recurrent HN cancers. In a cohort of 35 cases, they found that PS areas were $2.3 \times 10^4 \pm 5.8 \times 10^4$ for the newly diagnosed cancer group, $3.3 \times 10^4 \pm 1.7 \times 10^4$ for the recurrent cancer group, and $4.8 \times 10^4 \pm 8.1 \times 10^4$ for the posttreatment benign change group ($P = .031$); thereby concluding that this perfusion parameter showed promise in

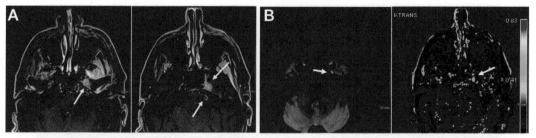

Fig. 1. (*A*) Axial T1+C FS, left image at level of foramen ovale and right image at the level of foramen rotundum and Meckel's cave, showing abnormal enhancement along left trigeminal branches and also it is a cisternal segment, features consistent with perineural tumor spread (PNTS) in this 67-year-old male with prior oral cavity SCCa. (*B*) Axial DWI in the same patient showing DWI hyperintense signal at the left foramen ovale. Ktrans also shows increased "permeability" at the left foramen ovale. Features support anatomic imaging showing PNTS.

distinguishing primary and recurrent tumors from benign treatment-related sequela. Furukawa and colleagues,[29] in their semiquantitative assessment to determine the diagnostic efficacy of time–intensity curve analysis to characterize malignant lesions from treatment-related changes, showed that malignant lesions had a significantly prolonged time to peak (TTP), lower relative maximum enhancement (RME), and relative washout (RWO) ratios than benign lesions, whereas postradiation changes demonstrated longer TTP with only lower RWO compared to recurrent lesions. Receiving operator curves (ROCs) analysis showed that RWO had the highest accuracy among the 3

parameters studied in their cohort of patients. Further refinements in technique and assessment of the use of voxel-based color maps of the initial and final AUC values derived from DCI studies were carried out by Lee JY and colleagues.[30] In their retrospective study, these authors compared the results of MR perfusion studies with initial and final AUC curves generated at 90 seconds with conventional MR sequences in 28 cases of local recurrences and 35 cases of posttreatment changes. They concluded that dynamic contrast-enhanced MR imaging significantly increased the diagnostic accuracy for detecting local recurrence (48%–54% vs 87%–91%; $P = .05$).

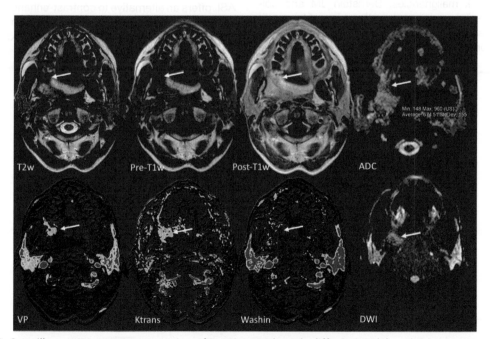

Fig. 2. Surveillance MRI, status postresection of invasive, moderately differentiated, keratinizing squamous cell carcinoma of the soft palate with negative margins. Patient declined adjuvant therapy. A T2 hypointense, T1 hypointense, enhancing area is seen in the right retromolar trigone with diffusion restriction. DCE perfusion images show increased VP and Ktrans values with minimally increased wash-in parameters. Biopsy was negative for carcinoma.

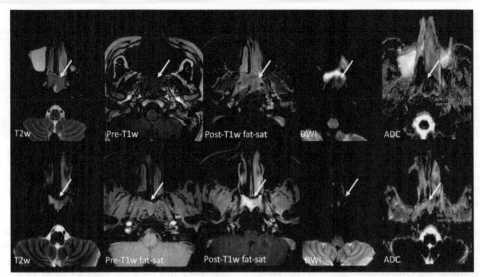

Fig. 3. EBV positive nasopharyngeal carcinoma before treatment (*arrows*, upper panel). Heterogeneous T1 and T2 isointense, enhancing mass with decreased ADC values. Effacement of fat planes between prevertebral muscles and the mass, suggestive of muscle invasion. Lower panel shows MRI images after combined chemotherapy and radiation therapy, demonstrating a decrease in mass size with increased ADC values. Interval increased T2 signal with decreased mass effect, suggestive of response to treatment. Biopsy was negative for carcinoma and showed only lymphoplasmacytic inflammation.

Given the range of parameters and values, perfusion MRI does show promise; however, lack of standardization limits more widespread acceptance of this technique in the assessment of treated head and neck malignancies. Bernstein JM and colleagues[25] present a systematic review of the applications of DCE as a biomarker to guide treatment and conclude that progress in the field requires the standardization of data, data sharing, and large multicenter collaborative validation studies.

Arterial Spin Labeling

ASL offers an alternative to contrast-enhanced MR perfusion studies. The technique uses the magnetization of inflowing arterial blood followed by a readout gradient-echo EPI with an excitation pulse

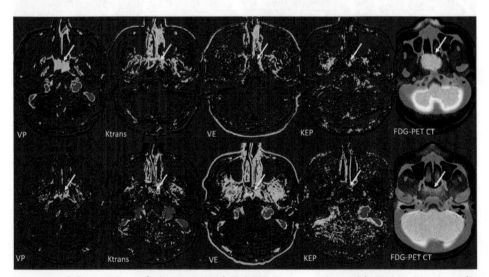

Fig. 4. Upper panel shows DCE perfusion maps and FDG-PET CT in a patient with EBV positive nasopharyngeal carcinoma before treatment. Prominently increased FDG uptake with increased Vp, Ktrans, Kep values are noted. Lower panel shows images after combined chemotherapy and radiation therapy. Interval normalized FDG uptake with decreased Vp, Ktrans, Kep values, and increased Ve values after treatment were demonstrated, representing treatment response.

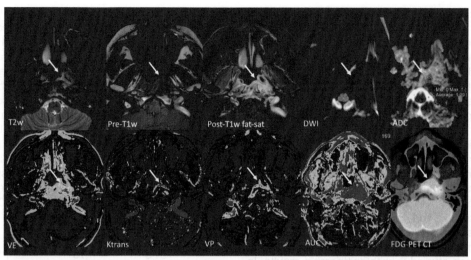

Fig. 5. One-year follow-up MRI after radiation therapy of nasopharyngeal adenoid cystic carcinoma. A T1 hyperintense, T2 hypointense lesion is seen in the left fossa of Rosenmuller with abnormal contrast enhancement and relatively high ADC values. Increased DCE perfusion parameters; Ve, Ktrans, Vp, AUC, and increased metabolic activity are seen on FDG-PET CT (lower panel), worrisome for recurrence and confirmed on biopsy.

of 30° for image acquisition. Control images without labeling are also required. Tumor blood flow (TBF) can then be calculated by the analysis of differences between the magnetized and control images.

Fujima and colleagues[31,32] evaluated the feasibility of ASL in an elegant study by the comparison of TBF measures before and after the treatment. TBF was also evaluated in the posttreatment period to assess the rate of change between the residual tumors and nonresidual tumors. Pre- and posttreatment mean TBF values were 121.4 ± 27.8 and 24.9 ± 14.9 mL/100 g/min, respectively. In 5 patients with residual tumors, posttreatment TBF was significantly higher (46.9 ± 7.1 mL/100 g/min) than the rest of the 17 patients in this cohort (18.4 ± 9.2 mL/100 g/min). The TBF reduction rate was significantly lower in

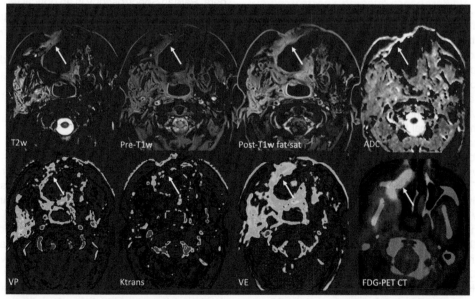

Fig. 6. Recurrent invasive keratinizing moderately differentiated squamous cell carcinoma of the maxilla. Increased thickness of right anterior maxillary sinus wall after free flap reconstruction with increased T2 signal and pathologic enhancement. ADC map is limited due to artifact. DCE perfusion maps showed patchy increased vascularization within the area (Vp, Ktrans, Ve). FDG-PET CT and biopsy confirmed recurrent disease.

patients with residual tumors (0.54 ± 0.12) than in those without (0.85 ± 0.06). The authors concluded that the technique may be useful for the noninvasive assessment of tumor viability in treated head and neck cancers.

A retrospective study of 47 patients with head and neck cancer, treated with radiotherapy and investigated with ASL and diffusion-weighted imaging, showed that TBF was significantly higher in recurrent tumors than in postradiation changes. Similar changes were observed in the ADC maps generated at this time with significantly lower ADC values in recurrent tumor than in postradiation changes. Accuracy for differentiating recurrent tumor and postradiation changes was increased by a combination of the TBF and ADC.[33]

Comparisons of ASL and DCE perfusion have also been studied [31] with comparable results. In this study, pseudocontinuous ASL technique for the entire tumor together with separate regional measurements in the central and peripheral portions of the tumor was compared with the results of the contrast-enhanced DCE perfusion studies carried out in a cohort of 18 patients. The ASL technique, however, underestimated the TBF in the central portion of the tumor. Moreover, the study underscored the importance of attention to the technique of the ASL studies, which was achieved by close attention to detail to ensure accurate image acquisition and subtraction of the control and flow images.

Magnetic Resonance Imaging Spectroscopy

Proton MRI spectroscopy is an established technique that primarily measures the concentration of metabolites in tissues and provides a snapshot of the biochemical structure of the area of interest. The application of MRI spectroscopy is limited in the head and neck because of the complex anatomy with an abundance of fat, irregular geometry of both the normal tissues, and of the commonest malignancies; and more importantly, the multiple interfaces of the air and soft tissues in the region.[4] In a systematic review and meta-analysis, van der Hoorn and colleagues[34] did not encounter any objective study which validated the diagnostic accuracy of MR spectroscopy. Recent studies have demonstrated elevated choline levels which are the hallmark for HNSCC and can act as a surrogate marker for the assessment of residual tumor in patients undergoing chemotherapy. In a series of 46 patients by King and colleagues,[35] all patients underwent 1H-MRS before treatment and the 30 patients with a posttreatment mass-like lesion underwent repeat 1H-MRS at 6 weeks posttreatment. The former group acted as a control for the assessment of cases in the latter group. The persistence of the choline peak in the posttreatment mass-like lesion was attributed to residual tumor with the caveat that the absence of such a peak does not exclude cancer. Therefore, the authors concluded that (1)H cannot be used as a substitute for clinical or conventional radiological follow-up. Alternate metabolites which were investigated on MRS included lactate levels. In a study by Le Q-T and colleagues,[35] 1H-MRS showed that lactate signal intensity, presumed to indicate tissue hypoxia, was not correlated with treatment response, locoregional control, or direct Po_2 measurements in node positive, resectable Stage 4 HNSCC.

Miscellaneous Techniques

BOLD imaging (blood oxygen level dependent intrinsic susceptibility-weighted MR imaging) is a unique MR technique that has been used to assess head and neck carcinomas. In summary, the sequence detects tissue hypoxia which may reduce the effectiveness of CRT. Relative tissue hypoxia can be measured by this technique which relies on the decrease in the signal intensity on $T2^*$ images due to the paramagnetic effects of deoxyhemoglobin. Feasibility of this technique in the clinical domain has been explored, although the technique has not received widespread acceptance.[36,37]

It is pertinent to note that spectroscopic techniques using the concept of Raman spectroscopy are now making inroads into the diagnosis and posttreatment assessment of head and neck cancers. Raman Spectroscopy is an optical technique capable of identifying chemical constituents based on a unique set of molecular vibrations. Noninvasive probes have been used in the intraoperative assessment of brain tumors and have shown potential in the assessment of head and neck malignancies as well.[38,39]

ADVANCED COMPUTED TOMOGRAPHIC TECHNIQUES
Computed Tomography Perfusion

Recent advances in CT technology have permitted a nuanced, validated, and replicable assessment of tumor vascularity by CT perfusion techniques (see Table 1). The underlying principle of CT perfusion is similar to MR perfusion in that a bolus of iodinated contrast is tracked in a tissue vascular bed through the arterial, capillary, and venous phases. CT perfusion is inherently superior to MR perfusion due to higher resolution, faster acquisition intervals, and relatively free from the presence of artifacts from blood products. The faster scan times also permit motion-free acquisitions which are particularly important in the head and neck whereby swallowing artifacts can delay and degrade images. CT perfusion also affords the ease of image acquisition bereft of the requirements of safe conduct of MR studies.[40]

Application of CT perfusion for the primary diagnosis of benign from malignant neck neoplasms,[41–43] estimation of the extent of head and neck cancers, evaluation of metastatic cervical nodes,[44] and guidance for optimal tissue sampling during biopsies[45] have been explored and described in the literature.

Assessment of increased vascularity can be a surrogate of angiogenesis. CT perfusion metrics were correlated with intratumoral microvessel density[46] estimated by CD31 antibodies staining of biopsies of head and neck cancers. In this study, there was a positive correlation with the vessel count and the BV ($P = .035$) with no significant correlation between the vessel count and BF ($P = .316$). No correlation between MTT and capillary permeability was noted. Similar correlations of negative correlation of capillary permeability on CT perfusion and EGFR expression were also noted. EGFR is a marker for local recurrence and disease-specific death.[47] Interleukin-8 is a biomarker of increased angiogenesis and has been positively correlated with relative BF, with no correlation between its expression to relative BV, relative capillary permeability, and relative MTT.[48] Two recent studies have elegantly summarized the utility of perfusion CT in the assessment of posttreatment sequelae in head and neck tumors. Dickerson and Srinivasan[49] in their review have underscored the similarity between MR perfusion studies and CT perfusion and have commented that CT-derived values tend to be lower in absolute terms especially when perfusion values rise; and that there is significant overlap between the literature for MR and CT perfusions. They have also highlighted that the reduction of patient radiation dose by advanced reconstruction models, reduced scanning peak voltages, and limiting the size of scanned regions have contributed to greater fidelity of data. Increased vascularity of tumors is reflected in increased perfusion that is associated with increased sensitivity to chemoradiation; however, larger incremental decrease in perfusion during the course of treatment is associated with better outcomes. Troeltzsch D and colleagues[50] have assessed perfusion parameters in recurrent HNSCC and have concluded that recurrent HNC can be differentiated from posttreatment tissue ($P<.05$) by measuring tissue perfusion by the single-input maximum slope algorithm at the area of interest and in normal uninvolved nuchal soft tissues. The method allowed delineating recurrent tumor tissue from benign nuchal tissue of reference ($P<.05$). Furthermore, the authors found that the data of patients with and without recurrent HNC are comparable as perfusion values of reference tissues in patients with and without HNC do not differ ($P>.05$).

Dual-Energy Computed Tomography

Aspects of tissue characteristics have been recently exploited by the technical advances in dual-energy CT. Dual-energy CT depends on the inherent differences in the propensity of materials to attenuate radiation based on the energy of the incident x-rays. A typical example is that of the polychromatic beam with an average energy of 80 kVp being closer to the k-edge of iodine that will be disproportionately attenuated by iodine in tissues than a beam of 140 kVp. Thus, scanners can perform sequential scans at 2 different energies to yield sets of data in images which can, for example, reduce metal artifacts, characterize, head and neck tumors, detect atherosclerotic plaques and parathyroid adenomas, and assess paranasal sinus ventilation.[51,52]

Studies specific to the posttreatment assessment of HNC have explored the fact that low-energy virtual monochromatic images enhance the visibility and contrast of soft tissues structures. In their study of a cohort of 16 patients with benign posttreatment changes and 24 cases with known malignancies including 7 recurrent tumors, Yamauchi and colleagues[53] had noted that malignant tissues were significantly different from benign posttreatment changes in spectral Hounsfield units at 40 keV ($P<.0001$), iodine concentration ($P<.0001$), and spectral Hounsfield units at 70 keV ($P = .0001$) with AUCs of 0.949, 0.943, and 0.858, respectively. They concluded that spectral Hounsfield units at 40 keV and iodine concentration may be superior to spectral Hounsfield units at 70 keV, which is similar to the multidetector CT detection of benign posttreatment sequelae from malignant tissues encountered in primary or recurrent head and cancers (**Fig. 7**).

Recent studies by Bahig and colleagues[54] have explored the role of dual-energy CT as a prognostic tool for the prediction of locoregional recurrence. Their data analyses involved measurements of the gross tumor volumes and gross nodal volumes. Iodine concentration maps in the segmented gross tumor volumes was then obtained using two material decomposition, resulting in a creation of quantitative histograms from the iodine concentration maps. This elaborate methodology underscores the versatility of the technique of dual-energy scanning. The results showed that the authors could predict locoregional recurrence in this cohort of patients with laryngeal and hypopharyngeal cancers.

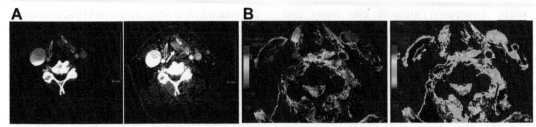

Fig. 7. (A) 77-year-old male with supraglottic laryngeal squamous cell carcinoma. Compare left image at 70 keV, with right image at 40 keV, both images have identical windowing (550:200). The left supraglottic lesion is more conspicuous at lower keV (*white arrow*). (B) Same patient with CT perfusion showing increased blood flow (left image) and blood volume (right image) at the left supraglottic lesion. Note that increased perfusion parameters are identifiable within the thyroid cartilage, and this makes the lesion at least a T3 category on these images, regardless of vocal cord mobility status.

Another unique application of dual-energy CT is in the assessment of the thyroid cartilage. The uneven and nonuniform ossification of the thyroid cartilage makes it challenging for the assessment of tumor infiltration and osteoradionecrosis in patients treated for HNC, especially in the laryngeal and hypopharyngeal region. Taking into consideration the energy dependent attenuation properties of the non-ossified and ossified portions of the thyroid cartilage, low energy virtual monochromatic images will accentuate the enhancing iodine-containing tissues such as enhancing tumor, whereas these changes will become less evident in the higher energy virtual monochromatic images with the enhancing tumor showing an attenuation similar to non-enhanced images.[52] Dual-energy CT studies have also been used as a research tool for distinguishing mandibular osteoradionecrosis based on the edema pattern in a porcine model.[55]

SUMMARY

Advanced MR and CT techniques are useful adjuncts to anatomic imaging and may assist in lesion discrimination and characterization. Diffusion MRI techniques help to identify highly cellular lesions and are sensitive to identifying malignant tissue in pre and posttherapeutic states. DCE (as well as many other advanced MRI techniques) can help identify aggressive features of head and neck neoplasms, which can assist in biopsy and therapy. DCE in the surveillance setting can be useful to identify persistent or recurrent disease. Ktrans is the most important DCE parameter, though several additional parameters can be helpful. DECT lower keV values can help increase lesion conspicuity. CTP can offer insight into tumoral vascularity and assess spread into adjacent spaces; rBF and rBV (as in the case of stroke imaging) are the most important maps. In conjunction with a good oncologic history and physical examination, these advanced CT and MR techniques can help add value to referring clinicians, enabling more effective, tailored management.

CLINICS CARE POINTS

- CT and MRI are the mainstay of disease assessment in head and neck cancer.
- Recurrent lesions tend to have lower ADC values than post treatment scarring.
- Recurrent lesions tend to have shorter TTP than radiation related changes.
- ASL is a noncontrast MR technique assessing blood flow, tumors (and recurrent lesions) tend to have higher relative blood flow.
- CT perfusion can identify regions of elevated blood volume to aid targeted biopsy in the post treatment neck. The maximum slope algorithm may be a useful single input marker to identify recurrent tumor.
- Dual energy CT has special application in increasing tissue contrast to identify malignant lesions and nodes at lower keV values. DECT is also useful in assessment of the thyroid cartilage.

DISCLOSURE

The authors have nothing to disclose.

REFERENCES

1. Lobert P, Srinivasan A, Shah GV, et al. Postoperative and postradiation changes on imaging. Otolaryngol Clin North Am 2012;45(6):1405–22.
2. Burri RJ, Kao J, Navada S, et al. Nonsurgical treatment of head and neck cancer. In: Som PM,

Curtin HD, editors. Head and neck imaging. St. Louis, MO: Mosby; 2011. p. 2893–914.

3. Ishikawa M, Anzai Y. MR imaging of lymph nodes in the head and neck. Neuroimaging Clin N Am 2004; 14(4):679–94.

4. Moore AG, Srinivasan A. Postoperative and postradiation head and neck: role of magnetic resonance imaging. Top Magn Reson Imaging 2015;24(1):3–13.

5. Blatt S, Ziebart T, Kruger M, et al. Diagnosing oral squamous cell carcinoma: how much imaging do we really need? A review of the current literature. J Craniomaxillofac Surg 2016;44(5):538–49.

6. Seeburg DP, Baer AH, Aygun N. Imaging of patients with head and neck cancer: from staging to surveillance. Oral Maxillofac Surg Clin North Am 2018; 30(4):421–33.

7. Conceptual guidelines for neck dissection classification. In: Deschler DG, Smith RV, editors. Quick reference guide to TNM staging of head and neck cancer and neck dissection classification. 4th edition. Alexandria, VA: American Academy of Otolaryngology–Head and Neck Surgery Foundation; 2014.

8. Colbert SD, Mitchell DA, Brennan PA. Woody hardness - a novel classification for the radiotherapy-treated neck. Br J Oral Maxillofac Surg 2015;53(4):380–3.

9. Hermans R. Posttreatment imaging in head and neck cancer. Eur J Radiol 2008;66(3):501–11.

10. Learned KO, Malloy KM, Loevner LA. Myocutaneous flaps and other vascularized grafts in head and neck reconstruction for cancer treatment. Magn Reson Imaging Clin N Am 2012;20(3):495–513.

11. Wang J, Takashima S, Takayama F, et al. Head and neck lesions: characterization with diffusion-weighted echo-planar MR imaging. Radiology 2001;220(3):621–30.

12. Varoquaux A, Rager O, Dulguerov P, et al. Diffusion-weighted and PET/MR imaging after radiation therapy for malignant head and neck tumors. Radiographics 2015;35(5):1502–27.

13. de Bondt RB, Nelemans PJ, Hofman PAM, et al. Detection of lymph node metastases in head and neck cancer: a meta-analysis comparing US, USgFNAC, CT and MR imaging. Eur J Radiol 2007;64(2):266–72.

14. Paulus P, Sambon A, Vivegnis D, et al. 18FDG-PET for the assessment of primary head and neck tumors: clinical, computed tomography, and histopathological correlation in 38 patients. Laryngoscope 1998;108(10):1578–83.

15. Vandecaveye V, De Keyzer F, Nuyts S, et al. Detection of head and neck squamous cell carcinoma with diffusion weighted MRI after (chemo)radiotherapy: correlation between radiologic and histopathologic findings. Int J Radiat Oncol Biol Phys 2007;67(4):960–71.

16. Abdel Razek AAK, Kandeel AY, Soliman N, et al. Role of diffusion-weighted echo-planar MR imaging in differentiation of residual or recurrent head and neck tumors and posttreatment changes. AJNR Am J Neuroradiol 2007;28(6):1146–52.

17. Brenet E, Barbe C, Hoeffel C, et al. Predictive value of early post-treatment diffusion-weighted MRI for recurrence or tumor progression of head and neck squamous cell carcinoma treated with chemo-radiotherapy. Cancers (Basel) 2020;12(5):1234.

18. Kim S, Loevner L, Quon H, et al. Diffusion-weighted magnetic resonance imaging for predicting and detecting early response to chemoradiation therapy of squamous cell carcinomas of the head and neck. Clin Cancer Res 2009;15(3):986–94.

19. Vandecaveye V, Dirix P, De Keyzer F, et al. Diffusion-weighted magnetic resonance imaging early after chemoradiotherapy to monitor treatment response in head-and-neck squamous cell carcinoma. Int J Radiat Oncol Biol Phys 2012;82(3):1098–107.

20. Tshering Vogel DW, Zbaeren P, Geretschlaeger A, et al. Diffusion-weighted MR imaging including bi-exponential fitting for the detection of recurrent or residual tumour after (chemo)radiotherapy for laryngeal and hypopharyngeal cancers. Eur Radiol 2013;23(2):562–9.

21. Jansen JFA, Parra C, Lu Y, et al. Evaluation of head and neck tumors with functional MR imaging. Magn Reson Imaging Clin N Am 2016;24(1):123–33.

22. Newbold K, Castellano I, Charles-Edwards E, et al. An exploratory study into the role of dynamic contrast-enhanced magnetic resonance imaging or perfusion computed tomography for detection of intratumoral hypoxia in head-and-neck cancer. Int J Radiat Oncol Biol Phys 2009;74(1):29–37.

23. Shukla-Dave A, Lee NY, Jansen JFA, et al. Dynamic contrast-enhanced magnetic resonance imaging as a predictor of outcome in head-and-neck squamous cell carcinoma patients with nodal metastases. Int J Radiat Oncol Biol Phys 2012;82(5):1837–44.

24. Baer AH, Hoff BA, Srinivasan A, et al. Feasibility analysis of the parametric response map as an early predictor of treatment efficacy in head and neck cancer. AJNR Am J Neuroradiol 2015;36(4):757–62.

25. Bernstein JM, Homer JJ, West CM. Dynamic contrast-enhanced magnetic resonance imaging biomarkers in head and neck cancer: potential to guide treatment? A systematic review. Oral Oncol 2014;50(10):963–70.

26. Ng SH, Lin CY, Chan SC, et al. Dynamic contrast-enhanced MR imaging predicts local control in oropharyngeal or hypopharyngeal squamous cell carcinoma treated with chemoradiotherapy. PLoS One 2013;8(8):e72230.

27. Agrawal S, Awasthi R, Singh A, et al. An exploratory study into the role of dynamic contrast-enhanced (DCE) MRI metrics as predictors of response in head and neck cancers. Clin Radiol 2012;67(9):e1–5.

28. Ishiyama M, Richards T, Parvathaneni U, et al. Dynamic contrast-enhanced magnetic resonance imaging in Head and Neck Cancer: differentiation of new H&N cancer, recurrent disease, and benign post-treatment changes. Clin Imaging 2015;39(4):566–70.

29. Furukawa M, Parvathaneni U, Maravilla K, et al. Dynamic contrast-enhanced MR perfusion imaging of head and neck tumors at 3 Tesla. Head Neck 2013;35(7):923–9.

30. Lee JY, Cheng KL, Lee JH, et al. Detection of local recurrence in patients with head and neck squamous cell carcinoma using voxel-based color maps of initial and final area under the curve values derived from DCE-MRI. AJNR Am J Neuroradiol 2019;40(8):1392–401.

31. Fujima N, Kudo K, Tsukahara A, et al. Measurement of tumor blood flow in head and neck squamous cell carcinoma by pseudo-continuous arterial spin labeling: comparison with dynamic contrast-enhanced MRI. J Magn Reson Imaging 2015;41(4):983–91.

32. Fujima N, Kudo K, Yoshida D, et al. Arterial spin labeling to determine tumor viability in head and neck cancer before and after treatment. J Magn Reson Imaging 2014;40(4):920–8.

33. Abdel Razek AAK. Arterial spin labelling and diffusion-weighted magnetic resonance imaging in differentiation of recurrent head and neck cancer from post-radiation changes. J Laryngol Otol 2018;132(10):923–8.

34. van der Hoorn A, van Laar PJ, Holtman GA, et al. Diagnostic accuracy of magnetic resonance imaging techniques for treatment response evaluation in patients with head and neck tumors, a systematic review and meta-analysis. PLoS One 2017;12(5):e0177986.

35. Le QT, Koong A, Lieskovsky YY, et al. In vivo 1H magnetic resonance spectroscopy of lactate in patients with stage IV head and neck squamous cell carcinoma. Int J Radiat Oncol Biol Phys 2008;71(4):1151–7.

36. King AD, Thoeny HC. Functional MRI for the prediction of treatment response in head and neck squamous cell carcinoma: potential and limitations. Cancer Imaging 2016;16(1):23.

37. Panek R, Welsh L, Dunlop A, et al. Repeatability and sensitivity of T2* measurements in patients with head and neck squamous cell carcinoma at 3T. J Magn Reson Imaging 2016;44(1):72–80.

38. Devpura S, Barton KN, Brown SL, et al. Vision 20/20: the role of Raman spectroscopy in early stage cancer detection and feasibility for application in radiation therapy response assessment. Med Phys 2014;41(5):050901.

39. Nooij RP, Hof JJ, van Laar PJ, et al. Functional MRI for treatment evaluation in patients with head and neck squamous cell carcinoma: a review of the literature from a radiologist perspective. Curr Radiol Rep 2018;6(1):2.

40. Davis AJ, Rehmani R, Srinivasan A, et al. Perfusion and permeability imaging for head and neck cancer: theory, acquisition, postprocessing, and relevance to clinical Imaging. Magn Reson Imaging Clin N Am 2018;26(1):19–35.

41. Tawfik AM, Abdel Razek AAK, Elsorogy LG, et al. Perfusion CT of head and neck cancer: effect of arterial input selection. AJR Am J Roentgenol 2011;196(6):1374–80.

42. Srinivasan A, Mohan S, Mukherji SK. Biologic imaging of head and neck cancer: the present and the future. AJNR Am J Neuroradiol 2012;33(4):586–94.

43. Hermans R, Op de beeck K, Van den Bogaert W, et al. The relation of CT-determined tumor parameters and local and regional outcome of tonsillar cancer after definitive radiation treatment. Int J Radiat Oncol Biol Phys 2001;50(1):37–45.

44. Trojanowska A, Trojanowski P, Bisdas S, et al. Squamous cell cancer of hypopharynx and larynx - evaluation of metastatic nodal disease based on computed tomography perfusion studies. Eur J Radiol 2012;81(5):1034–9.

45. Miles KA, Griffiths MR, Perfusion CT. a worthwhile enhancement? Br J Radiol 2003;76(904):220–31.

46. Ash L, Teknos TN, Gandhi D, et al. Head and neck squamous cell carcinoma: CT perfusion can help noninvasively predict intratumoral microvessel density. Radiology 2009;251(2):422–8.

47. Hoefling NL, McHugh KB, Light E, et al. Human papillomavirus, p16, and epidermal growth factor receptor biomarkers and CT perfusion values in head and neck squamous cell carcinoma. AJNR Am J Neuroradiol 2013;34(5):1062–6. S1–2.

48. Jo SY, Wang PI, Nör JE, et al. CT perfusion can predict overexpression of CXCL8 (interleukin-8) in head and neck squamous cell carcinoma. AJNR Am J Neuroradiol 2013;34(12):2338–42.

49. Dickerson E, Srinivasan A. Advanced Imaging Techniques of the Skull Base. Radiol Clin North Am 2017; 55(1):189–200.

50. Troeltzsch D, Niehues SM, Fluegge T, et al. The diagnostic performance of perfusion CT in the detection of local tumor recurrence in head and neck cancer. Clin Hemorheol Microcirc 2020;76(2):171–7.

51. Ginat DT, Mayich M, Daftari-Besheli L, et al. Clinical applications of dual-energy CT in head and neck imaging. Eur Arch Otorhinolaryngol 2016;273(3):547–53.

52. Forghani R. An update on advanced dual-energy CT for head and neck cancer imaging. Expert Rev Anticancer Ther 2019;19(7):633–44.

53. Yamauchi H, Buehler M, Goodsitt MM, et al. Dual-energy CT-based differentiation of benign posttreatment changes from primary or recurrent malignancy of the head and neck: comparison of spectral hounsfield units at 40 and 70 keV and iodine concentration. AJR Am J Roentgenol 2016;206(3):580–7.

54. Bahig H, Lapointe A, Bedwani S, et al. Dual-energy computed tomography for prediction of loco-regional recurrence after radiotherapy in larynx and hypopharynx squamous cell carcinoma. Eur J Radiol 2019;110:1–6.

55. Poort LJ, Stadler AAR, Ludlage JHB, et al. Detection of bone marrow edema pattern with dual-energy computed tomography of the pig mandible treated with radiotherapy and surgery compared with magnetic resonance imaging. J Comput Assist Tomogr 2017;41(4):553–8.

Imaging of Treated Thyroid and Parathyroid Disease

Kalen Riley, MD, MBA[a],*, Yoshimi Anzai, MD, MPH[b]

KEYWORDS

- Thyroid cancer • Thyroidectomy • Radioactive iodine (RAI) • Ultrasound (US)
- Computed tomography (CT) • Magnetic resonance imaging (MRI)

KEY POINTS

- The thyroid and parathyroid glands are endocrine structures located closely together within the neck. Pathologies affecting these glands include endocrine disorders of glandular function as well as malignancy.
- Thyroid cancer and potential treatment-related complications are commonly followed with imaging. Ultrasound is the imaging modality of choice for the follow-up of thyroid cancer with more advanced modalities including CT, MRI, and PET/CT reserved for more advanced disease states.
- Treated hyper and hypothyroidism are not commonly followed with imaging. However, these patients may be imaged for other reasons and treatment-related sequelae or complications are incidentally observed.
- Primary hyperparathyroidism (PHPT) is the most common parathyroid disease and also is not routinely followed with imaging. Complicated and/or recurrent cases may be evaluated with imaging and the initial posttreatment changes may be visible.

INTRODUCTION

The thyroid and parathyroid glands are endocrine structures located in the visceral space of the infrahyoid neck. Thyroid malignancy has seen a growing incidence over the last several decades without increasing mortality rate, presumably due to increasing diagnosis. Thyroid cancer is primarily treated surgically with or without adjuvant radioactive iodine (RAI) ablation. Imaging plays a critical role in the evaluation of patients with thyroid cancer, both in the pre and posttreatment setting. Disorders of thyroid function, that is, hyperthyroidism and hypothyroidism, are also fairly common, although imaging utilization is less frequent with these conditions. Parathyroid dysfunction results in disordered calcium metabolism. Imaging is frequently applied in the preoperative assessment of these patients undergoing parathyroidectomy, however, routine imaging in the postoperative setting is uncommon. Parathyroid carcinoma is rare; however, imaging may be used in the pre and posttreatment setting.

Knowledge of the expected posttreatment imaging appearances of these disease states as well as potential posttreatment complications is critical for the interpreting radiologist. This article reviews the most commonly observed imaging appearances of the thyroid and parathyroid glands after treatment for these various disease states as well as multiple possible complications.

THYROID CANCER
Epidemiology and histology subtypes

Within the United States, the incidence of thyroid cancer has been reported up to 15.7 cases per 100,000 people.[1] Over the last several decades, this reported incidence has increased nearly 3-fold and is largely thought to be secondary to

[a] Department of Radiology and Imaging Sciences, Indiana University School of Medicine, 550 N. University Boulevard, Room 0663, Indianapolis, IN 46202, USA; [b] Department of Radiology and Imaging Sciences, University of Utah School of Medicine, 30 North 1900 East #1A071, Salt Lake City, UT 84132, USA
* Corresponding author.
E-mail address: riley9@iupui.edu
Twitter: @KRileyMD (K.R.); @yoshimianzai (Y.A.)

Neuroimag Clin N Am 32 (2022) 145–157
https://doi.org/10.1016/j.nic.2021.08.014

neuroimaging.theclinics.com

increased detection rather than a true increase in disease incidence.[2] There is an approximately 3:1 female/male ratio and a median age of 51 at diagnosis.[1,2] Most thyroid cancers are well-differentiated tumors with the papillary subtype representing the vast majority (approximately 84%) of cases followed by the follicular subtype at 10% of cases.[3] Papillary and follicular thyroid cancers are grouped as differentiated thyroid cancer (DTC), as the clinical management of these entities is similar.

Medullary thyroid cancer (MTC) arises from parafollicular C cells of thyroid glands and produces calcitonin. MTC is primarily sporadic, however, does occur in a hereditary pattern in around 25% of cases.[4,5] The hereditary form of MTC is often associated with multiple endocrine neoplasia (MEN) type 2, which is linked to mutations in the RET proto-oncogene.[6] MEN type 2 has subclassification whereby Type 2A includes MTC, parathyroid adenoma or hyperplasia, and pheochromocytoma, whereas Type 2B includes MTC, pheochromocytoma, and mucosal neuroma. MTC is more aggressive than DTC and has a worse prognosis. Anaplastic thyroid cancer (ATC) is the most poorly differentiated of thyroid cancers. Although its incidence is lowest (1%–2% of all thyroid cancers), it accounts for 14% to 50% of cancer-related mortality of thyroid cancers with a median survival of 3 to 6 months.[7]

Surgical treatment of differentiated thyroid cancer

Surgery is the mainstay of treatment for differentiated thyroid cancer (DTC) with total thyroidectomy being the most common procedure (**Fig. 1**). The goals of total thyroidectomy are to remove the entire tumor laryngeal while minimizing procedure-related complications. Near-total thyroidectomy is also performed which is the removal of all thyroid tissue except for a small amount of posterior thyroid capsule to avoid recurrent nerve injury. More recently, thyroid lobectomy has become an acceptable treatment option for patients with smaller primary tumors (<1 cm) confined to one thyroid lobe (**Figs. 2** and **3**) and no nodules on the contralateral lobe.[8] Lobectomy is generally a safer procedure that avoids the risk of injury to structures within the contralateral neck. In properly selected patients, there is no significant difference in recurrence rates or survival for lobectomy versus total thyroidectomy.[9–11]

The primary benefits of total thyroidectomy over lobectomy are: 1) option to undergo RAI therapy for adjuvant therapy and 2) measurement of serum thyroglobulin for the surveillance of cancer recurrence. The main drawback is that patients will need to take thyroid hormone replacement medication for the rest of their life. Central or lateral compartment lymph node dissection may also be performed depending on the presence of nodal involvement (see **Fig. 1**). RAI therapy after total thyroidectomy may also be administered to ablate potential remnant thyroid tissue in intermediate or high-risk patients by American Thyroid Association (ATA) critieria.[12]

Complications of thyroid surgery include postoperative hematoma, vocal cord dysfunction, and hypoparathyroidism resulting in hypocalcemia, and typically do not result in any imaging. Vocal cord dysfunction due to postoperative recurrent laryngeal nerve injury, however, has been reported to be permanent in approximately 2.3% of patients (**Fig. 4**).[13,14] Patients with long-standing vocal cord paralysis may go on to have surgical therapy involving the injection of any number of implants or injectable materials which may be visualized on later cross-sectional imaging (**Fig. 5**).[15] Hypoparathyroidism is also a serious potential complication of total thyroidectomy. Patients may present with muscle pain, tingling, or twitching of fingers or toes, irritability, depression, and dry skin. Therefore, the parathyroid glands must be actively identified during the total thyroidectomy and preserved to avoid this complication.

Posttreatment surveillance

After receiving therapy, patients are followed with serial monitoring of thyroglobulin levels as well as neck ultrasound. Ultrasonography (US) has emerged as the imaging modality of choice in monitoring these patients given its relatively low cost, lack of ionizing radiation, and high accessibility as well as high accuracy in detecting nodal and thyroid bed recurrences.[12,16–18] The optimal sonographic technique will use a high-frequency ($\geq$10 MHz) linear probe to achieve high resolution. The ATA recommends US 6 to 12 months after surgery to evaluate the thyroid bed as well as the central and lateral nodal compartments for recurrent disease.[12] Subsequent follow-up intervals will vary among patients depending on individual risk factors. For patients who do receive thyroid remnant ablation, the ATA does recommend a posttherapy whole-body nuclear medicine scan to further assess staging and evaluate any remaining structural disease (**Fig. 6**).[12]

The recurrence of DTCs is fairly common and has been reported to occur in up to 30% of cases.[19] Locoregional recurrences are often non-palpable, making imaging follow-up extremely important. Ultrasound and possible ultrasound-

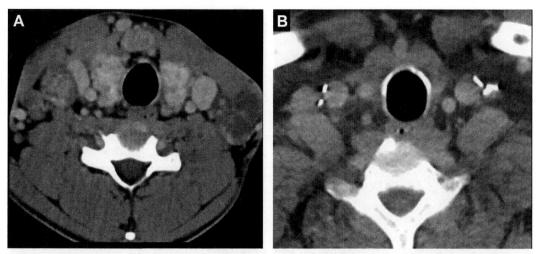

Fig. 1. Patient with papillary thyroid carcinoma and bilateral metastatic cervical lymphadenopathy (A). The patient underwent total thyroidectomy and bilateral lymph node dissections (B).

guided fine-needle aspiration (FNA) biopsy have been found to be accurate in detecting recurrences within the thyroidectomy bed, even when serum thyroglobulin is undetectable. Thyroidectomy bed recurrences are most likely to appear as irregular hypoechoic nodules with internal vascularity (Fig. 7).[20,21] However, many benign nodules within the postoperative bed may also appear hypoechoic, so FNA is often necessary to confirm the diagnosis. Cervical lymph node recurrences are also common and on imaging appear similar to pretreatment metastatic nodes. Typical sonographic features include abnormal rounded shape, hypoechogenicity, loss of the fatty hilum, and microcalcifications.[17,22]

Radioiodine whole-body scintigraphy (WBS) had historically been performed in the postoperative setting and had some utility in the detection of iodine avid disease. Currently, WBS is recommended in the immediate post–RAI setting to help with disease staging and potentially detect previously unknown sites of disease. Posttherapy WBS may change the disease staging and management strategy in 8% to 9% of patients as well as to detect previously unknown sites of disease.[23,24] WBS traditionally yields planar images, which do not offer detailed anatomic information and will not be helpful in aiding preoperative planning. WBS in conjunction with fused SPECT/CT may offer improved anatomic localization as well as

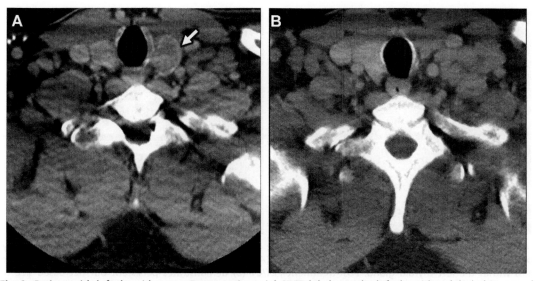

Fig. 2. Patient with left thyroid cancer. Preoperative axial CECT (A) shows the left thyroid nodule (white arrow). Axial postoperative CECT (B) shows uncomplicated left hemithyroidectomy.

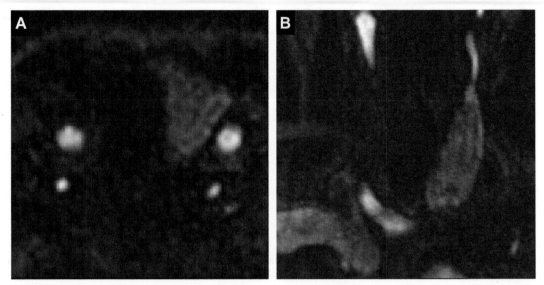

Fig. 3. Patient with right thyroid cancer status post right hemithyroidectomy. Axial (*A*) and coronal (*B*) postcontrast MRA of the neck shows uncomplicated postoperative appearance of the right thyroid lobe.

the detection of disease resulting in altered prognostic estimates.[25,26]

In the case of long-term follow-up, compared to serum thyroglobulin assays and new imaging modalities such as US, WBS is fairly insensitive in the detection of DTC metastases or recurrences.[18,27] Furthermore, I-131 WBS will not detect a tumor that does not avidly take up iodine or is dedifferentiated. As a result of these limitations, WBS has largely fallen out of favor in routine postoperative surveillance for patients with thyroid cancer. The ATA does not recommend routine follow-up WBS

in patients who had a posttherapy scan showing no uptake outside the thyroidectomy bed.

Computed tomography (CT), magnetic resonance imaging (MRI), and positron emission tomography/computed tomography (PET/CT) are also not routinely used in posttreatment surveillance of DTC, however, may play a role in cases of distant metastatic disease, recurrences that are invading adjacent structures, or other situations such as widespread nodal disease in which US may be inadequate for full disease mapping. Patients presenting with concerning symptoms

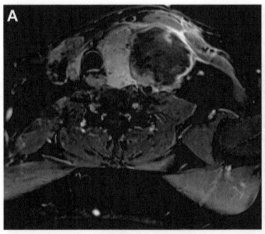
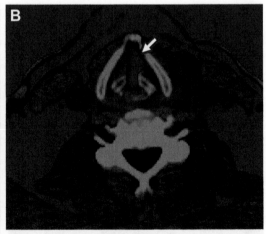

Fig. 4. Patient with anaplastic thyroid carcinoma of the left thyroid gland status post subtotal thyroidectomy. Axial post-contrast MRI after subtotal thyroidectomy (*A*) demonstrates a large, heterogeneously enhancing mass within the left thyroid gland. Post-treatment PET/CT (*B*) demonstrates persistent but decreased size of the left thyroid mass as well as enlargement of the left laryngeal ventricle (*white arrow*) consistent with vocal cord paralysis. The vocal cord paralysis was confirmed on flexible laryngoscopy.

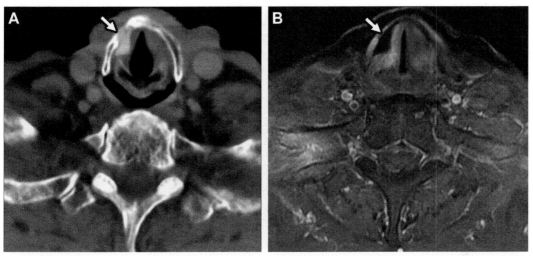

Fig. 5. Patient with a history of papillary thyroid carcinoma status postthyroidectomy. The postoperative course was complicated by right vocal cord paralysis and the patient later underwent placement of an implant into the vocal fold via a window in the thyroid cartilage (*white arrows*). Axial CECT (*A*) demonstrates a hyperdense implant within the right vocal fold with correlating hypointense appearance on T1 postcontrast MRI (*B*). Post-implant placement there is subsequent medialization of the vocal fold.

such as hoarseness, dysphagia, or a rapidly growing neck mass also warrant further evaluation with CT or MRI to assess for locoregional invasion (**Fig. 8**).

CT is often considered first-line in these situations due to its widespread availability, quickness, and lower cost than MRI. The ATA recommends

the consideration of contrast-enhanced CT (CECT) in patients with rising thyroglobulin and negative neck US.[12] One of the main concerns regarding CECT in imaging patients with DTC is the fact iodinated contrast media may saturate thyroid tissue and ultimately interfere with RAI uptake in an attempted future ablation. Patients who

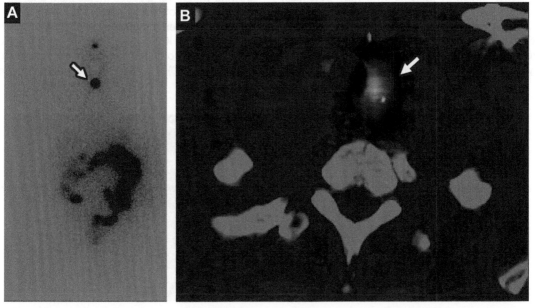

Fig. 6. Patient with papillary thyroid carcinoma status post total thyroidectomy, bilateral lymph node dissections, and RAI ablation. Post-RAI WBS obtained seven days after therapy (*A*) demonstrates focal uptake within the left thyroidectomy bed consistent with mild residual thyroid tissue (*white arrow*). Fused SPECT/CT (*B*) demonstrates the radiotracer avid tissue within the left thyroidectomy bed (*white arrow*).

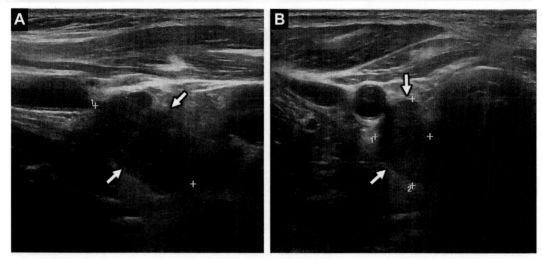

Fig. 7. Patient with papillary thyroid carcinoma status post thyroidectomy. Postoperative US images (*A, B*) reveal a hypoechoic nodule in the thyroidectomy bed (*white arrows*) concerning disease recurrence. Fine-needle aspiration biopsy was consistent with recurrent papillary carcinoma.

are candidates for future RAI ablation that do receive iodinated contrast media will need to wait 4 to 8 weeks before undergoing any therapy to allow the plasma iodine concentrations to normalize and minimize any risk of competitive inhibition.[28] MRI is also effective at detecting nodal recurrences within the neck as well as mapping the extent of locoregional invasion.[29-34] MRI has one advantage over CT in that it does not use iodinated contrast material, and therefore may be a better option in patients who may potentially receive RAI ablation therapy.

One interesting pattern of recurrent nodal disease that has been observed in patients with thyroid cancer is metastatic retropharyngeal lymphadenopathy, particularly in patients with a history of prior neck dissection (**Fig. 9**). It has been postulated that neck dissection disrupts the normal lymphatic drainage pattern of the neck, resulting in the unusual pattern of retropharyngeal nodal metastases.[35-39] These nodal recurrences are best evaluated with CECT or MRI as the retropharyngeal space is not well evaluated with physical examination or US.[30,35,36]

PET/CT using ^{18}F-FDG is not routinely used in the pretreatment setting as DTC is often slow growing with lower glucose metabolism and, as a result, does not avidly take up ^{18}F-FDG.[40,41] PET/CT, however, may play a role in the posttreatment setting as it has been shown to be sensitive in the detection of recurrent and distant metastatic disease (**Fig. 10**).[41-45] The ATA recommends the

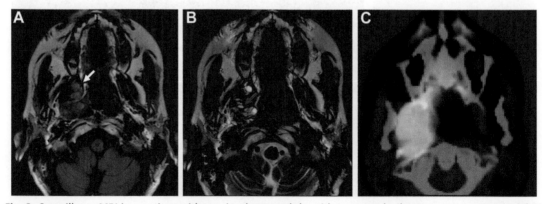

Fig. 8. Surveillance MRI in a patient with previously treated thyroid cancer and subsequent recurrence. Axial T1 (*A*) and axial T2 (*B*) show a heterogeneous signal mass with areas of intrinsic T1 hyperintensity (*white arrow*) and fluid-hematocrit levels (*red arrow*) involving the right parapharyngeal space and medial pterygoid muscle. The mass is markedly hypermetabolic on FDG PET/CT (*C*).

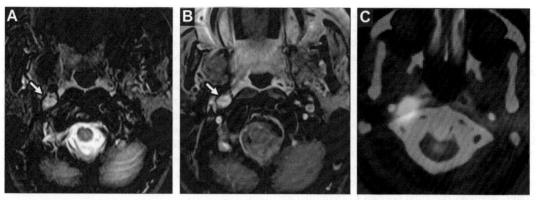

Fig. 9. Patient with a history of thyroid malignancy status posttotal thyroidectomy. Follow-up MRI was performed and axial T2 (*A*) and T1 post (*B*) demonstrate a recurrent right retropharyngeal lymph node metastasis. This node was noted to be hypermetabolic on PET/CT (*C*). The patient also had multiple other cervical lymph node metastases (not shown).

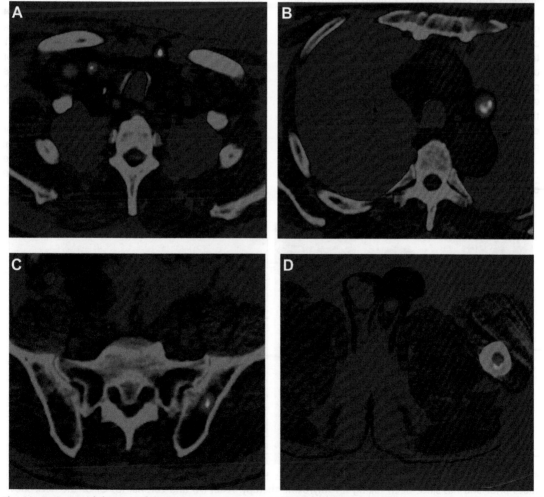

Fig. 10. Patient with history of thyroid cancer status post total thyroidectomy and RAI ablation. Follow-up PET/CT demonstrates multifocal hypermetabolic nodal (*A*, *B*, *C*, *D*) and skeletal metastases.

consideration of PET/CT in patients with elevated thyroglobulin more than 10 ng/mL. FDG PET/CT may also be useful in cases of more aggressive or de-differentiated thyroid cancers that show increased glucose metabolism.

Thyroid dysfunction

Disorders of thyroid hormone function, that is, hypothyroidism/hyperthyroidism are common and more frequently seen in older and female patients.[46–48] Common examples of hyperthyroidism include Graves' disease and toxic multinodular goiter, whereas common causes of hypothyroidism include Hashimoto's thyroiditis and drug/toxin-mediated causes. Although imaging may occasionally play a role in the diagnosis of these conditions, it is infrequently used in the posttreatment phase of these disorders.

Graves' disease is the most common cause of hyperthyroidism and is the result of circulating antibodies that bind to thyroid gland receptors and result in the excess production of thyroid hormone.[49] The condition may be treated with medications, RAI ablation, or in some cases thyroidectomy. In terms of imaging, a radioiodine uptake scan is often performed in the diagnostic phase; however, after definitive treatment imaging does not play an important role in the monitoring of these patients. Treatment-related sequelae may occasionally be seen incidentally on imaging examinations performed for other reasons (**Fig. 11**).

Graves' disease does have one main extrathyroidal manifestation known as Graves' ophthalmopathy (GO), thyroid eye disease (TED), or thyroid-associated orbitopathy (TAD). GO is characterized by the inflammation of the extraocular muscles and is seen in just over one-quarter of patients with Graves' disease.[50] Most cases of GO are mild; however, severe cases can result in compressive neuropathy of the optic nerve and threaten the patient's vision. Advanced cases may be treated with decompressive surgery to alleviate elevated intraocular pressure.[51] Patients who have undergone surgical treatment of GO may be imaged postoperatively to evaluate the decompressive appearance (**Fig. 12**).

Parathyroid diseases

Primary hyperparathyroidism (PHPT) is the most common parathyroid disorder and the third most common endocrine disorder overall. The incidence of the disorder increases with age and women are affected twice as frequently as men.[52] PHPT is the most common cause of hypercalcemia and results from the excess secretion of parathyroid hormone (PTH) by at least one of the 4 parathyroid glands. A single parathyroid adenoma is the most commonly observed cause of PHPT (75%–85%) with multiglandular adenoma and/or parathyroid gland hyperplasia being much less common.[52] PHPT is typically diagnosed by discovering elevated serum calcium levels on blood work.

Surgical resection is the mainstay of therapy for PHPT and is the only curative treatment. Bilateral neck exploration and examination of each of the 4 parathyroid glands had historically been the standard of care for the surgical management of

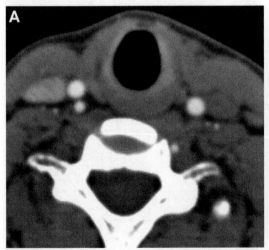
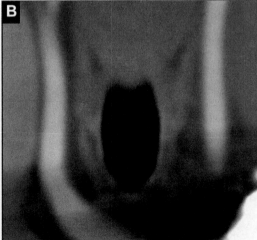

Fig. 11. Young female patient with a history of Graves' hyperthyroidism treated with RAI ablation nearly 2 decades prior and has since been taking levothyroxine therapy. Axial (*A*) and coronal (*B*) CT of the neck shows near-complete absence of the thyroid gland with faint residual tissue present. No surgical procedure was performed.

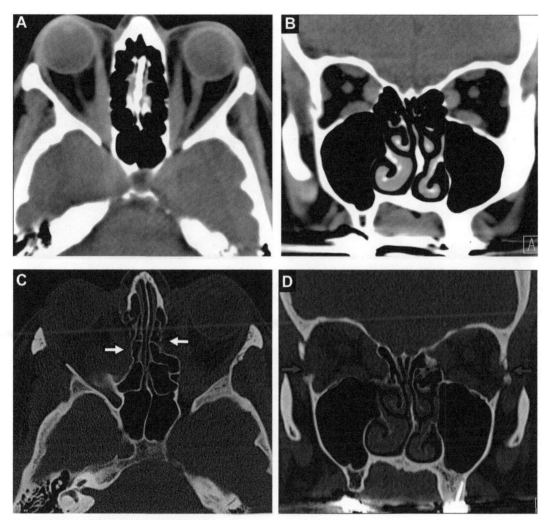

Fig. 12. Patient with Graves' ophthalmopathy. Axial (*A*) and coronal (*B*) noncontrast CT images of the orbits show enlarged extraocular muscles bilaterally, most pronounced within the inferior and medial rectus muscles. There is also associated moderate proptosis of the globe. Axial (*C*) and coronal (*D*) noncontrast images obtained after surgical decompression of the lamina papyracea (*white arrows*) and lateral orbital walls (*red arrows*).

PHPT (**Fig. 13**).[53] However, developments in minimally invasive surgical techniques now allow endocrine surgeons to target single parathyroid glands with equally effective procedures using smaller incisions and resulting in shorter operating times, shorter hospitalizations, and decreased costs.[53,54] Effective minimally invasive surgery, however, requires accurate preoperative localization of a presumed single parathyroid adenoma. Novel imaging techniques including 4D CT and fused single-photon emission computed tomography/computed tomography (SPECT/CT) can accurately localize parathyroid adenomas, allowing the surgeon to effectively take a minimally invasive surgical approach.[55,56] Bilateral neck exploration is still necessary for the scenario of

multiglandular disease or nonlocalization of an adenoma on preoperative imaging. Imaging does not play a role in the routine postoperative follow-up of these patients and is typically only used in cases of failed parathyroidectomy whereby the patients may require a subsequent surgery.[57]

Patients with recurrent PHPT despite surgical therapy or who are poor surgical candidates may also undergo US-guided percutaneous ethanol ablation of the parathyroid tissue/glands for control of their hypercalcemia. This procedure has been shown to be safe and effective for the control of hypercalcemia in these challenging clinical situations, and although recurrent hypercalcemia is common, subsequent re-ablations can be safely performed.[58,59] Parathyroid adenomas are

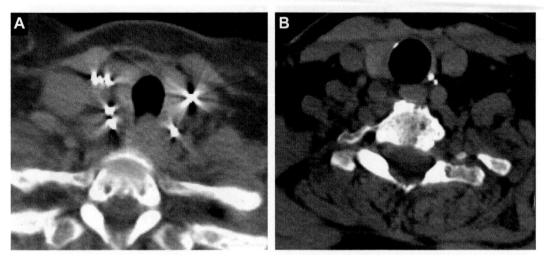

Fig. 13. Patient with PHPT with bilateral neck explorations and 3-gland resection. Axial CT (*A*) shows multiple surgical clips bilaterally related to prior gland resection. Second patient with left parathyroidectomy for hyperparathyroidism (*B*). Incidental note of left hemithyroidectomy for papillary thyroid carcinoma in the second patient.

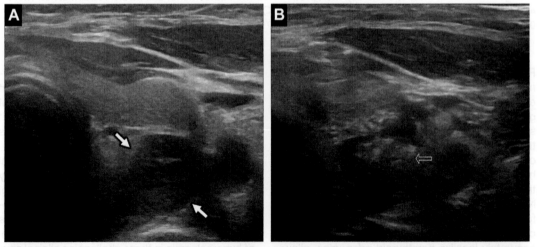

Fig. 14. Patient with prior failed parathyroidectomies, multiple medical comorbidities precluding subsequent parathyroid surgery. US image (*A*) showing a hypoechoic left superior parathyroid adenoma (*white arrows*). Ethanol ablation of the lesion was performed with postprocedure image (*B*) showing increased echogenicity of the lesion (*black arrow*) related to the alcohol injection.

typically hypoechoic on US, and after ethanol ablation, the lesion will seem more hyperechoic (Fig. 14).

SUMMARY

Disorders of the thyroid and parathyroid glands are fairly common and are frequently imaged after treatment. Multiple imaging modalities including US, CT, MRI, and nuclear medicine studies are used in the evaluation of these patients. Knowledge of the expected posttreatment appearance of these conditions as well as potential complications of these treatments will allow the interpreting radiologist to make timely and accurate diagnoses and contribute to the care of these patients.

CLINICS CARE POINTS

- Papillary thyroid carcinoma is by far the most common subtype of thyroid cancer, accounding for greater than 80% of cases.

- Imaging is an important part of post-treatment thyroid cancer surveillance and ultrasound is the most frequently employed modality.

- Thyroid cancer recurrence typically appears as a hypoechoic nodule with internal vascularity on ultrasound.

- Advanced modalities including CT, MRI, and PET/CT may be utilized as problem-solving tools in cases of more aggressive disease.

- Retropharyngeal nodal disease is an unusual but not uncommonly seen pattern of spread seen with recurrent thyroid cancer, particularly in those patients with a history of prior neck dissection.

- Imaging does not play a routine role in the post-treatment follow-up of thyroid dysfunction or hyperparathyroidism.

DISCLOSURE

The authors have nothing to disclose.

REFERENCES

1. SEER Cancer Stat Facts: Thyroid Cancer. National Cancer Institute. Bethesda, MD, Available at: https://seer.cancer.gov/statfacts/html/thyro.html. Accessed April 27, 2021.

2. Davies L, Welch HG. Current thyroid cancer trends in the United States. JAMA Otolaryngol Head Neck Surg 2014;140(4):317–22.

3. Aschebrook-Kilfoy B, Ward MH, Sabra MM, et al. Thyroid cancer incidence patterns in the United States by histologic type, 1992-2006. Thyroid 2011;21(2):125–34.

4. Ganeshan D, Paulson E, Duran C, et al. Current update on medullary thyroid carcinoma. AJR Am J Roentgenol 2013;201(6):W867–76.

5. Pacini F, Castagna MG, Cipri C, et al. Medullary thyroid carcinoma. Clin Oncol (R Coll Radiol) 2010; 22(6):475–85.

6. Eng C, Clayton D, Schuffenecker I, et al. The relationship between specific RET proto-oncogene mutations and disease phenotype in multiple endocrine neoplasia type 2. International RET mutation consortium analysis. Jama 1996;276(19): 1575–9.

7. Nagaiah G, Hossain A, Mooney CJ, et al. Anaplastic thyroid cancer: a review of epidemiology, pathogenesis, and treatment. J Oncol 2011;2011:542358.

8. Burns WR, Zeiger MA. Differentiated thyroid cancer. Semin Oncol 2010;37(6):557–66.

9. Adam MA, Pura J, Gu L, et al. Extent of surgery for papillary thyroid cancer is not associated with survival: an analysis of 61,775 patients. Ann Surg 2014;260(4):601–5.

10. Nixon IJ, Ganly I, Patel SG, et al. Thyroid lobectomy for treatment of well differentiated intrathyroid malignancy. Surgery 2012;151(4):571–9.

11. Vaisman F, Shaha A, Fish S, et al. Initial therapy with either thyroid lobectomy or total thyroidectomy without radioactive iodine remnant ablation is associated with very low rates of structural disease recurrence in properly selected patients with differentiated thyroid cancer. Clin Endocrinol (Oxf) 2011;75(1):112–9.

12. Haugen BR, Alexander EK, Bible KC, et al. 2015 American Thyroid Association Management Guidelines for Adult Patients with Thyroid Nodules and Differentiated Thyroid Cancer: The American Thyroid Association Guidelines Task Force on Thyroid Nodules and Differentiated Thyroid Cancer. Thyroid 2016;26(1):1–133.

13. Jeannon JP, Orabi AA, Bruch GA, et al. Diagnosis of recurrent laryngeal nerve palsy after thyroidectomy: a systematic review. Int J Clin Pract 2009;63(4): 624–9.

14. Patel KN, Yip L, Lubitz CC, et al. The American Association of Endocrine Surgeons Guidelines for the definitive surgical management of thyroid disease in adults. Ann Surg 2020;271(3):e21–93.

15. Vachha BA, Ginat DT, Mallur P, et al. "Finding a Voice": imaging features after phonosurgical procedures for vocal fold paralysis. AJNR Am J Neuroradiol 2016;37(9):1574–80.

16. Aiken AH. Imaging of thyroid cancer. Semin Ultrasound CT MR 2012;33(2):138–49.

17. Johnson NA, Tublin ME. Postoperative surveillance of differentiated thyroid carcinoma: rationale, techniques, and controversies. Radiology 2008;249(2):429–44.

18. Frasoldati A, Pesenti M, Gallo M, et al. Diagnosis of neck recurrences in patients with differentiated thyroid carcinoma. Cancer 2003;97(1):90–6.

19. Mazzaferri EL, Jhiang SM. Long-term impact of initial surgical and medical therapy on papillary and follicular thyroid cancer. Am J Med 1994; 97(5):418–28.

20. Kamaya A, Gross M, Akatsu H, et al. Recurrence in the thyroidectomy bed: sonographic findings. AJR Am J Roentgenol 2011;196(1):66–70.

21. Ko MS, Lee JH, Shong YK, et al. Normal and abnormal sonographic findings at the thyroidectomy sites in postoperative patients with thyroid malignancy. AJR Am J Roentgenol 2010;194(6): 1596–609.

22. Kumbhar SS, O'Malley RB, Robinson TJ, et al. Why Thyroid Surgeons Are Frustrated with Radiologists: Lessons Learned from Pre- and Postoperative US. Radiographics 2016;36(7):2141–53.

23. Fatourechi V, Hay ID, Mullan BP, et al. Are posttherapy radioiodine scans informative and do they influence subsequent therapy of patients with differentiated thyroid cancer? Thyroid 2000;10(7): 573–7.

24. Souza Rosário PW, Barroso AL, Rezende LL, et al. Post I-131 therapy scanning in patients with thyroid carcinoma metastases: an unnecessary cost or a relevant contribution? Clin Nucl Med 2004;29(12): 795–8.

25. Grewal RK, Tuttle RM, Fox J, et al. The effect of posttherapy 131I SPECT/CT on risk classification and management of patients with differentiated thyroid cancer. J Nucl Med 2010;51(9):1361–7.

26. Maruoka Y, Abe K, Baba S, et al. Incremental diagnostic value of SPECT/CT with 131I scintigraphy after radioiodine therapy in patients with well-differentiated thyroid carcinoma. Radiology 2012; 265(3):902–9.

27. Pacini F, Molinaro E, Castagna MG, et al. Recombinant human thyrotropin-stimulated serum thyroglobulin combined with neck ultrasonography has the highest sensitivity in monitoring differentiated thyroid carcinoma. J Clin Endocrinol Metab 2003;88(8): 3668–73.

28. Padovani RP, Kasamatsu TS, Nakabashi CC, et al. One month is sufficient for urinary iodine to return to its baseline value after the use of water-soluble iodinated contrast agents in post-thyroidectomy patients requiring radioiodine therapy. Thyroid 2012; 22(9):926–30.

29. Gross ND, Weissman JL, Talbot JM, et al. MRI detection of cervical metastasis from differentiated thyroid carcinoma. Laryngoscope 2001;111(11 Pt 1):1905–9.

30. Kaplan SL, Mandel SJ, Muller R, et al. The role of MR imaging in detecting nodal disease in thyroidectomy patients with rising thyroglobulin levels. AJNR Am J Neuroradiol 2009;30(3):608–12.

31. Takashima S, Sone S, Takayama F, et al. Papillary thyroid carcinoma: MR diagnosis of lymph node metastasis. AJNR Am J Neuroradiol 1998;19(3): 509–13.

32. Toubert ME, Cyna-Gorse F, Zagdanski AM, et al. Cervicomediastinal magnetic resonance imaging in persistent or recurrent papillary thyroid carcinoma: clinical use and limits. Thyroid 1999;9(6):591–7.

33. Wang J, Takashima S, Matsushita T, et al. Esophageal invasion by thyroid carcinomas: prediction using magnetic resonance imaging. J Comput Assist Tomogr 2003;27(1):18–25.

34. Wang JC, Takashima S, Takayama F, et al. Tracheal invasion by thyroid carcinoma: prediction using MR imaging. AJR Am J Roentgenol 2001;177(4):929–36.

35. Harries V, McGill M, Tuttle RM, et al. Management of Retropharyngeal Lymph Node Metastases in Differentiated Thyroid Carcinoma. Thyroid 2020;30(5): 688–95.

36. Otsuki N, Nishikawa T, Iwae S, et al. Retropharyngeal node metastasis from papillary thyroid carcinoma. Head Neck 2007;29(5):508–11.

37. Hartl DM, Leboulleux S, Vélayoudom-Céphise FL, et al. Management of retropharyngeal node metastases from thyroid carcinoma. World J Surg 2015; 39(5):1274–81.

38. Togashi T, Sugitani I, Toda K, et al. Surgical management of retropharyngeal nodes metastases from papillary thyroid carcinoma. World J Surg 2014; 38(11):2831–7.

39. Wang XL, Xu ZG, Wu YH, et al. Surgical management of parapharyngeal lymph node metastasis of thyroid carcinoma: a retrospective study of 25 patients. Chin Med J (Engl) 2012;125(20):3635–9.

40. Marcus C, Whitworth PW, Surasi DS, et al. PET/CT in the management of thyroid cancers. AJR Am J Roentgenol 2014;202(6):1316–29.

41. Shammas A, Degirmenci B, Mountz JM, et al. 18F-FDG PET/CT in patients with suspected recurrent or metastatic well-differentiated thyroid cancer. J Nucl Med 2007;48(2):221–6.

42. Chung JK, So Y, Lee JS, et al. Value of FDG PET in papillary thyroid carcinoma with negative 131I whole-body scan. J Nucl Med 1999;40(6):986–92.

43. Dong MJ, Liu ZF, Zhao K, et al. Value of 18F-FDG-PET/PET-CT in differentiated thyroid carcinoma with radioiodine-negative whole-body scan: a meta-analysis. Nucl Med Commun 2009;30(8):639–50.

44. Miller ME, Chen Q, Elashoff D, et al. Positron emission tomography and positron emission tomography-CT evaluation for recurrent papillary thyroid carcinoma: meta-analysis and literature review. Head Neck 2011;33(4):562–5.

45. Wang W, Macapinlac H, Larson SM, et al. [18F]-2-fluoro-2-deoxy-D-glucose positron emission tomography localizes residual thyroid cancer in patients with negative diagnostic (131)I whole body scans and elevated serum thyroglobulin levels. J Clin Endocrinol Metab 1999;84(7):2291–302.

46. Canaris GJ, Manowitz NR, Mayor G, et al. The Colorado thyroid disease prevalence study. Arch Intern Med 2000;160(4):526–34.

47. Hollowell JG, Staehling NW, Flanders WD, et al. Serum TSH, T(4), and thyroid antibodies in the United States population (1988 to 1994): National Health and Nutrition Examination Survey (NHANES III). J Clin Endocrinol Metab 2002;87(2):489–99.

48. Ross DS, Burch HB, Cooper DS, et al. 2016 American Thyroid Association Guidelines for Diagnosis and Management of Hyperthyroidism and Other Causes of Thyrotoxicosis. Thyroid 2016;26(10):1343–421.

49. Brent GA. Clinical practice. Graves' disease. N Engl J Med 2008;358(24):2594–605.

50. Tanda ML, Piantanida E, Liparulo L, et al. Prevalence and natural history of Graves' orbitopathy in a large series of patients with newly diagnosed graves' hyperthyroidism seen at a single center. J Clin Endocrinol Metab 2013;98(4):1443–9.

51. Jefferis JM, Jones RK, Currie ZI, et al. Orbital decompression for thyroid eye disease: methods, outcomes, and complications. Eye (Lond) 2018;32(3):626–36.

52. Fraser WD. Hyperparathyroidism. Lancet 2009;374(9684):145–58.

53. Wilhelm SM, Wang TS, Ruan DT, et al. The American Association of Endocrine Surgeons Guidelines for Definitive Management of Primary Hyperparathyroidism. JAMA Surg 2016;151(10):959–68.

54. Minisola S, Cipriani C, Diacinti D, et al. Imaging of the parathyroid glands in primary hyperparathyroidism. Eur J Endocrinol 2016;174(1):D1–8.

55. Bunch PM, Kelly HR. Preoperative Imaging Techniques in Primary Hyperparathyroidism: A Review. JAMA Otolaryngol Head Neck Surg 2018;144(10):929–37.

56. Bunch PM, Randolph GW, Brooks JA, et al. Parathyroid 4D CT: What the Surgeon Wants to Know. Radiographics 2020;40(5):1383–94.

57. Johnson NA, Tublin ME, Ogilvie JB. Parathyroid imaging: technique and role in the preoperative evaluation of primary hyperparathyroidism. AJR Am J Roentgenol 2007;188(6):1706–15.

58. Singh Ospina N, Thompson GB, Lee RA, et al. Safety and efficacy of percutaneous parathyroid ethanol ablation in patients with recurrent primary hyperparathyroidism and multiple endocrine neoplasia type 1. J Clin Endocrinol Metab 2015;100(1):E87–90.

59. Veldman MW, Reading CC, Farrell MA, et al. Percutaneous parathyroid ethanol ablation in patients with multiple endocrine neoplasia type 1. AJR Am J Roentgenol 2008;191(6):1740–4.

Imaging of the Postoperative Skull Base and Cerebellopontine Angle

Jeffrey Xi Yang, MD, Nafi Aygun, MD, Rohini Narahari Nadgir, MD*

KEYWORDS

- Cerebellopontine angle • Anterior craniofacial resection • Transsphenoidal • Postsurgical
- Postoperative • Skull base

KEY POINTS

- Knowledge regarding various approaches of skull base surgery, expected postoperative appearance, and common postsurgical complications can guide radiologic interpretation.
- Although there are predictable imaging changes following surgery, it is difficult to differentiate treatment change and residual disease at a single time point and immediate postsurgical imaging and follow-up imaging are often complementary.
- CSF leak is a common complication of skull base surgery. Other complications shared by multiple types of surgical approaches include infarct, vascular injury/thrombosis, and infection.

INTRODUCTION

For many pathologic conditions affecting the skull base and cerebellopontine angle (CPA), surgery is part of the treatment process. As surgical techniques and approaches have evolved through the years, imaging techniques have also advanced in a parallel manner to assess for residual disease, disease progression, and postoperative complications.[1] Complexity of skull base anatomy, small size of the relevant structures, lack of familiarity with surgical techniques, and postsurgical changes can confound radiologic evaluation. This article discusses the imaging techniques, surgical approaches, expected postoperative changes, and complications after surgery of the skull base, with emphasis on the CPA, anterior cranial fossa, and central skull base regions.

IMAGING TECHNIQUES

Computed tomography (CT) and MR imaging are mainstays in the imaging of the skull base and CPA. Modern multislice CT scanners can acquire images as thin as 0.5 mm with multiplanar evaluation in axial, coronal, sagittal, and oblique planes. CT covering the mastoid bones, temporal bones, and skull base without the administration of intravenous contrast is performed in postoperative assessment, primarily for evaluation of the bony integrity of the reconstructed skull base. In particular, CT can evaluate for osseous defects in cases of suspected cerebrospinal fluid (CSF) leak.[2] In cases where site of leak remains uncertain, CT imaging following injection of intrathecal contrast (CT cisternography) can aid in detection of subtle CSF leak, evidenced by abnormal accumulation of hyperattenuating CSF in the suspected anatomic compartment. CT angiography may be used in the emergency setting for assessment of intraoperative vascular injury or thrombosis, performed with bolus contrast injection in arterial and/or venous phase. Evaluation of the vasculature is enhanced with multiplanar maximum intensity projection and three-dimensional (3D) rotational reconstructions. When time is of the essence, conventional catheter angiography may be

The authors have no disclosures relevant to this article.

Division of Neuroradiology, Department of Radiology and Radiological Science, Johns Hopkins Hospital, 600 North Wolfe Street, Baltimore, MD 21287, USA

* Corresponding author.

E-mail address: rnadgir1@jhmi.edu

initiated instead of CT angiography for diagnosis and treatment purposes, including embolization or vessel sacrifice.

MR imaging is superior to CT for the evaluation of soft tissue lesions, with contrast-enhanced CT an alternative for patients with contraindications to MR imaging.[1] Whenever possible, this is done with higher magnetic strength at 3 T for improved soft tissue discrimination.[2] In addition to routine brain imaging, small field of view T1 precontrast and fat-suppressed T1 postcontrast sequences are obtained centered on the region of interest, be it the sella/central skull base, temporal bones, or orbit/face. Dedicated T2 images without and/or with fat suppression are also helpful in the postoperative analysis.

High-resolution precontrast and postcontrast T1 and T2 3D MR imaging of the skull base are especially helpful in identifying anatomic structures of the skull base because they provide excellent signal to noise ratio and high spatial resolution.[3,4] Typical 3D protocol involves precontrast and postcontrast T1 and T2 image acquisition with a slice thickness of 0.6 mm, matrix of 256 × 256, and field of view of 16.9 × 24.6.[5] 3D volumetric acquisition of the skull base is performed to encompass the region of interest, with subsequent creation of isotopic multiplanar reconstructions. Heavily T2-weighted images, such as constructive interference in steady-state (CISS, Siemens) or FIESTA (GE), provide excellent anatomic detail with respect to structures of interest and surrounding CSF fluid. 3D T1-weighted, non–fat saturated images before the administration of contrast allows for evaluation of intrinsic T1 signal.[6] Postcontrast T1 (MPRAGE or VIBE) and T2 images can help distinguish vessels, nerves, and pathologic tissue enhancement. Heavy T2 weighting also allows for detection of CSF with delineation of small skull base defects and areas of CSF leakage.[4,7] A 3D T2-weighted sequence with fat saturation, such as short tau inversion recovery, has the benefit for detecting intrinsic T2 signal abnormalities.[6]

Steady-state free precession, such as CISS, is limited by banding artifacts that present as linear bands of low signal that are most evident at the air-tissue interfaces caused by field inhomogeneities. Banding artifacts are ameliorated by alternating the field of the radiofrequency pulse by 180° and by keeping TR as low as possible.[8]

SURGICAL TECHNIQUES
Cerebellopontine Angle

Vestibular schwannomas are the most common intracranial tumor involving the CPA cistern, accounting for approximately 80% of all tumors in this location. Meningiomas and epidermoids account for a smaller percentage of tumors in the CPA, making up approximately 10% and 6%, respectively.[9] Other tumors of the CPA can include petroclival masses, such as chondrosarcoma, endolymphatic sac tumors, and paragangliomas. Excision of these lesions is the treatment of choice, by translabyrinthine, retrosigmoid (suboccipital), and middle cranial fossa approaches depending on the tumor size, location, patient's hearing status, and preference of the operating surgeon.[10] Similar approaches are considered with debulking of infectious or inflammatory diseases in these locations. In patients with trigeminal neuralgia, the retrosigmoid approach is used for microvascular decompression of the trigeminal nerve.

Translabyrinthine resection is preferred when the lesion is within the labyrinthine and cochlear structures, and in cases of larger CPA tumors. This approach involves a total mastoidectomy and labyrinthectomy with resection of the semicircular canals and portions of the vestibule with placement of a triangular fat graft over the mastoidectomy bed (Fig. 1). Hearing ability is often sacrificed during the surgery so this approach may also be used in cases of existing pronounced ipsilateral hearing loss.[10–12] The ossicles are sometimes removed and packing material, such as fat, fascia, or fibrin, is placed in the middle ear to limit occurrence of CSF leak.[11,13]

The retrosigmoid/suboccipital approach involves craniotomy or craniectomy with cranioplasty and dural incision from the superior margin of the transverse sinus to the sigmoid sinus ventrally (Fig. 2). The posterior mastoid air cells are often violated, but are promptly sealed with bone wax to prevent CSF leak. The posterior wall of the internal auditory canal (IAC) may be resected with or without internal labyrinthectomy to access the IAC fundus.[11–13] In the setting of trigeminal neuralgia, the retrosigmoid approach facilitates microvascular decompression of the trigeminal nerve in which a piece of shredded Teflon is placed between the offending vessel and the nerve (Fig. 3).[14]

A temporal craniotomy is performed for the middle cranial fossa approach resection with dissection of the dura over the petrous ridge and middle cranial fossa. The temporal lobe is then carefully retracted superiorly with a narrow exposure of the CPA cistern to limit the risk of temporal lobe injury.[12,13] Bone around the IAC is removed and the roof of the IAC is exposed.[13]

Anterior Craniofacial Resection

Most malignant tumors of the anterior skull base including squamous cell carcinoma, sinonasal

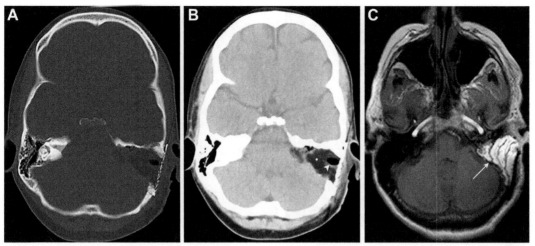

Fig. 1. Translabyrinthine resection. (*A*) Axial noncontrast CT image in bone window after translabyrinthine approach resection of vestibular schwannoma shows large left mastoidectomy defect with surgical absence of the internal auditory canal and semicircular canals and mesh cranioplasty hardware overlying the bone defect. (*B*) Soft tissue windows show fat attenuation within the fat graft at the resection site (*asterisk*). Small focus of residual gas is present within the graft in the immediate postoperative period (*arrowhead*). (*C*) Axial T1 unenhanced MR image in a different patient shows expected intrinsic T1 hyperintense fat graft material over the surgical bed (*arrow*).

undifferentiated carcinoma, adenocarcinoma, and esthesioneuroblastoma arise from the sinonasal cavity. The anterior skull base may also be involved through local invasion from tumors of the face, scalp, or orbits. Malignant tumors of the paranasal sinuses and nasal cavity account for 3% of head and neck tumors, with tumors of the ethmoid sinuses comprising 20% to 30% of paranasal sinus malignancies.[15] Surgery remains the gold standard for treatment. Ethmoid tumors

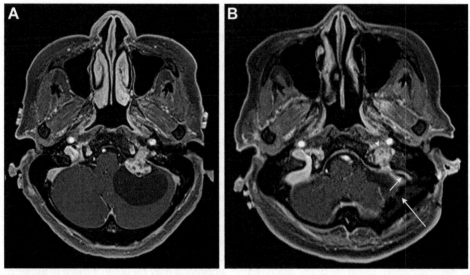

Fig. 2. Transmastoid/suboccipital approach for schwannoma resection. (*A*) Axial preoperative T1 fat-suppressed postcontrast axial image demonstrates an enhancing solid and cystic mass centered in the left jugular foramen projecting into the left cerebellar hemisphere. (*B*) Postoperative T1 fat-suppressed postcontrast axial image shows expected changes following tumor resection, including mesh cranioplasty hardware, extra-axial fluid, and air deep to the mesh (*long arrow*). After retrosigmoid resection, there is residual enhancing tumor in the jugular foramen (*arrowhead*), reactive dural-based enhancement, and nonocclusive filling defect consistent with thrombus within the left sigmoid sinus (*short arrow*).

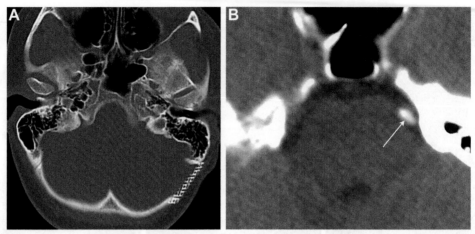

Fig. 3. Teflon graft. Axial noncontrast CT images following neurovascular decompression for left trigeminal neuralgia after left retrosigmoid approach with mesh cranioplasty (*A*) show hyperdense Teflon graft (*B*) inserted in the cerebellopontine angle between the trigeminal nerve and superior cerebellar artery (*arrow*).

invariably encroach on the cribriform plate, and anterior craniofacial resection is usually required for complete tumor resection.[15,16] This approach can also be taken for skull base revision following extensive craniofacial trauma or for surgical debridement of complex infections, such as in cases of acute sinusitis complicated by anterior frontal osteomyelitis and subperiosteal abscess (Pott puffy tumor).

Anterior craniofacial resection involves a combination of transcranial and transfacial techniques and is often combined with endonasal endoscopic approaches. The transcranial component is typically initiated with a bicoronal incision and low frontal craniotomy. The transfacial approach involves a lateral rhinotomy incision that is extended into a radical maxillectomy if more extensive maxillary resection is necessary.[16–18] Orbital exenteration may be performed if there is orbital tumor infiltration on preoperative imaging and vision is not salvageable. The anterior craniofacial technique allows exposure of the epidural space, sinonasal cavity, and anterior cranial fossa, allowing en bloc radical resection and has evolved to be the standard of care in anterior skull base malignancies.[18] In cases with dural or intradural involvement, the tumor is resected with microsurgical technique with placement of a dural patch graft. After resection, the floor of the anterior cranial fossa is reconstructed using a graft, such as metallic mesh, pedicled pericranial flap, osseous graft, or free flap.[11,16,18] In cases of extensive trauma, tumor, or infection involving the frontal sinuses, the frontal sinuses are often cranialized during surgery. This involves resection of the posterior wall of the frontal sinuses with removal of the sinus mucosa so that the frontal lobe dura lies adjacent to the floor and outer table of the frontal sinus, often accompanied by pericranial flap placement (**Fig. 4**).[19]

Transsphenoidal and Pterional Surgery

Endoscopic endonasal transsphenoidal approach surgery (**Fig. 5**) is a minimally invasive technique for the resection of sellar and parasellar tumors, and has been the standard surgical treatment of pituitary adenomas for decades. The technique can also be modified for the resection of other pathologies, such as anterior cranial fossa meningiomas and clival chordomas, with expanded transcribiform, transplanum, transsellar, and transclival approaches to gain a surgical window into the anterior cranial fossa, suprasellar space, or clivus.[20,21]

There are several traditional endonasal approaches that are considered for sellar surgery, including paraseptal, middle turbinectomy, and middle meatal approaches. In the paraseptal approach, a surgical window is created by fracturing and displacing the nasal septum and middle turbinate laterally from the ventral wall of the sphenoid sinus. The middle turbinectomy approach involves resection of the lower middle turbinate to open a narrowed nasal cavity. A middle meatal approach may be taken if there is tumor predominantly in the lateral sella or cavernous sinus with the surgical corridor between the middle turbinate and lateral nasal cavity wall.[20]

Once the rostrum of the sphenoid sinus is exposed, anterior sphenoidotomy is performed. A sphenoid septectomy is performed with osseous

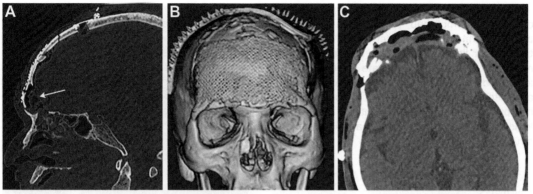

Fig. 4. Anterior craniofacial reconstruction. (*A*) Sagittal noncontrast CT and (*B*) 3D surface-rendered reconstructions of the skull and facial bones demonstrate craniofacial reconstruction following traumatic injury to the anterior skull base. These images show near anatomic alignment of the mesh cranioplasty with the native skull, and there is postoperative air subjacent to the new hardware. There has been cranialization of the frontal sinuses, with surgical absence of the posterior wall of the frontal sinuses (*arrow in A*). (*C*) On soft tissue windows, the cranialized appearance of the frontal sinuses is again shown, along with postoperative emphysema and pericranial flap placement within the reconstructed frontal sinuses.

fragments saved for later sellar reconstruction. The anterior sella wall is then located and opened. After tumor resection is completed, microdissective resection is performed at the interface of the tumor with normal pituitary tissue. A fat graft is then harvested from the periumbilical region and is placed in the resection bed in the situation of a large resection cavity or if intraoperative CSF leak is suspected. The anterior wall of the sella is then reconstructed using the previous saved fragments of bone. The anterior sellar reconstruction is supported with packing of the sphenoid sinuses

with absorbable gelatin sponge.[20–22] Other sealant materials include titanium mesh and DuraGen.[11,23] A vascular pedicle nasal septal mucoperiosteal flap covering the defect has helped decrease the incidence of CSF leaks in recent years. The flap is placed over fat or directly onto the dura, with graft fixation using a biologic glue, and nasal packing or a Foley balloon holding the balloon in place.[24]

Similar to clipping of anterior circulation aneurysms, a pterional approach resection is sometimes used for removal or biopsy of suprasellar

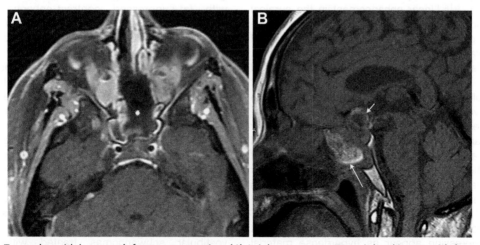

Fig. 5. Transsphenoidal approach for tumor resection. (*A*) Axial postcontrast T1-weighted image with fat suppression obtained following resection of planum sphenoidale meningioma shows transsphenoidal surgical approach, with resection of nasal septum and sphenoidotomy defect, fluid filled in the immediate postoperative setting (*asterisk*). (*B*) Sagittal T1-weighted image following pituitary adenoma resection shows focal defect at the anterior sella wall, with T1 hyperintense fat packing material in the sphenoid sinus (*long arrow*). T1 hyperintense blood products are present within the suprasellar surgical cavity (*short arrow*).

and parasellar lesions. After frontotemporal craniotomy is accomplished, retraction of the frontal and temporal lobes is preceded by opening of the anterior limb of the sylvian fissure, reducing retraction needed for adequate exposure. The arachnoid layers over the ipsilateral optic nerve and carotid artery dissected and the contralateral neurovascular structure are identified and pathologic tissue is carefully dissected away from these structures.[25]

EXPECTED POSTOPERATIVE IMAGING FINDINGS

General expected postsurgical changes after skull base tumor resection include scalp edema and subcutaneous emphysema, manifest as high T2 signal over the craniotomy site with scattered foci of susceptibility on MR imaging. Diffusion restriction along the margins of the surgical tract is seen, representing postoperative cytotoxic edema. Heterogeneous intensity material is visualized in the resection cavity, which can represent a combination of postsurgical hemorrhage, air, and packing material. T2 hyperintense extra-axial fluid collections are seen subjacent to the craniotomy site or over the brain convexities.

Cerebellopontine Angle

In the CPA, there is a characteristic flattened appearance of the lateral margin of the cerebellar hemisphere with prominence of the adjacent T2 hyperintense extra-axial CSF space as a result of retrosigmoid entry and cerebellar retraction (**Fig. 6**).[11,12] Linear enhancement in the surgical bed on early postoperative imaging is almost always present, likely reflecting a combination of granulation tissue and reactive dural thickening. Nodular enhancement is suspicious for residual tumor especially with subsequent enlargement on follow-up imaging, whereas postoperative reactive enhancement remains stable or decreases over time (**Fig. 7**).[12,13,26] For vestibular schwannoma resection via retrosigmoid approach, the IAC fundus is a frequent blind spot and therefore this area should be scrutinized for residual tumor. Residual tumor may sometimes be intentionally left behind for functional preservation of the facial nerve.[13,27]

Teflon grafts used in trigeminal neuralgia decompression appear as hyperdense material on CT. Rhizotomy is performed for trigeminal neuralgia, with postsurgical imaging exhibiting clumping, atrophy, and/or mild enhancement of the treated prepontine segment trigeminal nerve (**Fig. 8**).[28]

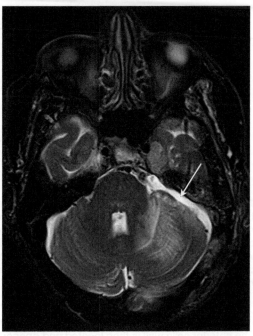

Fig. 6. Retrosigmoid approach tumor resection. Postsurgical axial fat-saturated T2 image after left suboccipital resection of a cerebellopontine angle meningioma shows a characteristic flattened appearance of the left cerebellar convexity with prominence of the overlying CSF space (*arrow*) and edema in the left cerebellar hemisphere.

Different surgical grafts can contribute to variable patterns of enhancement in the postsurgical setting. Fat grafts are best evaluated with fat-suppressed contrast-enhanced T1-weighted images, appearing as T1 hyperintense material that can enhance. Graft enhancement usually decreases over time because of tissue atrophy and fibrosis. Fat grafts can sometimes undergo necrosis with cystic change.[26] Rarely, disintegration and spread of the fat graft into the subarachnoid space can result in a lipoid meningitis.[11,12]

Stereotactic radiosurgery (SRS) is an alternative method for treating vestibular schwannomas, which involves administering high-concentrated doses of photon radiation to the residual lesion from multiple angles. Because of internal edema, 30% to 40% of lesions may temporarily increase in size immediately following SRS.[12,27] Most vestibular schwannomas treated with SRS decrease or remain stable in size on serial follow-up imaging. Central decreased enhancement is identified within 6 months after SRS. Cystic degeneration can occur in approximately 30% of cases within 1 year of treatment.[27]

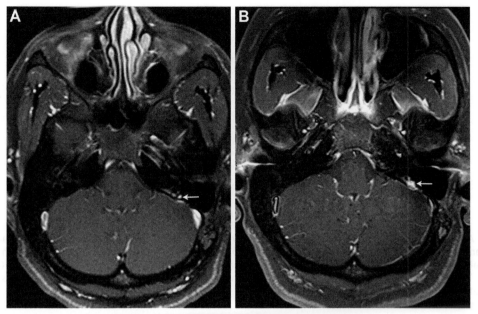

Fig. 7. Recurrent tumor. Postcontrast axial fat saturated T1-weighted images performed 1.5 years (*A*) and 4 years (*B*) after retrolabyrinthine resection of an endolymphatic sac tumor show enlargement of an enhancing focus along the posterior left temporal bone (*arrows*), suspicious for recurrent tumor.

Anterior Craniofacial Resection

Postsurgical MR imaging is generally obtained after surgery for its superior ability to discern various types of soft tissue following craniofacial reconstruction (**Fig. 9**). CT is useful in the immediate postoperative setting to evaluate for alignment of mesh and cranioplasty material with the native calvarium, often demonstrating scalp swelling and extra-axial air and fluid overlying the frontal lobes (see **Fig. 4**). On MR imaging, soft tissue is seen in the superior nasal cavity

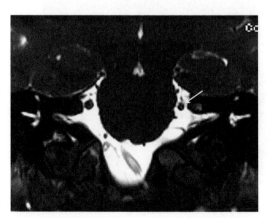

Fig. 8. Left rhizotomy for trigeminal neuralgia. Coronal CISS image shows expected postsurgical finding of diminished caliber of the prepontine segment of the left trigeminal nerve (*arrow*).

with variable signal intensity depending on the different graft materials used during the resection. Enhancing soft tissue is invariably present in the upper nasal cavity, usually representing granulation tissue, with serial follow-up imaging necessary to exclude residual disease.[29] Smooth enhancement along the floor of the anterior cranial fossa is seen with vascularized pericranial flaps used in the reconstruction of the anterior cranial fossa floor.[11]

Transsphenoidal and Pterional Surgery

Intraoperative MR imaging is occasionally implemented to assess for completeness of tumor resection during transsphenoidal surgery, with the option of additional resection after a second look of the operative bed. Evaluation is limited by drill artifacts from tiny metallic debris deposited from the surgical drill bit with susceptibility along the surgical tract, although this has improved with the introduction of porcelain-coated drills. Prominent blood products in the resection cavity can also obscure evaluation of residual tumor intraoperatively.[30]

Early postoperative MR imaging can show a surgical cavity of similar size to the presurgical sellar or suprasellar mass, albeit with different signal characteristics (**Fig. 10**). The cavity is uniformly fluid signal or with more heterogeneous signal intensity compared with preoperative imaging, which can represent a combination of postsurgical

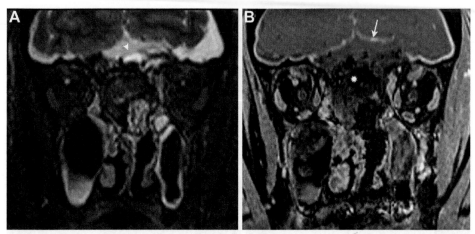

Fig. 9. Anterior craniofacial resection. (*A*) Coronal FS T2-weighted image and postcontrast T1-weighted image (*B*) after anterior craniofacial resection of an esthesioneuroblastoma show fluid, air, and packing material in the si-nonasal cavity (*asterisk*) and a T2 hyperintense extra-axial fluid collection in the anterior cranial fossa (*arrow-head*). There is expected pachymeningeal enhancement (*arrow*) without nodular enhancement to suggest residual tumor.

hemorrhage, fluid, and fat graft. Hemorrhage can present with varying signal intensity depending on the oxygenation stage of hemoglobin; fluid-fluid levels are sometimes present. There is variable enhancement in the resection bed. As postoperative hemorrhage and fluid is absorbed, there is progressive shrinkage of the surgical cav-ity with resolved mass effect on the optic chiasm and inferior frontal lobes with increase in

enhancement because of postoperative granula-tion tissue that becomes most prominent within a few months after surgery, at the time of first follow-up imaging study. Fat grafts in the resection cavity are clearly delineated as T1 and T2 bright material and regress over the first year after sur-gery.[23,31,32] Nasoseptal flaps appear as C-shaped area of enhancement adjacent to the surgical bed, which can demonstrate thicker enhancement on

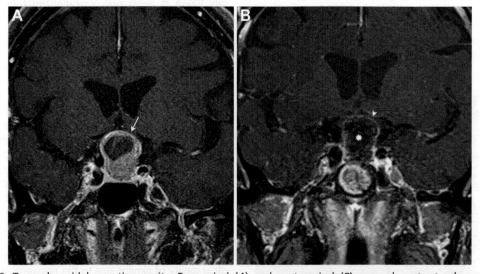

Fig. 10. Transsphenoidal resection cavity. Presurgical (*A*) and postsurgical (*B*) coronal contrast-enhanced T1-weighted images show an enhancing sellar/suprasellar pituitary adenoma impinging on the undersurface of the optic chiasm (*arrow*). Early after transsphenoidal resection, the resection cavity remains about the same size as the resected mass (*asterisk*), with absence of mass-like enhancement of the original tumor. There is persis-tent mass effect on the optic chiasm (*arrowhead*). These findings are expected, and size of the resection cavity and mass effect on the optic apparatus will decrease over time.

short-term follow-up MR imaging caused by increased vascularization (**Fig. 11**).[24]

It is difficult to discern normal pituitary tissue and pituitary infundibulum in the early postoperative setting, but the residual pituitary may be identified as tissue along the sellar floor or along the lateral sella adjacent to the cavernous sinus (**Fig. 12**). Precontrast T1-weighted images may show the bright posterior pituitary, if preserved, which can serve as a guide to the location of the anterior pituitary. Similarly, the infundibulum can point to the location of the residual anterior pituitary in the early postoperative setting. Subsequent follow-up MR imaging can show re-expansion of the normal pituitary gland, which can be mistaken for a recurrent mass. Careful comparison of early postoperative and first follow-up scans is necessary to resolve this issue. Endocrinologic evaluation is also helpful for the assessment of residual hormonally active pituitary adenomas.[23,31,32]

Although some argue, based on studies from 15 to 20 years ago, that routine acquisition of early postoperative MR imaging is not necessary, a recent study by Alhilali and colleagues[33] proposes that early MR imaging may have value because there is improved imaging quality with newer MR imaging techniques, such as high-resolution, fat-saturated, and volumetric imaging. In our opinion, early postoperative MR imaging performed within 48 hours of surgery is essential and serves as a baseline, particularly because of the frequent use of modern surgical hemostatic materials, such as GelFoam, which can incite enhancing granulation tissue after 3 months, leading to false positives on later MR imaging.[33]

POSTOPERATIVE COMPLICATIONS ON IMAGING
Cerebellopontine Angle

Prolonged retraction can result in diffusion restriction and ischemia acutely with atrophy of the cerebellar hemisphere on later follow-up imaging (**Fig. 13**). Middle cranial fossa approach resection with temporal lobe retraction can similarly lead to ischemia with temporal lobe atrophy and gliosis in the long-term, which can raise the risk of seizures.[13]

Early postsurgical complications of CPA surgery include CSF leak, meningitis, and vascular injury.[13,34] CSF leaks result from poor sealing of exposed mastoid air cells, poor wound closure, or increased intracranial pressure with no significant difference in incidence rates with different surgical approaches.[35] There is a wide range of postsurgical CSF leak rates ranging from 2% to 30%.[13] This can present as opacification of ipsilateral mastoid air cells and the middle ear cavity or as a pseudomeningocele adjacent to the craniotomy flap.[12,34] On CT, a focal osseous defect can reflect site of suspected leak. Correspondingly on MR imaging, T2 hyperintense meningeal or cerebral contents are visualized herniating through osseous defects. CT cisternography is sometimes used to diagnose occult CSF leaks, with extracranial extension of contrast demonstrated after cisternal injection of intrathecal contrast.

CSF leaks are also associated with an increased risk of postsurgical meningitis, prolonged hospital stay, and need for revision surgery.[27] Meningitis can result from direct infection in the surgical bed and contiguous spread of infection from superficial wound infection in the subcutaneous

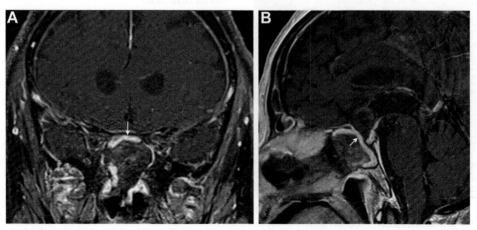

Fig. 11. Nasoseptal flap. Coronal FS postcontrast (*A*) and sagittal (*B*) T1-weighted images after transsphenoidal pituitary adenoma resection show an enhancing, C-shaped structure along the posterior margin and roof of the nasal cavity covering the sellar floor (*arrows*), compatible with a nasoseptal flap.

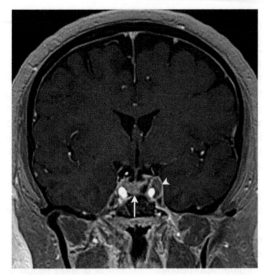

Fig. 12. Residual pituitary macroadenoma. Postsurgical contrast-enhanced coronal T1-weighted image shows residual tumor in the left cavernous sinus (*arrowhead*) after subtotal resection with normal enhancing pituitary tissue deviated to the right in the sella (*arrow*).

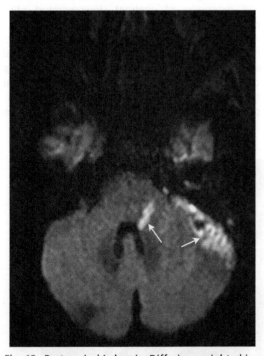

Fig. 13. Postsurgical ischemia. Diffusion-weighted image after left suboccipital resection shows diffusion restricting (ADC map not shown) cytotoxic edema in the left cerebellum and middle cerebellar peduncle from retraction and surgical manipulation (*arrows*).

soft tissues with intracranial extension. On MR imaging, meningitis appears as leptomeningeal enhancement with incomplete FLAIR suppression of CSF signal often with diffusion restriction in the affected sulci. If there is an associated organized infection, such a cerebral abscess or subdural empyema, it appears as a T2 hyperintense, peripherally enhancing fluid collection with internal diffusion restriction.

The most common vascular injury is dural sinus thrombosis (**Fig. 14**), which can occur after retraction or injury in the translabyrinthine and retrosigmoid approaches, with concomitant venous injury and parenchymal hemorrhage in a minority of cases.[12] The incidence rate was remarked to be 38.9% in a study of patients after translabyrinthine resection.[36] Arterial injury is rare, but the anterior inferior cerebellar artery is most at risk.[12,13]

Later complications of the CPA surgery include hearing loss and cerebellar and temporal lobe atrophy. The labyrinthine structures are difficult to identify in the retrosigmoid approach, increasing the risk of labyrinthine dehiscence, which presents with hearing loss.[15] Decreased signal in the labyrinthine structures on 3D CISS imaging is seen in the setting of membranous fenestration, microvascular injury to the cochlea, postsurgical hemorrhagic products, or labyrinthitis ossificans (**Fig. 15**).[12,13] An increase in T2 FLAIR signal in the labyrinthine structures can also be observed after vestibular schwannoma resection, possibly on the basis of increased protein content in endolymphatic fluid.[13] Enhancement of the labyrinthine structures can also be a sign of labyrinthitis ossificans and cochlear obliteration after surgery, which appears as sclerosis on CT. The translabyrinthine approach is associated with the highest incidence of cochlear obliteration after vestibular schwannoma resection.[37]

Anterior Craniofacial Resection

The most common postoperative complication is CSF leak.[16] This appears as a focal bony defect at the anterior skull base on CT and CSF signal at the site of defect on T2-weighted imaging can confirm the presence of leak (**Fig. 16**).

Pneumocephalus is also a frequent complication, appearing as intracranial air over the anterior frontal convexities. This is usually a benign entity of little to no clinical significance with self-resolution over time. Less commonly, air can be trapped intracranially from a "ball-valve" or "inverted pop bottle mechanism" leading to tension pneumocephalus and mass effect on the cerebral parenchyma, and is a life-threatening complication (**Fig. 17**).[38]

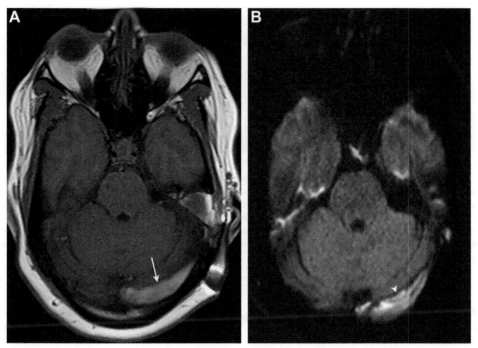

Fig. 14. Venous sinus thrombosis. (*A*) Axial noncontrast T1-weighted image after translabyrinthine schwannoma resection shows intrinsic high T1 signal in the left transverse sinus (*arrow*), indicating dural venous sinus thrombosis. (*B*) On diffusion-weighted imaging, there is corresponding diffusion restriction (ADC map not shown) along the course of the left transverse sinus (*arrowhead*) without ischemic change in the posterior fossa.

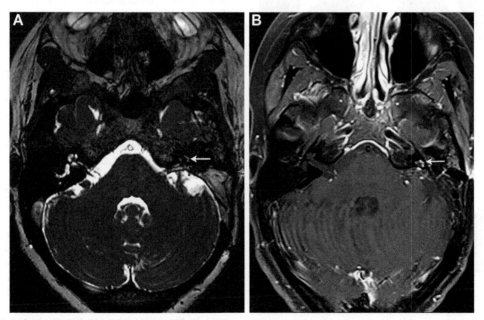

Fig. 15. Labyrinthitis. (*A*) Axial CISS and (*B*) postcontrast FS T1-weighted images 1 year after translabyrinthine vestibular schwannoma resection show loss of expected hyperintense signal and abnormal enhancement in the left cochlea (*arrows*), suggestive of labyrinthitis.

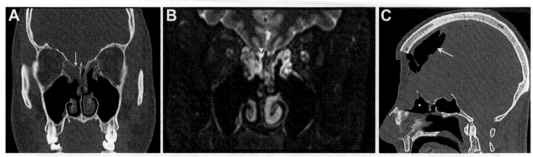

Fig. 16. Postoperative leak. (*A*) Coronal noncontrast CT and (*B*) T2-weighted MR imaging in a patient with CSF rhinorrhea after functional endoscopic sinus surgery reveals a focal defect in the right cribriform plate with adjacent fluid in the superior right ethmoid air cells and nasal cavity (*arrow*). On MR imaging, the right olfactory bulb is not well seen compared with the contralateral side (*arrowhead*) and may be herniated through this defect containing fluid contiguous with CSF. (*C*) Sagittal bone window CT in a different patient following anterior craniofacial reconstruction for skull base angiosarcoma resection shows air below the reconstructed skull base (*asterisk*) and extending over the frontal convexities (*arrow*), indicating air leak. Focal defects along the duroplasty are evident.

Meningitis and meningoencephalitis can result in leptomeningeal enhancement and signal changes in the subjacent frontal lobe parenchyma (**Fig. 18**). Frontal lobe ischemic change can sometimes be present on early postoperative imaging, depending on the degree of parenchymal retraction surgery. Encephaloceles can develop with brain tissue visualized herniating through a surgical osseous defect on MR imaging.[39,40]

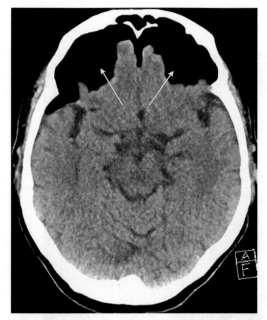

Fig. 17. Tension pneumocephalus. Axial noncontrast CT head after anterior craniofacial resection for nasal cavity melanoma shows extensive extra-axial pneumocephalus and mass effect over the bilateral frontal lobes (*arrows*) with a "Mount Fuji sign," suggestive of tension pneumocephalus.

Wound infections, epidural abscesses, and osteomyelitis of the bone flap are all potential complications of surgery. Wound and soft tissue infections are complicated by concomitant sinusitis. Some patients may develop nasocutaneous fistulas from wound infection and breakdown.

Transsphenoidal and Pterional Surgery

Similar to anterior craniofacial resection, CSF leak is the most common complication of transsphenoidal surgery, occurring at an incidence between 1% and 5%. It can occur with resection of pituitary microadenomas and larger macroadenomas, but seems to occur disproportionately in patients with larger tumors. If detected intraoperatively, this is repaired with fat or muscle grafting and fibrin glue. Low-volume CSF leakage and rhinorrhea noted postoperatively can sometimes resolve with lumbar drainage. Meningitis can also be a complication, occurring at an incidence between 0.4% and 2%, usually with a concomitant CSF leak that predisposes the patient to intracranial infection and is successfully treated with antibiotic therapy in most cases.[41–44]

Clinically significant intrasellar-suprasellar hemorrhage can present with progressively worsening vision and hematoma causing mass effect on imaging, often requiring surgical decompression.[42] Vascular injury can occur during the course of the surgery, because many vascular structures, such as the cavernous sinus, carotid arteries, anterior cerebral artery, anterior communicating artery, and their branches, course in close proximity to the sella. Injury to these structures can cause profuse intraoperative bleeding and delayed sequelae, such as pseudoaneurysm and

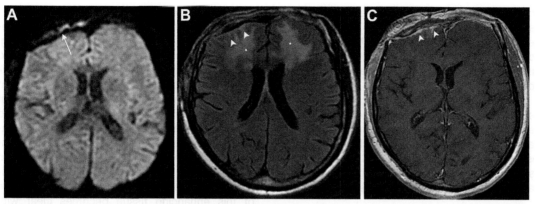

Fig. 18. Postsurgical infection. (*A*) Diffusion-weighted imaging in this patient presenting with drainage along incision site after anterior craniofacial resection for a right frontal sinus angiosarcoma shows a diffusion restricting extra-axial fluid collection (ADC not shown) over the right frontal convexity (*arrow*), concerning for abscess. (*B*) Axial FLAIR shows incomplete CSF signal suppression (*arrowheads*) over the right frontal convexity, and (*C*) postcontrast T1-weighted image shows leptomeningeal enhancement in this distribution, worrisome for meningitis. The purulent collection was confirmed surgically and the area was debrided. Imaging was complicated by confluence FLAIR signal abnormalities over the bilateral frontal lobes (*asterisks*), favored to represent postradiation change based evolution on subsequent imaging.

carotid-cavernous fistulas (**Fig. 19**).[41,45] Vasospasm is a rare complication with transsphenoidal surgery, possibly caused by violation of the leptomeninges with hemorrhagic products accumulating in the subarachnoid space.[45]

Patients may develop sphenoid sinusitis with an incidence rate of 0.5% to 5.7%, usually well-managed with medical treatment. Mucoceles can develop in the sphenoid sinus as a late complication, presenting as an expansile paranasal sinus

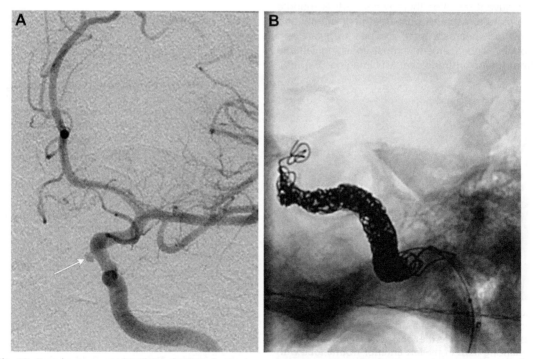

Fig. 19. Pseudoaneurysm. (*A, B*) Cerebral angiography performed emergently after internal carotid injury during transsphenoidal removal of a craniopharyngioma shows a 2.5-mm pseudoaneurysm (*arrow*) in the anterior genu of the cavernous segment of the cavernous internal carotid artery. The internal carotid artery was then coil embolized and sacrificed from the clinoidal to petrous segments.

mass with smooth thinning and remodeling of the surrounding bone, usually with mild peripheral enhancement and no internal enhancement. The density on CT and the T1/T2 intensity of the lesion is variable depending on the water and protein content of the lesion.[42,45]

Hydrocephalus is a rare complication after transsphenoidal surgery and is associated with the presence of intraoperative and postoperative CSF leak and CSF infection. The exact mechanism of action is unclear, but may be related to CSF infection and subarachnoid hemorrhage causing scarring of the arachnoid villi and poor CSF reabsorption.[45,46]

Residual/Recurrent Disease

Generally, residual and recurrent disease presents and nodular enhancement compared with the smooth and linear enhancement in expected reactive change. This is often difficult to discern in the early postoperative period because of postsurgical hemorrhage, and reactive soft tissue enhancement can confound assessment. Conversely, postoperative granulation tissue increases within a few months after the surgery and mimics recurrent tumor. Critical comparison of early postoperative and follow-up scans is necessary; increasing size and conspicuity of enhancement implies residual/recurrent tumor (see **Figs. 2** and **7**).

Adjuvant radiation therapy can further muddle the picture, because post-treatment effects and radiation necrosis can exhibit irregular and nodular enhancement almost indistinguishable from tumor on traditional MR imaging (**Fig. 20**).

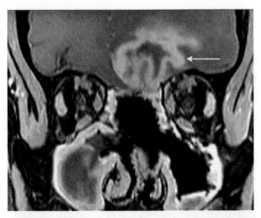

Fig. 20. Radiation necrosis. Coronal postcontrast T1-weighted image 1 year after anterior craniofacial resection of an esthesioneuroblastoma shows an enhancing mass in the left anterior frontal lobe with central necrosis (*arrow*), suggestive of recurrent tumor or radiation necrosis after adjuvant radiotherapy. There was decreased conspicuity of the lesion on follow-up imaging, favoring radiation necrosis.

PET-CT is often positive in radiation necrosis and MR imaging techniques, such as diffusion-weighted imaging, perfusion-weighted imaging, and spectroscopy, are often markedly limited because of susceptibility artifacts from the skull base. Review of the radiation fields is important in distinguishing radiation effect from recurrent tumor. The anterior inferior frontal lobes and mesial temporal lobes are frequent sites of radiation necrosis because extensive sinonasal cancers and central skull base tumors often necessitate inclusion of these regions in the radiation field for proper treatment. Often the nature of this enhancing tissue becomes clear with continued imaging surveillance, with the clinical picture shedding some insight because patients with radiation necrosis tend to be more well-appearing than those with tumor progression.

SUMMARY

Familiarity with the common surgical approaches used for skull base surgery procedures and recognition of the expected postoperative imaging findings for these surgeries can demystify the complex postoperative imaging appearance and improve detection of surgical complications and disease recurrence.

CLINICS CARE POINTS

- Post-operative imaging assessment following skull base surgery requires understanding of the various surgical approaches, the expected postoperative appearance, and awareness of common post-surgical complications.

- It can be difficult to differentiate treatment change and residual disease on immediate post-surgical imaging and follow-up imaging is often required.

- CSF leak is a common complication of skull base surgery. Other complications include infarct, vascular injury/thrombosis, and infection.

REFERENCES

1. Hudgins PA, Baugnon KL. Head and neck: skull base imaging. Neurosurgery 2018;82(3):255–67.
2. Prevedello LM. Advances in computed tomography evaluation of skull base diseases. Int Arch Otorhinolaryngol 2014;18(Suppl 2):S123–6.

3. Casselman JW, Kuhweide R, Deimling M, et al. Constructive interference in steady state-3DFT MR imaging of the inner ear and cerebellopontine angle. AJNR Am J Neuroradiol 1993;14(1):47–57.

4. Hingwala D, Chatterjee S, Kesavadas C, et al. Applications of 3D CISS sequence for problem solving in neuroimaging. Indian J Radiol Imaging 2011;21: 90–7.

5. Blitz AM, Northcutt B, Shin J, et al. Contrast-enhanced CISS imaging for evaluation of neurovascular compression in trigeminal neuralgia: improved correlation with symptoms and prediction of surgical outcomes. AJNR Am J Neuroradiol 2018;39(9): 1724–32.

6. Blitz AM, Aygun N, Herzka DA, et al. High resolution three-dimensional MR imaging of the skull base: compartments, boundaries, and critical structures. Radiol Clin North Am 2017;55:17–30.

7. Touska P, Connor SEJ. Recent advances in MRI of the head and neck, skull base and cranial nerves: new and evolving sequences, analyses and clinical applications. Br J Radiol 2019;92(1104):20190513.

8. Chavhan GB, Babyn PS, Jankharia BG, et al. Steady-state MR imaging sequences: physics, classification, and clinical applications. Radiographics 2008;28(4):1147–60.

9. Springborg JB, Poulsgaard L, Thomsen J. Nonvestibular schwannoma tumors in the cerebellopontine angle: a structured approach and management guidelines. Skull Base 2008;18(4):217–27.

10. Lee WJ, Isaacson JE. Postoperative imaging and follow-up of vestibular schwannomas. Otol Neurotol 2005;26(1):102–4.

11. Ginat DT, Horowitz PM, Moonis G, et al. Imaging of the postoperative skull base and cerebellopontine angle. Atlas of Postsurgical Neuroradiology. Springer; 2017. p. 311–50. https://doi.org/10.1007/978-3-319-52341-5_7.

12. Ginat DT, Martuza RL. Postoperative imaging of vestibular schwannomas. Neurosurg Focus 2012; 33(3):E18.

13. Silk PS, Lane JI, Driscoll CL. Surgical approaches to vestibular schwannomas: what the radiologist needs to know. Radiographics 2009;29(7):1955–70.

14. McLaughlin MR, Jannetta PJ, Clyde BL, et al. Microvascular decompression of cranial nerves: lessons learned after 4400 operations. J Neurosurg 1999; 90(1):1–8.

15. Cantù G, Riccio S, Bimbi G, et al. Craniofacial resection for malignant tumours involving the anterior skull base. Eur Arch Otorhinolaryngol 2006;263(7): 647–52.

16. Solero CL, DiMeco F, Sampath P, et al. Combined anterior craniofacial resection for tumors involving the cribriform plate: early postoperative complications and technical considerations. Neurosurgery 2000;47(6):1296–305.

17. Varshney S, Bist SS, Gupta N, et al. Anterior craniofacial resection: for paranasal sinus tumors involving anterior skull base. Indian J Otolaryngol Head Neck Surg 2010;62(2):103–7.

18. Albonette-Felicio T, Rangel GG, Martinéz-Pérez R, et al. Surgical management of anterior skull-base malignancies (endoscopic vs. craniofacial resection). J Neurooncol 2020;150(3):429–36.

19. Donath A, Sindwani R. Frontal sinus cranialization using the pericranial flap: an added layer of protection. Laryngoscope 2006;116(9):1585–8.

20. Jho HD. Endoscopic transsphenoidal surgery. J Neurooncol 2001;54:187–95.

21. Jho HD, Carrau RL. Endoscopic endonasal transsphenoidal surgery: experience with 50 patients. J Neurosurg 1997;87(1):44–51.

22. Cappabianca P, Cavallo LM, de Divitiis E. Endoscopic endonasal transsphenoidal surgery. Neurosurgery 2004;55(4):933–41.

23. Rajaraman V, Schulder M. Postoperative MRI appearance after transsphenoidal pituitary tumor resection. Surg Neurol 1999;52(6):592–8.

24. Kang MD, Escott E, Thomas AJ, et al. The MR imaging appearance of the vascular pedicle nasoseptal flap. AJNR Am J Neuroradiol 2009;30(4):781–6. Erratum in: AJNR Am J Neuroradiol. 2009 Aug; 30(7):E113.

25. Bohnstedt BN, Eads T, Weyhenmeyer J, et al. Transcranial approaches to the sellar and parasellar areas. In: Laws E Jr, Cohen-Gadol A, Schwartz T, et al, editors. Transsphenoidal surgery. Cham (Switzerland): Springer; 2017. p. 191–211.

26. Brors D, Schäfers M, Bodmer D, et al. Postoperative magnetic resonance imaging findings after transtemporal and translabyrinthine vestibular schwannoma resection. Laryngoscope 2003;113(3):420–6.

27. Lin EP, Crane BT. The management and imaging of vestibular schwannomas. AJNR Am J Neuroradiol 2017;38(11):2034–43.

28. Northcutt BG, Seeburg DP, Shin J, et al. High-resolution MRI findings following trigeminal rhizotomy. AJNR Am J Neuroradiol 2016;37(10):1920–4.

29. Schuster JJ, Phillips CD, Levine PA. MR of esthesioneuroblastoma (olfactory neuroblastoma) and appearance after craniofacial resection. AJNR Am J Neuroradiol 1994;15(6):1169–77.

30. Fahlbusch R, Ganslandt O, Buchfelder M, et al. Intraoperative magnetic resonance imaging during transsphenoidal surgery. J Neurosurg 2001;95(3): 381–90.

31. Kremer P, Forsting M, Ranaei G, et al. Magnetic resonance imaging after transsphenoidal surgery of clinically non-functional pituitary macroadenomas and its impact on detecting residual adenoma. Acta Neurochir (Wien) 2002;144(5):433–43.

32. Yoon PH, Kim DI, Jeon P, et al. Pituitary adenomas: early postoperative MR imaging after transsphenoidal

resection. AJNR Am J Neuroradiol 2001;22(6): 1097–104.

33. Alhilali LM, Little AS, Yuen KCJ, et al. Early postoperative MRI and detection of residual adenoma after transsphenoidal pituitary surgery. J Neurosurg 2020; 134(3):761–70. https://doi.org/10.3171/2019.11.JNS191845.

34. Betka J, Zvěřina E, Balogová Z, et al. Complications of microsurgery of vestibular schwannoma. Biomed Res Int 2014;2014:315952.

35. Mangus BD, Rivas A, Yoo MJ, et al. Management of cerebrospinal fluid leaks after vestibular schwannoma surgery. Otol Neurotol 2011;32(9):1525–9.

36. Guazzo E, Panizza B, Lomas A, et al. Cerebral venous sinus thrombosis after translabyrinthine vestibular schwannoma: a prospective study and suggested management paradigm. Otol Neurotol 2020;41(2):273–9.

37. Feng Y, Lane JI, Lohse CM, et al. Pattern of cochlear obliteration after vestibular schwannoma resection according to surgical approach. Laryngoscope 2020;130(2):474–81.

38. Clevens RA, Marentette LJ, Esclamado RM, et al. Incidence and management of tension pneumocephalus after anterior craniofacial resection: case reports and review of the literature. Otolaryngol Head Neck Surg 1999;120(4):579–83.

39. Richtsmeier WJ, Briggs RJ, Koch WM, et al. Complications and early outcome of anterior craniofacial resection. Arch Otolaryngol Head Neck Surg 1992; 118(9):913–7.

40. Gray ST, Lin A, Curry WT, et al. Delayed complications after anterior craniofacial resection of malignant skull base tumors. J Neurol Surg B Skull Base 2014;75(2):110–6.

41. Black PM, Zervas NT, Candia GL. Incidence and management of complications of transsphenoidal operation for pituitary adenomas. Neurosurgery 1987;20(6):920–4.

42. Cappabianca P, Cavallo LM, Colao A, et al. Surgical complications associated with the endoscopic endonasal transsphenoidal approach for pituitary adenomas. J Neurosurg 2002;97(2):293–8.

43. Charalampaki P, Ayyad A, Kockro RA, et al. Surgical complications after endoscopic transsphenoidal pituitary surgery. J Clin Neurosci 2009;16(6):786–9.

44. Halvorsen H, Ramm-Pettersen J, Josefsen R, et al. Surgical complications after transsphenoidal microscopic and endoscopic surgery for pituitary adenoma: a consecutive series of 506 procedures. Acta Neurochir (Wien) 2014;156(3):441–9.

45. Alzhrani G, Sivakumar W, Park MS, et al. Delayed complications after transsphenoidal surgery for pituitary adenomas. World Neurosurg 2018;109:233–41.

46. Sharma M, Ambekar S, Sonig A, et al. Factors predicting the development of new onset postoperative hydrocephalus following trans-sphenoidal surgery for pituitary adenoma. Clin Neurol Neurosurg 2013;115(10):1951–4.

Imaging of the Postoperative Temporal Bone

Paraag R. Bhatt, MD[a],*, Jennifer C. Alyono, MD[b], Nancy J. Fischbein, MD[a], Mrudula Penta, MD[a]

KEYWORDS

- Postoperative temporal bone • Tympanostomy • Mastoidectomy • Temporal bone resections
- IAC and CPA approaches • Superior semicircular canal dehiscence repair
- Sigmoid sinus wall reconstruction • Ossicular reconstruction

KEY POINTS

- Postoperative temporal bone image interpretation is challenging.
- Careful review of the patient's clinical and operative history is critical to identify expected postoperative appearance versus complications.
- Common surgical procedures involving the temporal bone include tympanostomy, mastoidectomy, temporal bone resections, internal auditory canal and cerebellopontine angle surgical approaches, superior semicircular canal dehiscence repair, sigmoid sinus wall reconstruction, ossicular reconstruction, and auditory implant placement.
- Common interpretive pitfalls include lack of knowledge regarding expected postsurgical anatomic alterations, appearance of otologic hardware, correct hardware positioning, as well as delayed recognition of postoperative complications.
- Common postoperative temporal bone complications include postoperative hemorrhage, excessive pneumocephalus, brain retraction injury, vascular injury, cerebrospinal fluid leak, hardware malposition or migration, and bone or ossicular dehiscence.

INTRODUCTION

Postsurgical changes of the temporal bone can be difficult for radiologists to interpret accurately. The combination of inherently complex native temporal bone anatomy with unique, region-specific postoperative change makes evaluation of this region challenging. Consideration of the most common types of temporal bone surgical procedures and the expected postoperative appearance is critical when reviewing these studies, because it is this fundamental understanding of the expected postoperative appearance that serves as the foundation to discern postsurgical disorder such as disease recurrence and postoperative complications. Ultimately, prompt recognition of postintervention temporal bone disorder helps improve patient care and helps to show the added value of radiological interpretation to referring clinicians.[1]

This article covers common temporal bone procedures, including tympanostomy, mastoidectomy, temporal bone resections, cerebellopontine angle (CPA) and internal auditory canal (IAC) approaches, superior semicircular canal dehiscence repair, sigmoid sinus wall reconstruction, ossicular reconstruction, and auditory implants. Several common postoperative complications are also covered. The discussion includes the specific clinical

[a] Department of Radiology, Stanford University, 300 Pasteur Drive, Room S047, Stanford, CA 94305, USA;
[b] Department of Otolaryngology, Head and Neck Surgery, Stanford University, 801 Welch Road, MC 5739, Stanford, CA 94305, USA
* Corresponding author.
E-mail address: paraagb@gmail.com

Neuroimag Clin N Am 32 (2022) 175–192
https://doi.org/10.1016/j.nic.2021.08.006
1052-5149/22/© 2021 Elsevier Inc. All rights reserved.

indications, as well as the unique surgical and imaging features, which help distinguish these procedures from one another.

TYMPANOSTOMY TUBE

Tympanostomy is a procedure in which a myringotomy (incision through the tympanic membrane) is made and a tube is placed through the myringotomy to maintain patency of the defect. Tympanostomy tubes are most commonly placed for chronic middle ear effusions and recurrent acute otitis media, but can also be placed for less common indications such as otitic barotrauma or patulous eustachian tube. Although tympanostomy tubes come in an assortment of sizes and shapes, they are most often seen as a tubular structure on thin-section high-resolution temporal bone computed tomography (CT) (Fig. 1). CT can help identify the presence of a tympanostomy tube, although it may not be obtained for that purpose. It is important to recognize tympanostomy and for radiologists not to misinterpret the tube as a foreign body, displaced ossicle, or other potential component of otologic hardware. In some cases, the tympanostomy tube can be difficult to visualize on CT, particularly if the tube is plastic and/or obscured by overlying attenuating debris or fluid.[2,3] When tympanostomy tubes are displaced, they typically fall out into the ear canal on their own, but they can become displaced medially into the middle ear (Fig. 2) and possibly result in conductive hearing loss, so a comment regarding tube position should be included in the imaging report.[3,4]

MASTOIDECTOMY

Mastoidectomy is a commonly performed temporal bone surgical procedure that varies in extent from cortical mastoidectomy to radical mastoidectomy. Although the most common indications for mastoidectomy include chronic otitis media and cholesteatoma, there are several additional potential indications, including coalescent mastoiditis, cochlear implantation, middle ear neoplasms, facial nerve exploration, and endolymphatic sac procedures.[1,3]

Canal Wall Up Mastoidectomy

Canal wall up (CWU) mastoidectomy (Fig. 3) involves removal of the lateral cortex of the mastoid bone as well as potentially all of the mastoid air cells extending from the borders of the tegmen mastoideum superiorly, to the sigmoid sinus posteriorly, and posterior wall of the external auditory canal anteriorly. The procedure preserves or leaves up the posterior wall of the external auditory canal. The extent of CWU mastoidectomy can vary from a cortical mastoidectomy, in which the Koerner septum is not traversed, to complete removal of all the mastoid air cells. Indications for CWU mastoidectomy include acute or chronic otitis media, mastoiditis, access for cochlear implantation, and access to the second genu and descending facial nerve segments.[1,5,6] Typically, the resultant mastoidectomy bowl should be aerated on CT. The presence of soft tissue attenuation in the postoperative setting may indicate benign disorder, such as fibrosis/scarring, or may represent granulation tissue or recurrent cholesteatoma in the appropriate clinical setting. Mastoidectomy cavities may also be opacified because of surgical obliteration: historically, a variety of surgical materials have been used to fill the mastoidectomy bowl, including bone, fat, cartilage, or nonautogenous material such as hydroxyapatite.[3,7] In these cases, review of the operative history is critical in determining whether this

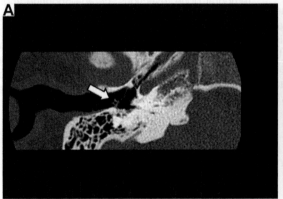
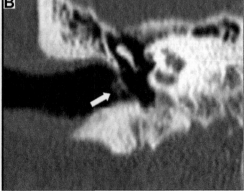

Fig. 1. Tympanostomy. Axial (*A*) and coronal (*B*) CT of the right temporal bone show an appropriately positioned tympanostomy tube (*arrows*), depicted as a focal tubular object straddling the tympanic membrane.

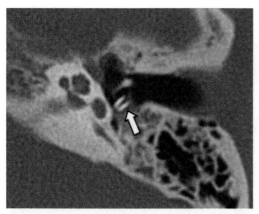

Fig. 2. Tympanostomy tube displacement. Axial CT of the left temporal bone shows a tympanostomy tube (*arrow*) that is displaced medially into the middle ear cavity.

material reflects disorder or expected postoperative change.

The facial recess approach can be performed as part of CWU mastoidectomy. As part of this procedure, bone lateral to the mastoid segment of the facial nerve and medial to the chorda tympani is removed to allow access to the middle ear cavity from the mastoid posteriorly. This procedure is also known as a posterior tympanotomy. This exposure is often used for cochlear implantation or for cholesteatoma resection, because the facial recess is often a site of disease recurrence.[1,6]

Canal Wall Down Mastoidectomy

Canal wall down (CWD) mastoidectomy (Fig. 4) involves removal of all the mastoid air cells and Koerner septum. In contrast with CWU mastoidectomy, CWD mastoidectomy also removes the posterior wall of the external auditory canal. There are several indications for which CWD mastoidectomy might be performed, including cholesteatoma that has already eroded the posterior canal wall, recurrent cholesteatoma, or for exteriorization/marsupialization of cholesteatoma matrix that cannot be fully resected.[1] Examples of marsupialization of cholesteatoma matrix might be cholesteatoma eroding into the lateral semicircular canal or other portion of the membranous labyrinth (especially in an only hearing ear), or dehiscence of the dura with thin cholesteatoma matrix that cannot be removed without dural resection.

The resultant mastoid cavity communicates with the external auditory canal and is thereby externalized. As in CWU mastoidectomy, material within the mastoidectomy bowl following CWD mastoidectomy may represent granulation tissue, postoperative material, or recurrent disease; therefore, clinical and operative correlation in these cases is critical.[3,7] Cerumen and epithelial debris may also fill the mastoid cavity, leading to an opacified appearance on imaging. Although at times this may appear concerning, if the material is lateral to the epithelial lining of the cavity, it can be addressed merely with an ear cleaning. Cholesteatoma would only be considered recurrent if it were trapped medial to the cavity's epithelial lining. CWD mastoidectomy can also be subdivided into modified radical and radical mastoidectomies.

Canal Wall Down Modified Radical and Radical Mastoidectomy

Radical mastoidectomy (Fig. 5) is a subcategory of CWD mastoidectomy in which the middle ear cavity, in addition to the mastoid, is effectively externalized. A radical mastoidectomy involves

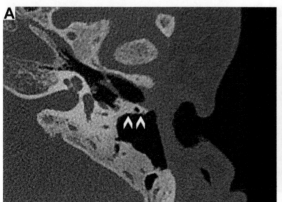
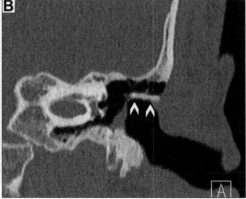

Fig. 3. CWU mastoidectomy. Axial (*A*) and coronal (*B*) CT of the left temporal bone show postoperative changes of CWU mastoidectomy for cholesteatoma resection. Note the preservation of the posterior wall of the external auditory canal (EAC) (*arrowheads*).

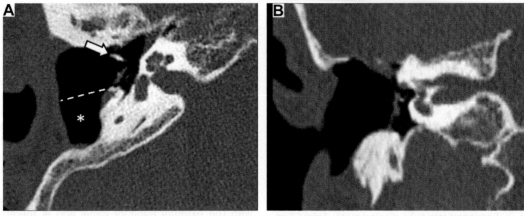

Fig. 4. CWD mastoidectomy. Axial (*A*) and coronal (*B*) CT of the right temporal bone show postoperative changes of CWD mastoidectomy for cholesteatoma resection. Note is made of absence of the mastoid air cells (*asterisk*) as well as the posterior wall of the EAC (*dotted line*). In addition, a partially imaged ossicular prosthesis is visualized (*arrow*).

removal of the tympanic membrane and the middle ear structures, including all the ossicles, without reconstruction. The eustachian tube and middle ear cavity remain exposed to the mastoidectomy defect.[1,8] Although currently infrequently performed, this procedure is typically reserved for very extensive middle ear disease processes, including unresectable cholesteatoma.[1,9,10]

Modified radical CWD mastoidectomy (**Fig. 6**) refers to those procedures that fall short of radical mastoidectomy.[1,8] In this case, the tympanic membrane and ossicles are either left in situ (ie, in a Bondy-type mastoidectomy, performed when there is no cholesteatoma involvement of the middle ear), or, if needed, the tympanic membrane can be reconstructed, with grafting.

TEMPORAL BONE RESECTION

Temporal bone resection is a broad term referring to several procedures that are typically performed for resection of malignant tumors involving the temporal bone. Lateral temporal bone resection (LTBR) (**Fig. 7**) refers to en bloc resection of the bony ear canal, ear canal skin, tympanic membrane, and lateral ossicles (malleus and incus). In this procedure, CWU mastoidectomy with opening of the facial recess is performed. Bone removal is then extended along the superior aspect of the bony canal to the zygomatic root. Inferiorly, bone between the inferior aspect of the tympanic ring and the descending facial nerve is removed. The incudostapedial joint is separated, and the incus is removed. The

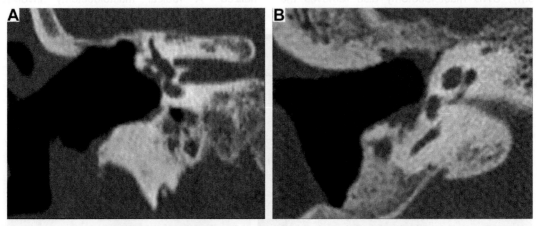

Fig. 5. CWD radical mastoidectomy. Axial (*A*) and coronal (*B*) CT of the right temporal bone show postoperative changes of radical mastoidectomy for recurrent infection, including absence of the mastoid air cells, posterior wall of the EAC, tympanic membrane (TM), as well as the ossicles. Note that the middle ear space has not been reconstructed in a radical mastoidectomy.

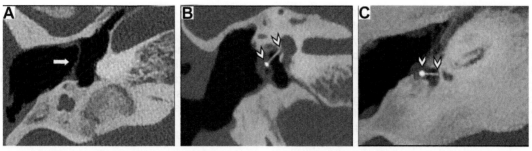

Fig. 6. CWD modified radical mastoidectomy and total ossicular replacement prosthesis (TORP). Axial (*A*), coronal (*B*), and axial (*C*) maximum intensity projection (MIP) CT of the right temporal bone show postoperative changes of modified radical mastoidectomy for cholesteatoma resection. Postoperative changes of TM reconstruction (*arrow*) as well as TORP, which extends from the TM to the oval window, are also depicted (*arrowheads*).

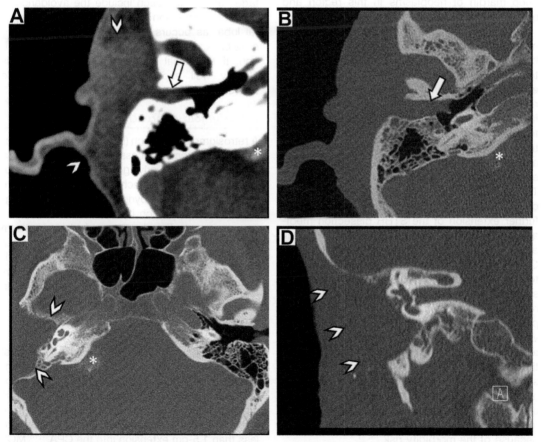

Fig. 7. LTBR. Preoperative axial soft tissue (*A*) and bone (*B*) kernel CT of the right temporal bone show an infiltrative mass (squamous cell carcinoma) involving the subcutaneous soft tissues underlying the right pinna (*arrowheads*). The mass is depicted extending deep into the EAC (*arrow*) and abutting the TM. Postoperative axial (*C*) and coronal (*D*) CT of the right temporal bone show postoperative changes of LTBR for tumor removal. Note is made of postsurgical changes of resection of the EAC and TM, mastoidectomy, and partial ossicular chain removal (incus and malleus). Nonspecific postoperative opacification (*arrowheads*) of the surgical cavity is related in part to a surgically placed temporalis flap. Incidental note is made of a right CPA partially calcified meningioma (*asterisk*) included in the field of view.

tensor tympani tendon is incised. In addition, with either digital pressure on the canal or with osteotomes, the bone of the anterior tympanic ring is fractured to allow removal of the bony ear canal, tympanic membrane, and malleus en bloc. The procedure may be combined with parotidectomy and/or neck dissection, depending on tumor subtype and extent. If there is significant adjacent soft tissue removal, or anticipated need for adjuvant radiation, a temporalis muscle flap or a microvascular free flap may be used for reconstruction. In contrast with LTBR, sleeve resection refers to a less extensive procedure that involves removal of the skin of the ear canal up to or including the tympanic membrane. In modern times, this type of procedure is typically reserved for tumors that only involve the cartilaginous portion of the canal, or for in situ noninvasive disease because of lack of adequate control of the deep margin of neoplasms in this region and resultant high recurrence rates.[11,12]

More extensive temporal bone resections for malignancy include subtotal and total temporal bone resections. Subtotal temporal bone resection (STBR) involves removal of elements of the external auditory canal, middle ear, bony labyrinth, and mastoid cavity. The procedure frequently begins with an LTBR, which is used to remove tumor in the ear canal and gain potential access to the middle ear, jugular foramen, and middle and posterior fossae with overall extent of bone removal tailored to tumor extent. Total temporal bone resection (TTBR) involves complete removal of the temporal bone with further extension of the STBR dissection medially to the petrous apex. As in STBR, overall extent of resection is tailored to tumor margins. Overall morbidity is greater with TTBR, with potential postoperative complications including stroke from carotid artery sacrifice (when required) as well as multiple lower cranial nerve palsies. Balloon test occlusion with neurointerventional radiology may be considered preoperatively when tumor is adjacent to or involving the carotid to determine the risk of ischemic stroke should the artery be violated. With the availability of adjuvant therapy (radiation, chemotherapy, immunotherapy), it is uncommon to intentionally sacrifice the internal carotid because of the morbidity risk.[12,13]

With regard to temporal bone resections, CT and magnetic resonance (MR) imaging play important and complementary roles in preoperative evaluation of tumor extent, surgical planning, and surgical guidance, as well as in the postoperative evaluation of complications and for ongoing tumor surveillance.

INTERNAL AUDITORY CANAL AND CEREBELLOPONTINE ANGLE APPROACHES

There are 3 main surgical approaches to access the IAC and CPA: translabyrinthine, retrosigmoid, and middle cranial fossa (MCF). The most common disorders addressed via these approaches are vestibular schwannoma and meningioma.

Translabyrinthine Approach

The translabyrinthine approach (**Fig. 8**) is used when hearing preservation is not a goal.[14] The technique involves mastoidectomy, labyrinthectomy, and removal of the bone overlying the middle and posterior fossae, as well as overlying the IAC. Reconstruction commonly involves obliteration of the mastoid cavity with fat and sealing off of the aditus ad antrum and/or eustachian tube to prevent cerebrospinal fluid (CSF) leak. Advantages of this approach include the avoidance of significant retraction on the cerebellum or temporal lobe, as occurs with other approaches, and ease of exposure of the fundus of the IAC. In addition, if the facial nerve requires grafting, it is already well exposed. Disadvantages include loss of hearing and a higher rate of CSF leak.[1,15]

Retrosigmoid Approach

A retrosigmoid approach (**Fig. 9**) involves a suboccipital craniotomy. Access to the IAC is afforded via drilling of the overlying bone from its posterior aspect. Because this technique does not require violation of the labyrinth, it is a hearing-preservation approach if the cochlear nerve can be preserved. Disadvantages include a more limited view of the fundus, the need for cerebellar retraction, and higher rates of postoperative headache if drilling is required, because drilling is performed intradurally (as opposed to extradurally in a translabyrinthine approach).[1,15–17]

Middle Cranial Fossa Approach

The MCF approach (**Fig. 10**) involves a temporal craniotomy and subsequent elevation of the temporal lobe off the petrous floor, which allows exposure of the IAC from its superior aspect. During this approach, the CPA is not well exposed; therefore, the MCF approach is reserved for IAC lesions with less than 1.5-cm extension into the CPA.[1,16] MCF approaches are also used to treat temporal lobe encephaloceles and superior semicircular canal dehiscence. With regard to using this approach for resection of vestibular schwannomas, the main advantage is its potential to preserve hearing. Disadvantages include the need for temporal lobe retraction, limitations of tumor size and

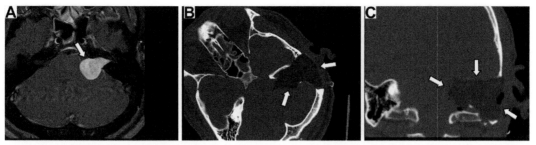

Fig. 8. Translabyrinthine approach. Preoperative axial (*A*) postcontrast MR imaging of the brain shows an enhancing presumed vestibular schwannoma (*arrow*) involving the left IAC and CPA. Postoperative axial (*B*) and coronal (*C*) head CT show left translabyrinthine approach with CWU mastoidectomy, resection of the semicircular canals, partial resection of the posterior wall of the IAC, and placement of fat graft (*arrows*).

location that can be removed, and risk of facial nerve paresis because the facial nerve is typically positioned superior to the tumor, between the surgical access and the tumor.[1,15]

Postoperative Imaging

Choosing the appropriate imaging modality when performing postoperative imaging depends on the specific clinical question being addressed. Contrast-enhanced fat-suppressed MR imaging can be obtained postoperatively on a routine basis to establish a postoperative baseline. Linear, non-masslike enhancement involving the IAC or labyrinth is a common postoperative finding, with presence of this enhancement remaining stable

or decreasing in conspicuity over time.[1,18] Therefore, serial imaging may be helpful in distinguishing postoperative from true pathologic enhancement, because increasing nodular, irregular, or masslike enhancement may indicate the presence of recurrent tumor in the setting of prior resection of an enhancing mass. Correlation with the patient's operative history is critical in these settings. CT may be performed on an urgent basis for mental status or other unexpected neurologic changes. In the immediate postoperative setting, this may reveal intracranial hemorrhage or tension pneumocephalus; in the subacute or chronic setting with mental status changes, this may reveal hydrocephalus.

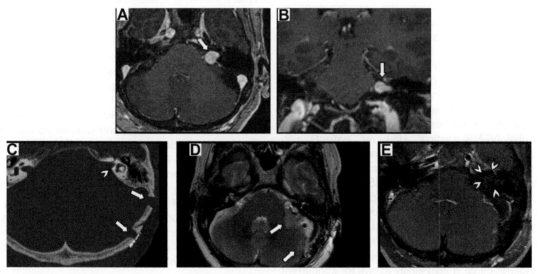

Fig. 9. Retrosigmoid approach. Preoperative axial (*A*) and coronal (*B*) postcontrast MR imaging show an enhancing (*arrow*) presumed vestibular schwannoma within the left IAC with associated widening of the left porus acusticus and extension into the CPA. Postoperative axial (*C*) head CT shows postsurgical changes of retrosigmoid approach with craniotomies posterior to the sigmoid sinus (*arrows*) as well as resection of the posterior wall of the IAC (*arrowhead*). Postoperative axial T2-weighted (*D*) and postcontrast (*E*) MR imaging of the brain show typical postoperative retraction injury (*arrows*) in the adjacent left cerebellum as well as expected non–masslike linear enhancement (*arrowheads*) involving the visualized membranous labyrinthine structures.

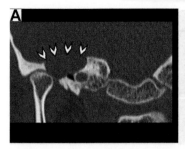 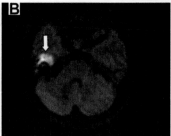 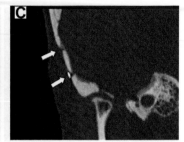

Fig. 10. MCF approach. Preoperative coronal (A) CT of the right temporal bone shows an erosive lesion (*arrow-heads*) of the right middle ear cavity that bulges into the MCF via a dehiscent tegmen tympani. Preoperative axial (B) diffusion-weighted image shows diffusion restriction (*arrow*) typical of a cholesteatoma. Postoperative coronal (C) CT of the right temporal bone shows postoperative changes of right MCF approach with craniotomies (*arrows*) located in the squamous temporal bone.

SUPERIOR SEMICIRCULAR CANAL DEHISCENCE REPAIR

The association of the radiological finding of superior semicircular canal dehiscence (SSCD) with clinical symptoms has only recently been described in the medical literature (1998 by Minor and colleagues).[19,20] SSCD can be identified on high-resolution CT scans in ~2% of the population but is identified in a much higher percentage of patients who present with referable symptoms.[21] Symptoms related to SSCD are variable but can include auditory and/or vestibular abnormalities such as vertigo or oscillopsia induced by pressure and sound, pulsatile tinnitus, aural fullness, or a pseudoconductive hearing loss. Diagnosis is made from the combination of audiometric and vestibular testing, imaging findings, and clinical assessment, because many individuals with SSCD are asymptomatic or do not require treatment. In addition, many more patients have radiographic dehiscence than have histopathologic dehiscence (as seen on postmortem temporal bone studies) or physiologic dehiscence (as evaluated on vestibular evoked myogenic potential [VEMP] testing). However, patients with debilitating symptoms may benefit from surgical intervention.[19,22] Multiple surgical techniques for treatment of symptomatic SSCD have been described, such as the MCF approach, transmastoid approach, and round window reinforcement.

The first approach described for SSCD repair (Fig. 11) was via the MCF. In addition to affording access to resurfacing or plugging of the dehiscent superior canal, it also easily allows for concurrent repair of any accompanying tegmen defects and/or encephaloceles, which are common in this patient population.[22] Disadvantages of this approach include the need for temporal lobe retraction, and difficulty accessing more medial dehiscences of the superior canal to the superior petrosal sinus.

The transmastoid approach does not require temporal lobe retraction or craniotomy, and may be preferable in patients prone to headache. This approach may also be advantageous if the superior canal is dehiscent medial to the superior petrosal sinus, which is more difficult to access via the middle fossa. In many transmastoid cases, the dehiscence is not visually confirmed before plugging. A low-hanging tegmen may preclude safe exposure of the canal. Preoperative thin-section CT imaging is helpful in determining the best approach.[22]

Once exposure of the dehiscence is achieved by either approach, resurfacing and/or plugging of the defect can be performed with a variety of materials, including autologous bone dust, bone wax, cartilage, or hydroxyapatite bone cement, which has bonelike density on postoperative CT imaging.[19,22]

Round window reinforcement or obliteration (with temporalis fascia, tragal cartilage, perichondrium, fat, or connective tissue) is performed via a tympanomeatal flap.[22] This surgery does not directly address the superior canal dehiscence. Instead, it removes the round window as one of the 3 open windows, leaving the SSCD and oval window patent. Compared with MCF and transmastoid approaches, fewer studies have examined the efficacy of round window surgery.[22,23]

Regardless of approach, postoperatively, thin-section CT in conjunction with VEMP testing may be useful if patient symptoms fail to improve in order to evaluate graft or plug positioning and to exclude recurrent or new dehiscence.

SIGMOID SINUS WALL RECONSTRUCTION

Sigmoid sinus wall anomalies are a common and potentially surgically correctable cause of pulsatile tinnitus of venous origin. Anomalies of the sigmoid sinus wall associated with venous pulsatile

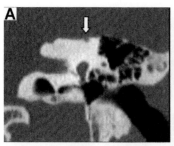
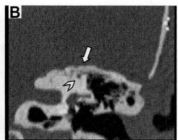
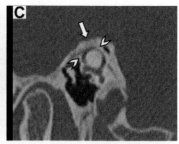

Fig. 11. SSCD repair. Preoperative coronal (*A*) CT of the left temporal bone shows dehiscence of the left superior semicircular canal (*arrow*). Postoperative coronal (*B*) and Pöschl projection (*C*) CT of the left temporal bone show postoperative changes of left MCF approach craniotomy (*asterisk*) with coverage of the superior semicircular canal (*arrowheads*) dehiscence with hydroxyapatite bone cement (*arrows*).

tinnitus include thinning and dehiscence of the sigmoid plate with or without associated venous diverticulum. Preoperative CT or MR imaging with or without dedicated dural venous vascular imaging has an essential role in identifying the presence of these anomalies in patients present with pulsatile tinnitus of venous origin (**Fig. 12**), but only CT can conclusively show bony dehiscence. In patients with significant symptoms, open surgical treatment with sigmoid sinus wall reconstruction is increasingly considered. Open surgical technique for sigmoid sinus wall reconstruction involves mastoidectomy followed by skeletonization of the sigmoid sinus. The affected area is identified and then is resurfaced with any of several materials, including autologous bone dust or cartilage, or hydroxyapatite cement. Critically, the goal is not to ligate or occlude the sinus, because this could lead to intracranial hypertension. The newly created hard exterior (bone cement or autologous bone dust) serves to

diminish transmissibility of venous vibrations from the previously exposed venous wall.[24,25] Postoperatively, in patients with concerning symptoms such as new or worsening headache, dural venous phase CT venography, contrast-enhanced MR imaging, or MR venography can be used to evaluate for appropriate positioning of postoperative material, including whether the deep soft tissue graft component results in excessive mass effect on the underlying sigmoid sinus or whether dural venous sinus thrombosis is present. In addition, postoperative imaging may also evaluate for residual or possibly untreated dehiscences in patients whose tinnitus fails to resolve following surgery.[24,25]

OSSICULAR RECONSTRUCTION

Ossicular reconstruction is a frequent finding on postoperative temporal bone CT. Ossicular reconstruction is typically performed in patients with a

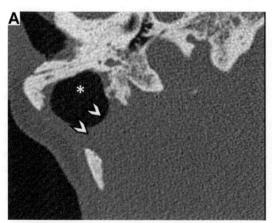
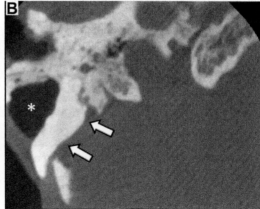

Fig. 12. Sigmoid sinus wall resurfacing. Preoperative axial (*A*) CT of the right temporal bone shows wide bony dehiscence (*arrowheads*) of the right sigmoid sinus plate secondary to osteoradionecrosis in a patient after mastoidectomy (*asterisk*) and radiation therapy for treatment of malignancy 10 years prior. Postoperative axial (*B*) CT of the right temporal bone shows reconstruction of the sigmoid sinus plate with hydroxyapatite bone cement (*arrows*) and coverage of the sigmoid sinus plate defect.

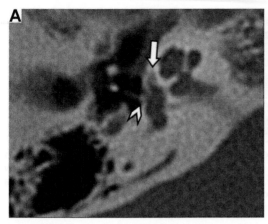 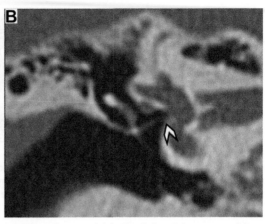

Fig. 13. Stapes surgery for otosclerosis. Postoperative axial (*A*) and coronal (*B*) CT of the right temporal bone show postoperative changes of stapes surgery with appropriately positioned piston-type stapes prosthesis with medial aspect of the prosthesis (*arrowheads*) in position at the oval window. Note is made of osseous lucency (*arrow*) involving the fissula ante fenestram consistent with fenestral otosclerosis.

history of ossicular erosion/destruction in the setting of cholesteatoma or chronic otitis media, as well as in the setting of otosclerosis and several congenital middle ear anomalies.[1,26] A wide variety of prostheses exist to help facilitate the particular needs of individual patients depending on the extent of disease and surgeon preference.[1,6] Thin-section CT is typically the study of choice to evaluate ossicular reconstruction, because CT can evaluate for graft and prosthesis malpositioning. In addition, CT can also evaluate for recurrent cholesteatoma, granulation tissue, or adhesions in patients who develop new/recurrent conductive hearing loss following ossicular reconstruction.[1,26] MR imaging may be complementary to CT in particular scenarios to help differentiate disorder (ie, recurrent cholesteatoma) from granulation tissue. MR imaging compatibility of implanted devices must always be considered in order to ensure patient safety, but most ossicular prostheses are safe under physiologic imaging conditions.[27] The most common ossicular reconstructive procedures include stapes surgery, partial ossicular replacement prosthesis, and total ossicular replacement prosthesis.

Stapes Surgery

Stapes surgery (Fig. 13) is typically performed for otosclerosis, in which abnormal bone formation and remodeling lead to immobility of the stapes, and encompasses both stapedotomy and stapedectomy, which appear similar on imaging.[1,8] The more commonly performed stapedotomy involves removal of the superstructure and opening of a fenestra into the oval window, through which a prosthesis can be placed. The less common

stapedectomy involves total or subtotal removal of the stapes footplate, in addition to the superstructure. The open oval window is then covered by a soft tissue graft, followed by placement of a prosthesis. Prostheses are affixed to a mobile lateral ossicular chain (typically to the long process of the incus) and extend to the oval window. A variety of prostheses are available, in different shapes (ie, bucket handle, piston, clip, wire loop) and of different materials (ie, plastic, nonmagnetic stainless steel, titanium, and nitinol).[1,5,27] In cases where there is a shortened long process of the incus, malleus to stapes footplate prostheses can be used. Conductive hearing loss after stapes surgery can be caused by several factors, including displacement of the prosthesis at its medial or lateral end, redevelopment of otosclerotic plaque surrounding the prosthesis, fracture of the incus, or adhesions within the middle ear.

Partial Ossicular Replacement Prosthesis

Partial ossicular replacement prosthesis (PORP) (Fig. 14) is the most common type of middle ear prosthesis used, and it is typically used in cases of cholesteatoma or chronic otitis media where there has been partial or complete erosion of the incus.[5] These prostheses typically span from the tympanic membrane or malleus handle laterally to an intact and mobile stapes medially, but they can also span from a shortened long process to the stapes head. In the postoperative period, new conductive hearing loss may indicate recurrent disorder, including cholesteatoma or granulation tissue, and high-resolution CT may be obtained. New conductive hearing loss may also be caused by hardware malposition or dislodgement, including prosthesis

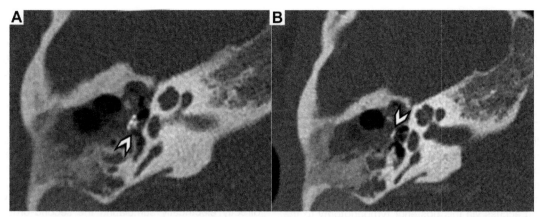

Fig. 14. PORP. Axial (*A*, *B*) CT of the right temporal bone shows a titanium Frisbee PORP placed following choles-teatoma resection. The prosthesis extends from the tympanic membrane laterally to the native stapes capitulum medially (*arrowheads*). The remaining native ossicles are surgically absent. Presumed postsurgical changes of nonspecific soft tissue in the middle ear cavity are also noted.

subluxation at its articulation with the stapes or prosthesis extrusion.[1,26]

Total Ossicular Replacement Prosthesis

Total ossicular replacement prostheses (TORPs) (see **Fig. 6**) are used in cases where the stapes superstructure is absent but there is an intact and mobile footplate. The prosthesis extends laterally from the undersurface of the tympanic membrane and/or malleus to the stapes footplate. As in the case of PORP, prosthetic subluxation, extrusion, and/or residual or recurrent disorder can produce new conductive hearing loss.[1,26]

Autologous Materials

In current practice, synthetic materials are more commonly used for ossiculoplasty. However, autologous cartilage or bone may also be used. Incus interposition (**Fig. 15**) is perhaps the best-known

variant, which typically involves reshaping of the body and short process of the incus to span from the malleus handle to an intact and mobile stapes. Graft subluxation and graft necrosis are potential complications and may also present as new conductive hearing loss.[1,26]

AUDITORY IMPLANTS

Hearing loss is a significant cause of patient morbidity affecting millions of people worldwide. A variety of implantable hearing devices exist to aid patients with this concern. Determination of the applicable device depends on several factors, including the type of hearing loss (conductive versus sensorineural), extent of hearing loss, anatomic considerations, and patient preference. Radiologists who interpret postoperative temporal bone imaging studies should familiarize themselves with common imaging features of these

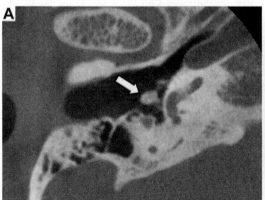
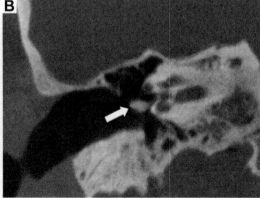

Fig. 15. Incus interposition. Axial (*A*) and coronal (*B*) CT images of the right temporal bone show postoperative changes of incus interposition with autograft (*arrows*) used for ossicular reconstruction. The graft extends from the tympanic membrane laterally to the stapes capitulum medially.

devices to help identify correct positioning and potential postoperative complications. Common devices discussed in this article include cochlear implant, osteointegrated bone conduction devices, and auditory brainstem implant.

Cochlear Implant

Cochlear implants (CIs) (Fig. 16) are used for patients with at least moderate to profound sensorineural hearing loss. Surgical placement of a CI begins with a CWU mastoidectomy and identification of the facial nerve in its descending segment.[1,5] The facial recess is then drilled, allowing access via this posterior tympanotomy to the middle ear and round window from the mastoid. The receiver-stimulator portion of the implant is typically placed subperiosteally posterosuperior to the mastoid cavity. The electrode is then threaded through the round window or through an adjacent bony cochleostomy into the cochlea (ideally within the scala tympani), with the interceding wire looping within the mastoid. The electrode array transmits impulses to the spiral ganglion cells of the cochlea to facilitate hearing.[1,28] On CT, the oblique reformation parallel to the cochlear turns (Stenvers view) allows the best evaluation of the insertion depth and location of the electrode array, which are important for the assessment of hearing and speech outcomes.[29]

Osseointegrated Bone Conduction Devices

Osseointegrated bone conduction devices (Fig. 17) are implanted for patients with either conductive hearing loss not amenable to conventional hearing aids (ie, patients with canal atresia or chronic otorrhea), or with single-sided deafness (SSD). The prosthesis typically consists of a titanium screw, which is inserted directly into the calvarium. It then connects either percutaneously with an abutment exiting the skin, or transcutaneously via magnets outside the skin, to a microphone and processor. In the case of SSD, the implant is placed ipsilateral to the side of hearing loss, and sound is conducted through the skull to the contralateral, normal-hearing cochlea.[30]

Auditory Brainstem Implant

For patients with profound sensorineural hearing loss and significant abnormalities of the cochlea and/or cochlear nerve who may not be candidates for a CI, an auditory brainstem implant (ABI) (Fig. 18) may be an option. The implant works by directly electrically stimulating the second-order neurons in the cochlear nucleus using a multichannel surface array and thereby bypasses the cochlear nerve. Surgery to place the ABI is typically performed via either a translabyrinthine or retrosigmoid craniotomy, with the approach directed through the foramen of Lushka at the level of the glossopharyngeal nerve (cranial nerve IX) to access the region of the cochlear nucleus. Postoperatively, CT imaging has a role to exclude potential complications, including hematoma, excessive pneumocephalus, or brain herniation.[31] This type of device has traditionally been used for patients with neurofibromatosis type 2 (NF2), with hearing compromised by vestibular schwannomas, but has also been used in patients without NF2 (ie, those born without a cochlear nerve or cochlea). Despite the restorative sound awareness potential of this device, overall outcomes remain modest relative to CI.[31]

POSTOPERATIVE COMPLICATIONS

Prompt recognition of postsurgical complications helps improve outcomes for patients and shows radiologist value to referring clinicians. Postoperative hemorrhage can be a complication of both

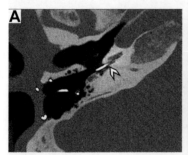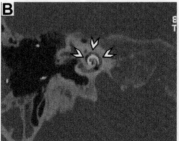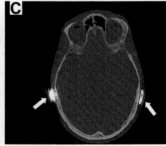

Fig. 16. Cochlear implant. Axial (*A*) CT image of the right temporal bone shows postsurgical changes of CWU mastoidectomy for cochlear implant with electrode array entering at the cochleostomy (*arrowhead*). Stenvers CT view (*B*) shows appropriate positioning of the electrode array (*arrowheads*) within the turns of the cochlea. Axial (*C*) head CT shows bilateral internal transmit and receiver implants (*arrows*) of the CIs embedded in the calvarium.

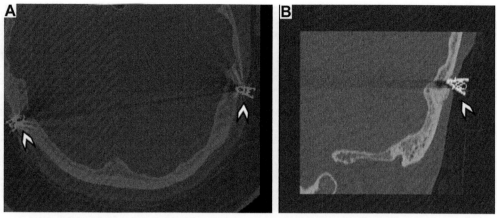

Fig. 17. Osteointegrated bone conduction device. Axial (*A*) and coronal (*B*) head CT show expected positioning of bilateral percutaneous bone conduction devices (*arrowheads*) inserted in the calvarium.

otologic and neuro-otologic temporal bone surgeries. In addition, excessive pneumocephalus and brain retraction injury with edema and/or infarction may occur following neuro-otologic surgery. Other postoperative temporal bone complications include CSF leak, vascular injury, hardware complications, and bone or ossicular dehiscence.[1]

In cases of mastoidectomy, inadvertent violation of the labyrinthine structures can occur, resulting in fistula between the surgical site and the cochlea or the semicircular canals.[1,26] In addition, if there is osseous tegmen dehiscence during mastoidectomy or other temporal bone surgery (which result from surgery or can be related to underlying disorder present at the time of surgery; ie, cholesteatoma), there may be resultant CSF leak should the dura be violated (**Fig. 19**), or, in the case of extension of brain parenchyma through the defect, encephalocele formation (**Fig. 20**).[1]

Vascular injury is a rare but potentially severe complication of temporal bone surgery, especially complex surgeries that require access to the IAC and CPA. In such procedures, tumor dissection from adjacent neurovascular structures can injure the anterior inferior cerebellar artery or other segments of the vertebrobasilar circulation and result in downstream ischemia and/or infarction. In addition, in cases in which dural venous sinus manipulation and/or compression is performed, such as in sigmoid sinus wall reconstruction as well as translabyrinthine and retrosigmoid approach surgeries, venous thrombosis (**Fig. 21**) can occur and should be assessed for in the appropriate postoperative setting. Venous thrombosis may also be complicated by subsequent dural arteriovenous fistula formation (**Fig. 22**).[1]

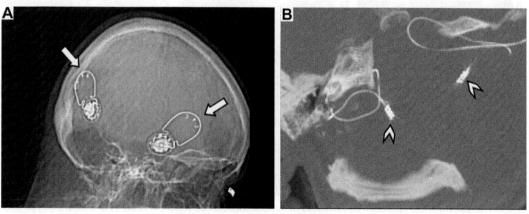

Fig. 18. ABI. Lateral scout image (*A*) of the head shows bilateral internal transmit and receiver implants (*arrows*) for bilateral ABI. Axial (*B*) MIP CT head image shows bilateral electrode arrays (*arrowheads*) related to bilateral ABI placed for sensorineural hearing loss in a patient with neurofibromatosis type 2.

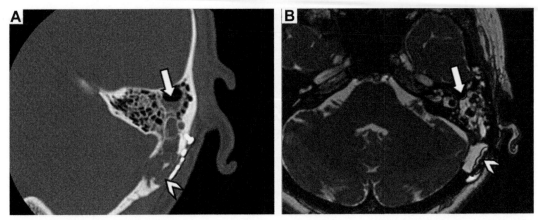

Fig. 19. Retrosigmoid approach complicated by CSF leak. Axial (*A*) CT and axial (*B*) FIESTA (fast imaging employing steady-state acquisition) MR imaging of the left temporal bone show postoperative changes of retrosigmoid approach but also with fluid signal consistent with CSF at the craniotomy site (*arrowhead*) and the adjacent left mastoid air cells (*arrow*).

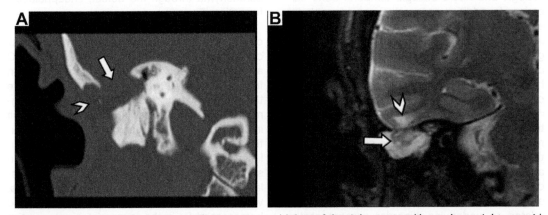

Fig. 20. Encephalocele following mastoidectomy. Coronal (*A*) CT of the right temporal bone shows right mastoidectomy (*arrowhead*) complicated by wide bony dehiscence (*arrow*) of the tegmen mastoideum. Coronal (*B*) T2-weighted fat-saturated MR imaging of the brain shows a right temporal encephalocele (*arrow*) protruding inferiorly via the tegmen defect. Associated signal changes (*arrowhead*) are noted in the herniated left temporal subcortical white matter.

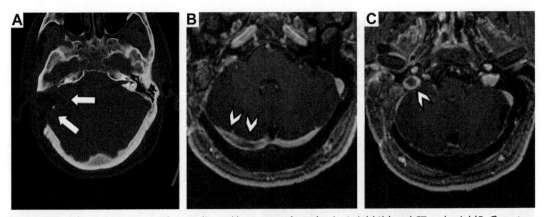

Fig. 21. Translabyrinthine approach complicated by venous thrombosis. Axial (*A*) head CT and axial (*B, C*) postcontrast brain MR imaging show postoperative changes related to prior right translabyrinthine approach (*arrows*) complicated by venous thrombosis involving the right transverse sinus extending downstream into the right internal jugular vein (*arrowheads*).

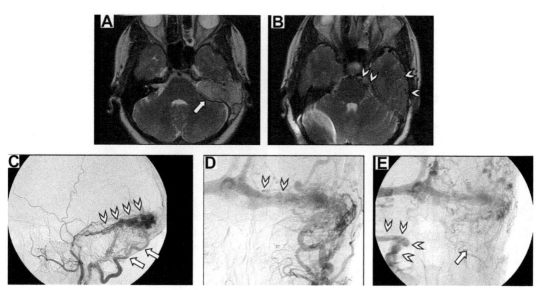

Fig. 22. Translabyrinthine approach complicated by venous thrombosis and subsequent dural arteriovenous fistula (DAVF) formation. Sequential axial T2-weighted brain MR imaging shows expected postoperative (*A*) appearance following translabyrinthine approach (*arrow*) for vestibular schwannoma resection with subsequent follow-up imaging (*B*) showing multiple new enlarged serpiginous veins (*arrowheads*) within the left prepontine cistern and MCF concerning for DAVF formation. Lateral (*C*) and frontal (*D*) fluoroscopic projections following contrast injection of the left EAC during cerebral angiogram confirm presence of DAVF arising in part from the left occipital artery (*arrows*) extending into the left transverse sinus (*arrowheads*) with early drainage into the dural venous sinuses. Subsequent venous phase frontal projection (*E*) shows extensive filling defect of the left sigmoid sinus and internal jugular vein (*arrow*) compared with the right (*arrowheads*), consistent with internal thrombus.

Hardware complications are also important for radiologists to be aware of, notably prosthesis malpositioning (**Fig. 23**). For example, in the case of stapes prosthesis placement, although some penetration through the oval window into the vestibule is expected, entry of the prosthesis deep into the vestibule should raise concern for malposition (**Fig. 24**), especially if there is a clinical history of significant vertigo. Ultimately, clinical correlation with patient symptoms is critical because prosthesis malpositioning can present with worsening or new conductive hearing loss.[1,6,26]

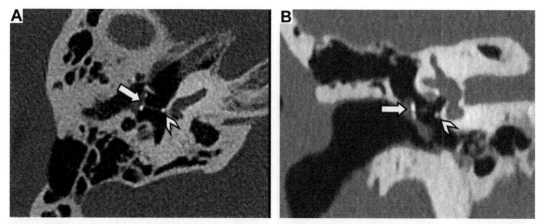

Fig. 23. TORP malpositioning. Axial (*A*) and coronal (*B*) CT of the right temporal bone show a malpositioned titanium TORP in this patient who presented with new hearing loss. The lateral end of the prosthesis (*arrow*) is apposed to the tympanic membrane as expected; however the medial end of the prosthesis (*arrowhead*) is positioned at the cochlear promontory and appears inferiorly displaced from the oval window.

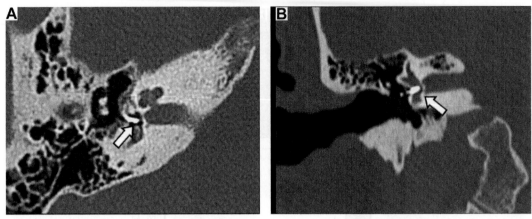

Fig. 24. Stapes prosthesis malpositioning. Axial (*A*) and coronal (*B*) CT of the right temporal bone show a malpositioned stapes prosthesis (*arrows*) that penetrates too deeply into the vestibule. Patient reported worsened hearing and dizziness.

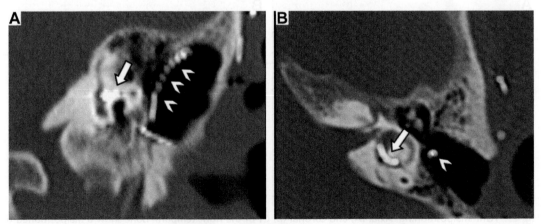

Fig. 25. CI electrode malpositioning. Coronal (*A*) and axial (*B*) CT of the left temporal bone show a CI with wires (*arrowheads*) traversing the mastoid cavity. However, the CI electrode array (*arrows*) has been malpositioned into the vestibule instead of the cochlea and terminates within the lateral semicircular canal.

With regard to CI placement, several hardware complications can occur, including electrode extrusion (in which the electrode is seen backing out of the cochlea) and electrode array malpositioning (ie, into the vestibule, semicircular canal, or possibly the IAC) (Fig. 25), which can manifest as decreasing device performance. Thin-section temporal bone CT remains the study of choice to evaluate for such hardware complications.[1]

SUMMARY

Imaging of the postoperative temporal bone is challenging. Recognition of common temporal bone surgical procedures and their potential complications is essential for accurate radiological interpretation. Greater knowledge in this area will ultimately serve patients and referring providers with prompt diagnosis and improved patient outcomes.

CLINICS CARE POINTS

- Postoperative temporal bone imaging interpretation can be difficult for all but the most experienced radiologists.

- Careful review of patient clinical and operative history is critical to identify potential postoperative disorders and/or complications.

- Serial imaging in the postoperative setting may be helpful in distinguishing postoperative from true pathologic enhancement because progressive/increasing nodular, irregular, and/or masslike enhancement may indicate the presence of recurrent tumor in the setting of prior enhancing mass resection on MR imaging.

- Common interpretative pitfalls include lack of knowledge regarding expected postsurgical anatomic changes, wide variety of otologic hardware, correct hardware positioning, as well as delayed recognition of postoperative complications.

- Common surgical procedures involving the temporal bone include tympanostomy, mastoidectomy, temporal bone resection, IAC and CPA surgical approaches, SSCD repair, sigmoid sinus wall reconstruction, ossicular reconstruction, and auditory implant placement.

- Postoperative temporal bone complications include postoperative hemorrhage, excessive pneumocephalus, brain retraction injury, vascular injury, CSF leak, hardware complications, and bone or ossicular dehiscence.

- Correlation with patient's symptoms is useful because auditory implant and ossicular prosthetic-related complications often present with new/increasing hearing loss.

DISCLOSURE

The authors have no relevant commercial or financial disclosures.

REFERENCES

1. Penta M, Pinho MC, Isaacson B, et al. Postsurgical temporal bone: a pictorial essay of commonly encountered neuro-otologic surgical approaches and postoperative imaging appearance. Neurographics 2016. https://doi.org/10.3174/ng.3160152.

2. Klein MA, Kelly JK, Eggleston D. Recognizing tympanostomy tubes on temporal bone CT: typical and atypical appearances. Am J Roentgenol 1988. https://doi.org/10.2214/ajr.150.6.1411.

3. Juliano AF, Ginat DT, Moonis G. Imaging review of the temporal bone: Part II. traumatic, postoperative, and noninflammatory nonneoplastic conditions. Radiology 2015. https://doi.org/10.1148/radiol.2015140800.

4. Groblewski JC, Harley EH. Medial migration of tympanostomy tubes: an overlooked complication. Int J Pediatr Otorhinolaryngol 2006. https://doi.org/10.1016/j.ijporl.2006.05.015.

5. Mukherji SK, Mancuso AA, Kotzur IM, et al. CT of the temporal bone: findings after mastoidectomy, ossicular reconstruction, and cochlear implantation. Am J Roentgenol 1994. https://doi.org/10.2214/ajr.163.6.7992748.

6. Larson TL, Wong ML. Imaging of the mastoid, middle ear, and internal auditory canal after surgery: what every radiologist should know. Neuroimaging Clin N Am 2009. https://doi.org/10.1016/j.nic.2009.06.005.

7. Mehta RP, Harris JP. Mastoid obliteration. Otolaryngol Clin North Am 2006. https://doi.org/10.1016/j.otc.2006.08.007.

8. Powitzky ES, Hayman LA, Chau J, et al. High-resolution computed tomography of temporal bone: Part IV: coronal postoperative anatomy. J Comput Assist Tomogr 2006;30(3):548–54.

9. Lambert PR. Mastoidectomy. In: Cummings otolaryngology - head and neck surgery. Elsevier; 2010. p. 2009–16. https://doi.org/10.1016/B978-0-323-05283-2.00143-9.

10. Chole R, Brodie H, Jacob A. Surgery of the mastoid and Petrosa. 4th edition. Philadelphia: Lippincott Williams & Wilkins; 2014. p. 2080–111.

11. Medina JE, Park AO, Neely JG, et al. Lateral temporal bone resections. Am J Surg 1990;160(4):427–33.

12. Paul G. Temporal bone resection. In: Kountakis SE, editor. Encyclopedia of otolaryngology, head and neck surgery. Springer Berlin Heidelberg; 2013. p. 2737–9. https://doi.org/10.1007/978-3-642-23499-6_767.

13. Gidley PW, DeMonte F. Subtotal and total temporal bone resection. In: Gidley PW, DeMonte F, editors. Temporal bone Cancer. Springer International Publishing; 2018. p. 245–53. https://doi.org/10.1007/978-3-319-74539-8_18.

14. Nickele CM, Akture E, Gubbels SP, et al. A stepwise illustration of the translabyrinthine approach to a large cystic vestibular schwannoma. Neurosurg Focus 2012. https://doi.org/10.3171/2012.7.FOCUS12208.

15. Silk PS, Lane JI, Driscoll CL. Surgical approaches to vestibular schwannomas: what the radiologist needs to know. Radiographics 2009;29(7):1955–70.

16. Brackmann DE, Arriaga MA. Neoplasms of the Posterior Fossa. In: Cummings Otolaryngology - head and neck surgery. 2010. https://doi.org/10.1016/b978-0-323-05283-2.00178-6.

17. Forbes JA, Carlson ML, Godil SS, et al. Retrosigmoid craniotomy for resection of acoustic neuroma with hearing preservation: a video publication. Neurosurg Focus 2014. https://doi.org/10.3171/2014.V1.FOCUS13451.

18. Weissman JL, Hirsch BE, Fukui MB, et al. The evolving MR appearance of structures in the internal auditory canal after removal of an acoustic neuroma. AJNR Am J Neuroradiol 1997;18(2):313–23.

19. Chung LK, Ung N, Spasic M, et al. Clinical outcomes of middle fossa craniotomy for superior semicircular canal dehiscence repair. J Neurosurg 2016;125(5):1187–93.

20. Minor LB, Solomon D, Zinreich JS, et al. Sound- and/or pressure-induced vertigo due to bone dehiscence of the superior semicircular canal. Arch Otolaryngol Head Neck Surg 1998;124(3):249–58.

21. Berning AW, Arani K, Branstetter BF 4th. Prevalence of superior semicircular canal dehiscence on high-resolution CT imaging in patients without vestibular or auditory abnormalities. AJNR Am J Neuroradiol 2019;40(4):709–12.

22. Palma Diaz M, Cisneros Lesser JC, Vega Alarcón A. Superior semicircular canal dehiscence syndrome - diagnosis and surgical management. Int Arch Otorhinolaryngol 2017;21(2):195–8.

23. Silverstein H, Kartush JM, Parnes LS, et al. Round window reinforcement for superior semicircular canal dehiscence: a retrospective multi-center case series. Am J Otolaryngol 2014;35(3):286–93.

24. Raghavan P, Serulle Y, Gandhi D, et al. Postoperative imaging findings following sigmoid sinus wall reconstruction for pulse synchronous tinnitus. Am J Neuroradiol 2016;37(1):136–42.

25. Zeng R, Wang G-P, Liu Z-H, et al. Sigmoid sinus wall reconstruction for pulsatile tinnitus caused by sigmoid sinus wall dehiscence: a single-center experience. PLoS One 2016;11(10):e0164728.

26. Stone JA, Mukherji SK, Jewett BS, et al. CT evaluation of prosthetic ossicular reconstruction procedures: what the otologist needs to know. Radiographics 2000. https://doi.org/10.1148/radiographics.20.3.g00ma03593.

27. Syms MJ. Safety of magnetic resonance imaging of stapes prostheses. Laryngoscope 2005;115(3):381–90.

28. Witte RJ, Lane JI, Driscoll CLW, et al. Pediatric and Adult Cochlear Implantation. Radiographics 2003. https://doi.org/10.1148/rg.235025046.

29. Colby CC, Todd NW, Harnsberger HR, et al. Standardization of CT depiction of cochlear implant insertion depth. Am J Neuroradiol 2015;36(2):368 LP–371.

30. Ghossaini SN, Roehm PC. Osseointegrated auditory devices: bone-anchored hearing aid and PONTO. Otolaryngol Clin North Am 2019. https://doi.org/10.1016/j.otc.2018.11.005.

31. Barber SR, Kozin ED, Remenschneider AK, et al. Auditory brainstem implant array position varies widely among adult and pediatric patients and is associated with perception. Ear Hear 2017. https://doi.org/10.1097/AUD.0000000000000448.

Imaging of the Postoperative Eye and Orbit

Daniel T. Ginat, MD, MS

KEYWORDS

• Eye • Orbit • Postoperative • Imaging

KEY POINTS

- There is a wide array of eye and orbit surgeries, ranging from eyelid, refractive, retinal, nasolacrimal drainage, and oncologic procedures.
- The effects of many of these surgeries can be observed on CT and MRI through the presence of various implants and altered anatomy.
- Imaging can be useful for assessing surgical complications, such as device malposition or migration.

INTRODUCTION

There is a plethora of surgical procedures that are performed in the eye and orbit. Although ultrasound and optical coherence tomography are often performed for ophthalmic imaging, conventional computed tomography (CT) and MR imaging scans are useful for the postoperative assessment of the eye and orbit. The consequences of these procedures can often be observed on diagnostic imaging through the presence of various implants and altered anatomy. The expected postoperative changes in the eye and orbit, the impact of implants on image quality and safety, and potential associated complications are reviewed in this article.

IMAGING PROTOCOLS
Computed Tomography

A suggested orbit CT protocol consists of 3-mm slice thickness soft tissue and 1-mm slice thickness bone window images with multiplanar reformats. Intravenous contrast is generally not necessary for assessing implant positioning or evaluating the altered bony anatomy, but is useful for cases of suspected tumor or infection. Implementation of metal artifact reduction software is useful for patients with implants that tend to produce streak artifact, as indicated in subsequent sections of this article.

MR Imaging

A typical MR imaging obit protocol consists of multiplanar T1-weighted and T2-weighted sequences with up to 3-mm slice thickness. As for CT, intravenous contrast can be administered with MR imaging scans particularly when tumor or infection is suspected and there are no contraindications. The use of fat-suppressed sequences is particularly useful for postcontrast T1-weighted sequences. Degradation of the fat-suppressed images by artifacts from some implants is mitigated using the Dixon method. For example, although surgically implanted metal devices are generally safe and compatible with MR imaging, selecting lower field strength scanners can also help minimize susceptibility artifacts.

Department of Radiology, Section of Neuroradiology, University of Chicago, 5841 South Maryland Avenue, Chicago, IL 60637, USA
E-mail address: dtg1@uchicago.edu

Neuroimag Clin N Am 32 (2022) 193–202
https://doi.org/10.1016/j.nic.2021.08.007

neuroimaging.theclinics.com

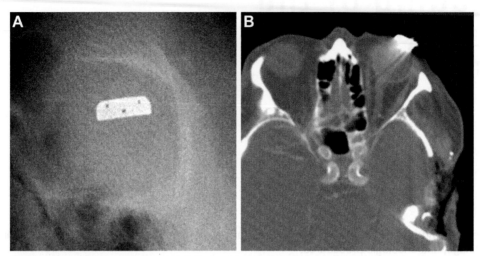

Fig. 1. Eyelid weight. Frontal radiograph (A) and axial CT (B) show a rectangular metal implant in the upper eyelid. There are small suture holes in the eyelid weight. The implant produces streak artifact on CT.

IMAGING FINDINGS
Eyelid Weight and Spring

Palpebral weights and springs are used to reanimate the eyelid to prevent corneal injury in patients with facial nerve paralysis.[1–3] These devices are MR imaging safe and are encountered incidentally as part of the imaging work-up for recurrent tumors. The eyelid weights appear as slightly curved plates with holes for securing the implant and can produce substantial beam hardening artifact on CT (Fig. 1). The eyelid springs do not produce substantial beam hardening on CT and consists of a prong secured to the superior orbital rim and

another prong positioned in the upper eyelid (Fig. 2).

Keratoprosthesis

Alloplastic implants are used to treat cases of complicated corneal blindness.[4] For example, Boston keratoprostheses are used in conjunction with corneal donor grafts. On CT, the keratoprosthesis plastic front plate that functions as a lens appears as soft tissue attenuation alongside the higher attenuation titanium locking back plate and locking ring (Fig. 3). These prostheses are MR imaging compatible and do not produce any significant

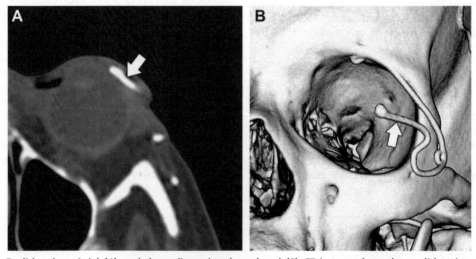

Fig. 2. Eyelid spring. Axial (A) and three-dimensional rendered (B) CT images show the eyelid spring prongs secured to the superior orbital rim and the upper eyelid (arrows).

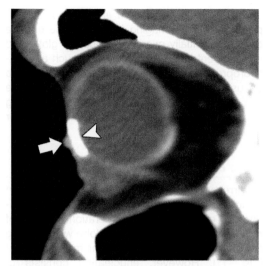

Fig. 3. Sagittal CT image shows a type 1 Boston KPro in the anterior globe, consisting of a plastic front plate that functions as a lens and appears as soft tissue attenuation (*arrow*) alongside the higher attenuation titanium locking back plate and locking ring (*arrowhead*).

artifacts. An alternative option for corneal reconstruction is the osteo-odonto-keratoprosthesis, which comprises a portion of the tooth.

Intraocular Lens Implant

Artificial intraocular lens implants are used to substitute a diseased lens, most commonly from cataracts. The lens implants are comprised of a refractive optic component and haptics that secure the implant to the capsular bag. The optic portions of intraocular lens implants are generally visible on routine clinical CT and MR imaging scans, whereas the haptic portions are not discernible on clinical images.[5] In particular, the implants appear as thin hyperattenuating

structures on CT and low signal on T2-weighted MR imaging sequences (**Fig. 4**). The implants are MR imaging compatible and do not produce any significant artifacts.

Glaucoma Drainage Implants

The excess intraocular pressure is reduced in patients with glaucoma using aqueous drainage devices, such as the Ahmed and Baerveldt shunts, among others. These devices are usually positioned along the superotemporal aspect of the globe and can accumulate variable amounts of fluid in the reservoirs, forming filtration blebs. The blebs are visible on imaging along the periphery of the implants (**Fig. 5**). The size of the bleb correlates with the preoperative intraocular pressure and there is associated compression of the lacrimal gland.[6] Alternatively, the stainless steel Ex-PRESS mini glaucoma filtration device is used to drain the aqueous humor. The device is positioned in the anterior chamber of the globe and is MR imaging compatible with negligible artifact on CT or MR imaging (**Fig. 6**).[7]

Scleral Buckling

Retinal detachment is treated by encircling the globe with a band, which applies pressure to the sclera and helps reappose the retina. The scleral bands are partially or completely circumferential and indent the globe. The bands are often composed of high-attenuation silicone rubber or low-attenuation silicone sponge, both of which have low signal on all MR imaging sequences (**Fig. 7**).[8] In the past, hydrogel scleral buckles were used, but were subsequently avoided because of their propensity for excessive swelling and fragmentation. The swollen hydrogel scleral bands display nearly fluid attenuation on CT and fluid signal on MR imaging and sometimes develop rim calcifications (**Fig. 8**).[9]

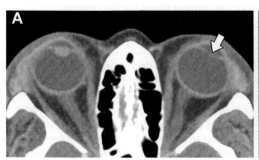
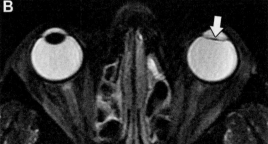

Fig. 4. Intraocular lens implant. Axial CT (*A*) and T2-weighted MR image (*B*) show the hyperattenuating and low signal implant in the left globe in cross-section (*arrows*). The implant is much thinner than the native lens.

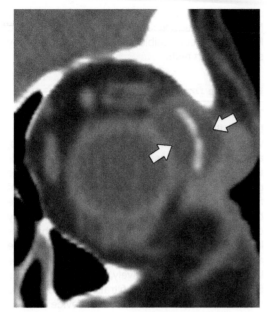

Fig. 5. Ahmed glaucoma drainage device. Coronal CT image shows a fluid-filled bleb (*arrows*) surrounding the hyperattenuating reservoir footplate in the superotemporal orbit.

Intraocular Tamponade

Vitrectomy with silicone oil tamponade is performed for mechanical apposition of the retina in patients with rhegmatogenous retinal detachment. The silicone oil demonstrates high attenuation on CT, but unlike hemorrhage, the material floats

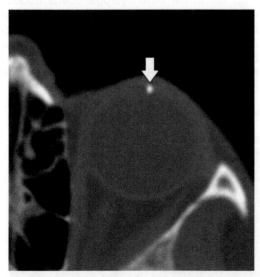

Fig. 6. EX-PRESS mini glaucoma shunt. Axial CT image shows a punctate metallic drainage device in the anterior chamber (*arrow*).

and displays chemical shift artifact and fat suppression on MR imaging (**Fig. 9**).[10] The silicone oil can potentially migrate beyond the globe and into the ventricular system. Gases, such as octafluoropropane and sulfur hexafluoride, can also be used for retinal tamponade and display the same imaging characteristics as air on imaging (**Fig. 10**). The gases can persist within the eye for up to a few weeks.

Globe Evisceration and Enucleation

An irreversibly damaged eye, such as from trauma or certain tumors, is removed by enucleation or evisceration.[11] Evisceration consists of removing the contents of the globe while leaving the scleral shell and extraocular muscles intact (**Fig. 11**). However, enucleation consists of removing the entire globe, while leaving the other orbital and periorbital tissues intact. The resulting anophthalmic socket is filled using an implant, which is often fitted with a prosthetic shell for cosmetic purposes. There is a variety of materials that are used for globe implants (**Fig. 12**). Of note, porous implants, such as MEDPOR (Stryker Corp, Kalamazoo, MI), can display internal enhancement because of fibrovascular ingrowth (**Fig. 13**).[12]

Orbital Exenteration

Exenteration of the orbit, which consists of removing the eye globe and surrounding tissues, is most often indicated for malignant tumors. The resulting defect is usually filled with a free flap. For example, myocutaneous flaps consist of adipose tissue and muscle components. The muscle component can demonstrate enhancement on imaging,[13] but typically displays a striated pattern and can atrophy (**Fig. 14**). Recurrent tumors following orbital exenteration and free flap reconstruction demonstrate a wide range of imaging appearances, but most often appear as a soft tissue mass often similar in appearance to the primary tumor and arising along the flap margin.[14]

Orbital Decompression

Endoscopic orbital decompression is a treatment option for patients with thyroid eye disease complicated by proptosis and optic neuropathy.[15] The procedure may involve orbital wall and fat resection via various approaches. The orbital contents tend to protrude through the defects into the adjacent sinus and can sometimes obstruct drainage (**Fig. 15**). The extraocular muscles can enlarge follow the decompression surgery.

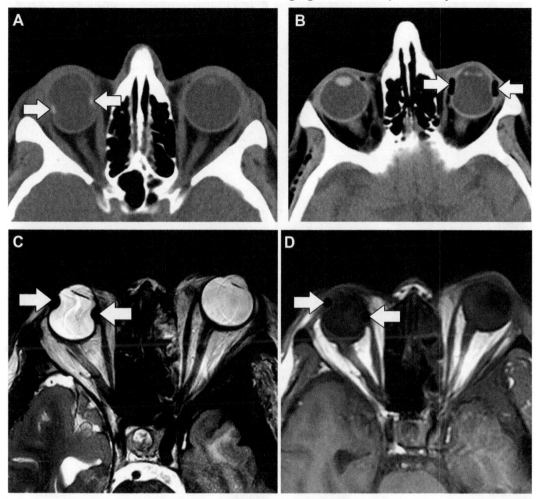

Fig. 7. Silicone scleral bands. Axial CT (*A*) shows a hyperattenuating right silicone rubber scleral band that indents the globe (*arrows*). Axial CT (*B*) shows the nearly air attenuation silicone sponge scleral buckle that partially encircles the left globe (*arrows*). Axial T2-weighted (*C*) and T1-weighted (*D*) MR images show a right silicone scleral buckle with low intensity on both sequences (*arrows*). There are also bilateral lens implants on the MR imaging.

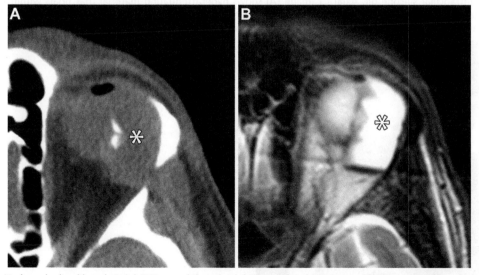

Fig. 8. Hydrogel scleral band. Axial CT image (*A*) and axial T2-weighted MR image (*B*) show a swollen rectangular strip of the scleral band with fluid attenuation and signal (*asterisk*). There are also small dystrophic calcifications along the medial edge of the scleral band.

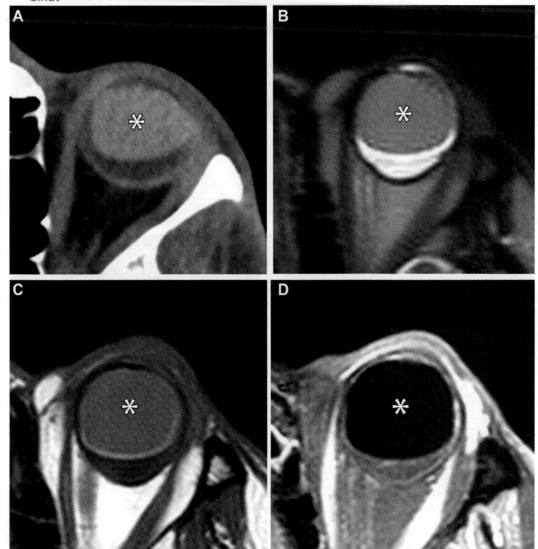

Fig. 9. Intraocular silicone oil. Axial CT image (*A*) shows hyperattenuating material that floats within the left globe (*asterisk*). Axial T2-weighted (*B*), T1-weighted (*C*), and postcontrast fat-suppressed T1-weighted (*D*) MR images show that the silicone oil (*asterisk*) displays chemical shift artifact and fat suppression.

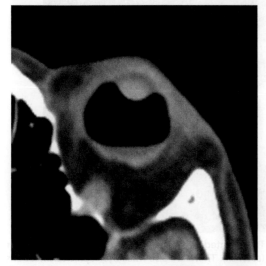

Fig. 10. Pneumatic retinopexy. Axial CT image shows gas in the vitreous chamber of the globe.

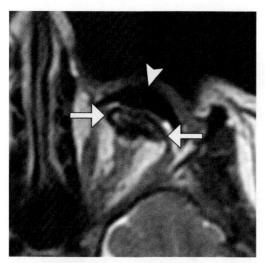

Fig. 11. Evisceration. Axial T2-weighted MR image shows a collapsed low T2 signal scleral shell (*arrows*). There is also an eye prosthesis (*arrowhead*).

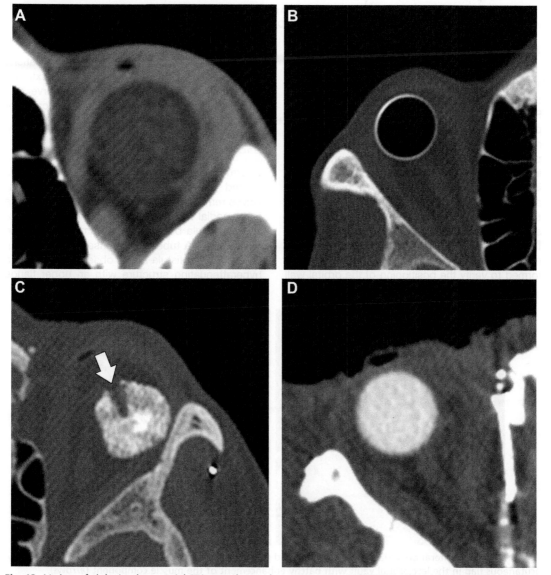

Fig. 12. Variety of globe implants. Axial CT image shows a low-attenuation MEDPOR implant (*A*). Axial CT image shows a hollow glass shell implant (*B*). Axial CT image shows a hyperattenuating hydroxyapatite implant with a groove (*arrow*) for the peg of an accompanying eye prosthesis (*C*). Axial CT image shows a hyperattenuating silicone implant (*D*).

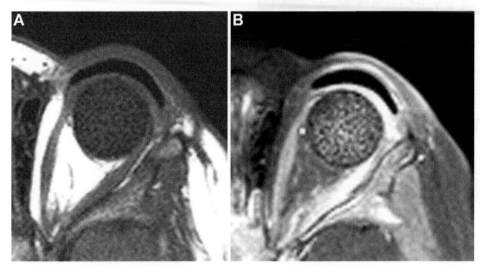

Fig. 13. Globe implant with fibrovascular ingrowth. Axial T1-weighted (*A*) and postcontrast fat-suppressed T1-weighted (*B*) MR images show enhancement of a MEDPOR globe implant.

Orbital Wall Reconstruction

Trauma and tumor resection can lead to defects in the orbital walls that require surgical repair. Reconstruction of orbital wall defects is accomplished using a variety of materials, such as titanium mesh, porous polyethylene sheet, silicone plate, and bone graft. For example, polyethylene implants have soft tissue attenuation on CT, which is difficult to distinguish from hemorrhage, although the implants have a rectilinear configuration (**Fig. 16**). These materials do not produce any significant artifact on CT or MR imaging. Ideally, the implanted material should closely reapproximate the native bone contours. CT is often performed to verify the positioning of the orbital wall reconstruction implants. Potential complications of the surgery include impingement of the extraocular muscles (**Fig. 17**) or the optic nerve and encroachment of the infraorbital nerve canal or nasolacrimal duct.[16]

Dacryocystorhinostomy

Obstruction of the lacrimal drainage system is treated via dacryocystorhinostomy.[17] This involves removing a small portion of bone from the inferomedial orbital wall and creating a new passage or fistula between the lacrimal sac and the nasal cavity. A tube is often inserted to maintain patency of the fistula and is observed on CT as a hyperattenuating structure with an upper flange

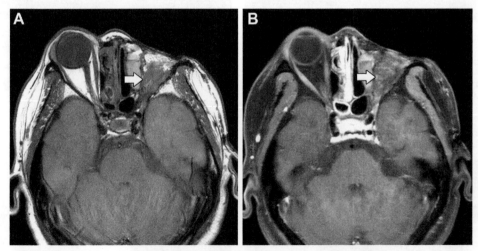

Fig. 14. Orbital exenteration. Axial T1-weighted (*A*) and postcontrast fat-suppressed T1-weighted (*B*) show a myocutaneous flap in the left orbital vault with patchy enhancement of the muscle component (*arrows*).

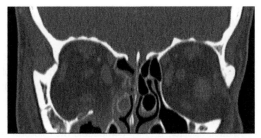

Fig. 15. Orbital wall decompression for thyroid eye disease. Coronal CT image shows right inferior and medial orbital wall defects with protrusion of the orbital contents into the adjacent sinonasal cavities, where there are obstructed secretions and mucosal thickening.

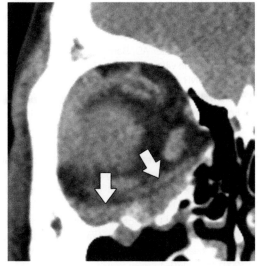

Fig. 16. Orbital wall reconstruction. Coronal CT image shows the intermediate-attenuation low-profile Omnipore sheet implants (arrows) in the inferior orbit for orbital floor reconstruction.

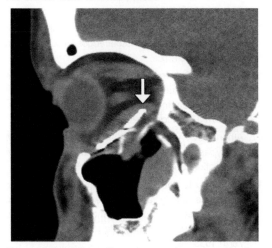

Fig. 17. Orbital wall reconstruction complication. Sagittal CT image shows impingement of the inferior rectus muscle by a malpositioned titanium mesh (arrow) in a patient with associated vertical diplopia.

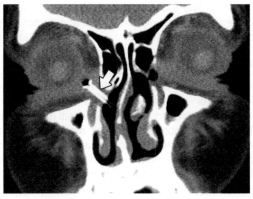

Fig. 18. Dacryocystorhinostomy. Coronal CT image shows a flanged tube (arrow) that traverses a defect in the inferomedial right orbital wall.

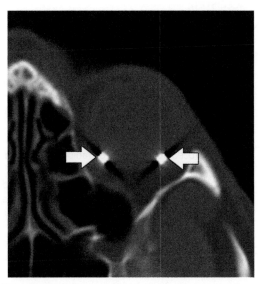

Fig. 19. Tantalum markers. Axial CT image shows small metal structures (arrows) along the posterior aspect of the globe with beam hardening artifact.

(Fig. 18). The tubes used for this procedure are generally MR imaging compatible and do not produce significant artifact.

Tantalum Markers

Implantation of ocular tantalum markers is performed for planning proton radiation therapy, which is a standard treatment of uveal melanoma. The markers appear as small metal structures along the surface of the globe and produce mild beam hardening artifact (Fig. 19). The presence of the markers is not a contraindication for MR imaging and the markers produce minor artifact.[18]

CLINICS CARE POINTS

- CT is a useful imaging modality for delineating various surgical implants and anatomic alterations from surgeries involving the eye and orbit.

- Although some implants can cause artifacts that undermine image quality, most eye and orbit surgical implants are amenable to MR imaging.

- Familiarity with potential imaging manifestations of eye and orbit surgeries is important to avoid misconstruing expected findings as abnormal.

DISCLOSURE

None.

REFERENCES

1. Marra S, Leonetti JP, Konior RJ, et al. Effect of magnetic resonance imaging on implantable eyelid weights. Ann Otol Rhinol Laryngol 1995;104(6): 448–52.
2. Ginat DT, Bhama P, Cunnane ME, et al. Facial reanimation procedures depicted on radiologic imaging. AJNR Am J Neuroradiol 2014;35(9):1662–6.
3. Levine RE, Shapiro JP. Reanimation of the paralyzed eyelid with the enhanced palpebral spring or the gold weight: modern replacements for tarsorrhaphy. Facial Plast Surg 2000;16(4):325–36.
4. Nonpassopon M, Niparugs M, Cortina MS. Boston type 1 keratoprosthesis: updated perspectives. Clin Ophthalmol 2020;14:1189–200.
5. Kuo MD, Hayman LA, Lee AG, et al. In vivo CT and MR appearance of prosthetic intraocular lens. AJNR Am J Neuroradiol 1998;19(4):749–53.
6. Ferreira J, Fernandes F, Patricio M, et al. Magnetic resonance imaging study on blebs morphology of Ahmed valves. J Curr Glaucoma Pract 2015;9(1): 1–5.
7. Mabray MC, Uzelac A, Talbott JF, et al. Ex-PRESS glaucoma filter: an MRI compatible metallic orbital foreign body imaged at 1.5 and 3T. Clin Radiol 2015;70(5):e28–34.
8. Lane JI, Watson RE Jr, Witte RJ, et al. Retinal detachment: imaging of surgical treatments and complications. Radiographics 2003;23(4):983–94.
9. Ginat DT, Singh AD, Moonis G. Multimodality imaging of hydrogel scleral buckles. Retina 2012;32(8): 1449–52.
10. Mathews VP, Elster AD, Barker PB, et al. Intraocular silicone oil: in vitro and in vivo MR and CT characteristics. AJNR Am J Neuroradiol 1994;15(2):343–7.
11. Kord Valeshabad A, Naseripour M, Asghari R, et al. Enucleation and evisceration: indications, complications and clinicopathological correlations. Int J Ophthalmol 2014;7(4):677–80.
12. De Potter P, Duprez T, Cosnard G. Postcontrast magnetic resonance imaging assessment of porous polyethylene orbital implant (MEDPOR). Ophthalmology 2000;107(9):1656–60.
13. Chong J, Chan LL, Langstein HN, et al. MR imaging of the muscular component of myocutaneous flaps in the head and neck. AJNR Am J Neuroradiol 2001;22(1):170–4.
14. Lee PS, Sedrak P, Guha-Thakurta N, et al. Imaging findings of recurrent tumors after orbital exenteration and free flap reconstruction. Ophthal Plast Reconstr Surg 2014;30(4):315–21.
15. Metson R, Pletcher SD. Endoscopic orbital and optic nerve decompression. Otolaryngol Clin North Am 2006;39(3):551, ix.
16. Reiter MJ, Schwope RB, Theler JM. Postoperative CT of the orbital skeleton after trauma: review of normal appearances and common complications. AJR Am J Roentgenol 2016;206(6):1276–85.
17. Athanasiov PA, Madge S, Kakizaki H, et al. A review of bypass tubes for proximal lacrimal drainage obstruction. Surv Ophthalmol 2011;56(3):252–66.
18. Oberacker E, Paul K, Huelnhagen T, et al. Magnetic resonance safety and compatibility of tantalum markers used in proton beam therapy for intraocular tumors: a 7.0 Tesla study. Magn Reson Med 2017; 78(4):1533–46.

Imaging of the Postoperative Jaws and Temporomandibular Joints

Dania Tamimi, BDS, DMSc[a],*, Michael Gunson, DDS, MD[b]

KEYWORDS

- Dentoalveolar surgery • Dental implants • Orthognathic surgery • Total joint replacement

KEY POINTS

- Preoperative imaging is important for determining the extent of a lesion and the normal anatomic configuration of the structures.
- Obtaining a baseline image immediately postoperatively is crucial for evaluation of progress and recurrence.
- Benign lesions with high recurrence rate, such as keratocysts and ameloblastomas, should be followed up long term radiographically because recurrences may occur several years later.
- It takes about 6 to 8 weeks for the first signs of bony healing to be radiographically visible.
- Nonunion of bony segments after about 3 months may indicate fibrous union or infection. Healed bony margins may be sclerotic (must be differentiated from early osteonecrosis if history of antiresorptive drugs is present).

INTRODUCTION

Surgical procedures in the oral cavity and maxillofacial complex are diverse and involve multiple tissues unique to this region. These procedures are used to remove pathology and infection, but can also restore temporomandibular joint (TMJ) and masticatory function, optimize jaw and occlusal relationships, prosthetically replace teeth and TMJs, improve esthetics, and increase upper respiratory tract dimensions. Procedures in the oral cavity are often complicated by infection stemming from the naturally occurring oral flora because the procedures often expose the underlying bone to the microorganisms that reside within the oral cavity, but can also be complicated iatrogenically. This article introduces the reader to the more commonly encountered surgical procedures through examination of the indications, anatomy to consider, and the radiographic imaging of success and failure of these procedures. The imaging of postsurgical malignant neoplasia is not included in this article.

DENTOALVEOLAR SURGERY
Extraction of Impacted Teeth

Indication

Most teeth erupt into the oral cavity normally without incident. The teeth that erupt last into the oral cavity (the third molars) tend to have a higher incidence for impaction. There are several presentations for these impacted third molars that are named for their alignment in relation to the dental midline and arch. Third molars are mesioangularly, distoangularly, buccoangularly, linguoangularly, and vertically impacted, with any of these being superficial or deep in the bone (**Fig. 1**). Other teeth

a Private Practice in Oral and Maxillofacial Radiology, Orlando, FL, USA; b Private Practice in Oral and Maxillofacial Surgery, 334 South Patterson Avenue, Santa Barbara, CA 93111, USA
* Corresponding author.
E-mail address: daniatamimi@hotmail.com

Neuroimag Clin N Am 32 (2022) 203–229
https://doi.org/10.1016/j.nic.2021.08.010
1052-5149/22/© 2021 Elsevier Inc. All rights reserved.

neuroimaging.theclinics.com

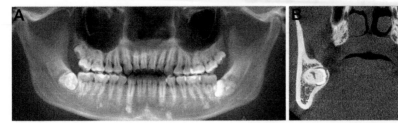

Fig. 1. Cone-beam computed tomography (CBCT) panoramic and coronal reformations showing different angulation types of third molars impactions. (*A*) Panoramic shows a transversely oriented right third molar and horizontally impacted left third molars. These are further evaluated on the coronal view (*B*) to show the linguoangular orientation of the right third molar with a thin lingual alveolar plate (high risk for injuring the lingual nerve) and the contact between the left inferior alveolar nerve (IAN) canal and the left third molar (*arrow*). (*Courtesy of* J Schaumberg, DDS, Fort Lauderdale, FL.)

can also be impacted, but the third molars are by far the most commonly impacted teeth. The deeper the tooth is embedded in bone, the more complicated the surgical procedure and the more likely the development of postsurgical complications.

Radiographic anatomy to consider
Mandibular third molars
- *Inferior alveolar nerve (IAN) canal:* The contents of this canal can be injured during extraction of an impacted third molar if the tooth is in contact with it and more so the more intimate its relationship with the canal. A surgeon and radiologist should evaluate the relationship of the tooth with the canal before extraction. The canal is located buccally, lingually, or apically to the tooth. It is compressed by the roots, in slight contact with them, or not in contact at all. A canal may present passing through the furcation area of the root and even with the roots of the tooth developing around it (**Fig. 2**).[1] Injury of the nerve within this canal can result in numbness and paresthesia. The lingual nerve

is also an important structure for the surgeon to identify clinically and to protect during the procedure, but this is not readily identifiable on computed tomography (CT) or cone-beam CT (CBCT) because it is not encased in bone.[2]

Maxillary third molars
- *Maxillary sinus and infratemporal fossa:* Maxillary third molars can be deeply impacted and displaced into the maxillary sinuses (**Fig. 3**) (especially in the case of an associated benign mass) or may be positioned more laterally in relation to the maxilla with a thin bony separation between it and the infratemporal fossa. Evaluation of the proximity of the tooth to these structures is important to minimize the risk of displacement, which in many cases necessitates another surgical procedure for retrieval.

Imaging of success
A tooth extraction site that has not been complicated by infection heals by deposition of immature (woven) bone on the internal surface of the socket

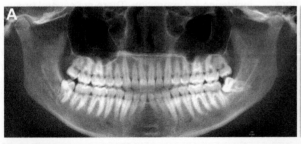
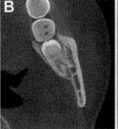
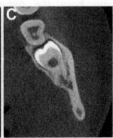

Fig. 2. CBCT panoramic reconstruction (*A*) shows distoangular orientation of the mandibular right third molar and mesioangular orientation of the left third molar. The image of the IAN canal is seen overlapping over the roots. (*B*) Axial view of the same tooth shows the IAN canal in contact with the root and partially passing through the furcation. (*C*) Axial view of a different horizontally impacted third molar with the IAN canal passing through the furcation of the roots. The risk of injury to the nerve with surgical removal of the tooth is high. (*Courtesy of* J Schaumberg, DDS, Fort Lauderdale, FL.)

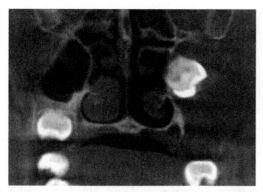

Fig. 3. Coronal CBCT shows a maxillary impacted third molar that has been displaced into the left maxillary sinus by a benign odontogenic lesion that occupies the entire sinus. (*Courtesy of* M Noujeim, DDS MS, San Antonio, TX)

that starts to become radiographically visible by 6 to 8 weeks (**Fig. 4**). This gives the appearance of bone filling from the outside in. Eventually, the socket becomes filled with bone and faint outline of the higher density lamina dura of the socket can persist or resorb beyond 6 months (see **Fig. 4**).

Imaging of complications

Tooth extraction is complicated by infection, fracture of the tooth or alveolus, or by violation of the adjacent anatomy. Osteomyelitis should be ruled out in these areas of recent extraction if the patient presents with any clinical signs of infection (eg, pain, swelling, pus). The CT and CBCT radiographic appearance is a delayed organization of the bone within the socket (when compared with other extraction sites of teeth that were removed at the same time), interruption of the bony cortex of the mandible, and periosteal reaction (**Fig. 5**).[3]

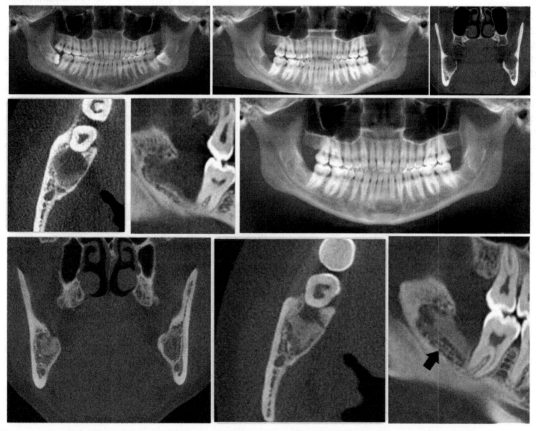

Fig. 4. A series of CBCT reformations showing the normal healing after third molar extraction made on the day of tooth extraction (*A*), 3 months postoperative (*B–E*), and 7 months postoperative (*F–I*). At 3 months, a thin layer of immature bone is seen lining the walls of the sinus. At 7 months, the right side shows the formation of dense bone filling the socket and effacement of the lamina dura borders of the socket (*arrow*). The left side is organizing but at a slower pace, indicating follow-up to rule out possible complication preventing the healing from progressing at the same rate as the opposite side. (*Courtesy of* J Schaumberg, DDS, Fort Lauderdale, FL.)

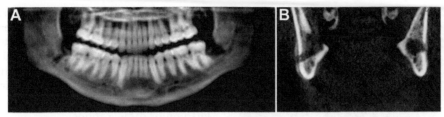

Fig. 5. Panoramic (A) and coronal CBCT (B) shows bilateral third molar extractions that have been complicated by osteomyelitis. The socket does not show bone deposition within it and there is interruption of the cortices of the mandible with overlying periosteal reaction noted bilaterally.

MR imaging findings include loss of T1 signal because fatty marrow is replaced by exudate in acute cases and marked hyperintensity on STIR because of edema or hyperemia. The surrounding soft tissue inflammation has high signal on STIR and T1 contrast-enhanced and fat-saturated images (Fig. 6).

Dental Implant Surgery

Indications

Dental implants have quickly become a mainstream method of replacing missing teeth. Successful osseointegration of these implants depends on the lack of infection, the vitality of the bone following the osteotomy, the presence of adequate bone to support the implant in all dimensions, and a biomechanically sound configuration of the implant and crown replacing the tooth. Evaluation of adequate bone height and width and the proximity to anatomy should be evaluated before implant placement to avoid

violating important anatomic structures and to ensure the success of the dental implant.

Radiographic anatomy to consider
Maxilla
- *Maxillary sinuses:* The maxillary sinuses tend to pneumatize the maxillary posterior alveolar processes, notably after the loss of the posterior teeth. This creates inadequate bone height and volume for the placement of implants. Such sinuses could be grafted using particulate graft, which should not be confused for fibro-osseous pathology (Fig. 7).
- *Anterior superior alveolar canal and incisive canal:* These canals are in the anterior region of the maxilla. The incisive (nasopalatine) canal is in the midline posterior to the central incisors and, together with bone loss on the facial aspect of the alveolar process, can minimize the amount of bone available of an anterior tooth implant (Fig. 8). The anterior

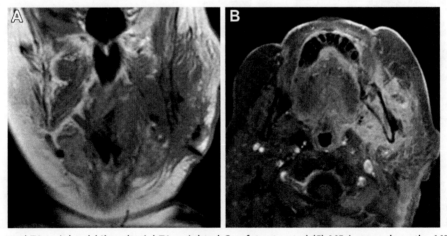

Fig. 6. Coronal T1-weighted (A) and axial T1-weighted C + fat-saturated (B) MR images show the MR imaging appearance of osteomyelitis in the mandible. The high fatty marrow signal has been replaced on T1-weighted (A), and T1-weighted C + fat saturation shows diffuse enhancement of the marrow space with masticator space enhancement. (*From* Koenig L, Tamimi D, Petrikowski G, Perschbacher S. Mandible-Maxilla Osteomyelitis. In: Koenig L, Tamimi D, Petrikowski G, Perschbacher S, editors. Diagnostic Imaging: Oral and Maxillofacial, 2nd Edition. USA: Elsevier; 2018. p. 387-390; with permission)

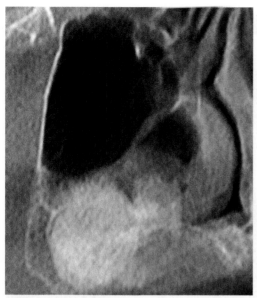

Fig. 7. Custom sagittal oblique CBCT view shows the high-density granular appearance of a particular sinus graft in a "sinus lift" maxillary posterior alveolar process ridge augmentation. (*Courtesy of* A Schetritt, DDS.)

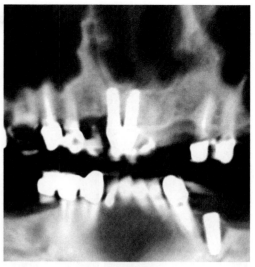

Fig. 9. CBCT panoramic reformation shows an anterior dental implant in contact with the anterior superior alveolar canal.

superior alveolar canal branches off of the infraorbital nerve before its emergence through the infraorbital foramen. It descends along the lateral walls of the nasal cavity then converges toward the midline. This more horizontal terminal portion may be injured by canine or lateral incisor implants (**Fig. 9**).[4]

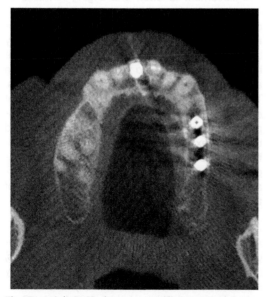

Fig. 8. Axial CBCT shows a maxillary central incisor implant that is in contact with the incisive canal.

Mandible

- *Inferior alveolar canal (IAC):* Implants should avoid contacting the canal because its violation may result in paresthesia. This canal can bifurcate and have multiple branches, which should be detected before implant placement (**Fig. 10**).
- *Mental foramen:* The IAC canal travels slightly anterior to the mental foramen in the mandible before making a U-turn to partially emerge from this foramen. This U-turn is called the "anterior loop of the IAC" and should be located to avoid injury.
- *Incisive canal:* After partially emerging from the mental foramen, the IAC continues anteriorly to the midline in the incisive canal and should be identified in the case of anterior implant placement (**Fig. 11**).
- *Lingual canal and foramen:* This is a midline structure that runs from the lingual surface of the anterior mandible to the center of the basal bone in this sagittal plane. The lingual artery enters through this foramen. Injury by an implant should be avoided.
- *Submandibular fossa:* With disuse atrophy of the mandibular posterior alveolar process, the alveolar process becomes more lingually (medially) positioned while the basal bone remains in its original position. This results in a deepening of the submandibular gland fossa on the medial aspect of the mandible, making the vertical height of the alveolar process available for implant placement shorter. This should be considered because violations of

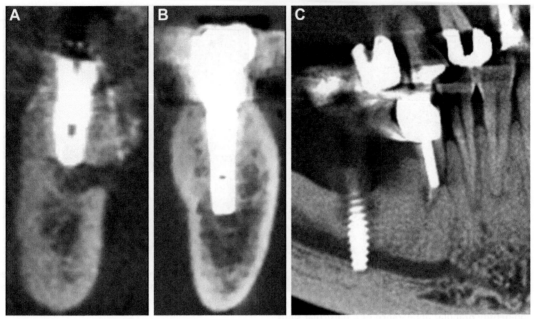

Fig. 10. Coronal (*A, B*) and sagittal (*C*) CBCT shows varying degrees of inferior alveolar nerve canal violation.

the submandibular gland and fossa may occur (**Fig. 12**).

Alveolar processes
- *Disuse atrophy of the alveolar processes:* The primary purpose of the alveolar bone is to support teeth. With the loss of teeth, the

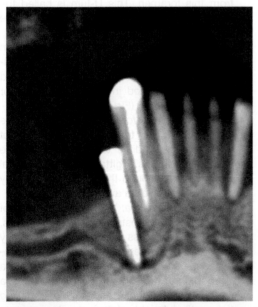

Fig. 11. CBCT panoramic reformation shows a dental implant in contact with the mandibular incisive canal (anterior branch of the IAN canal).

bone recedes, making the placement of an adequately long and ideally positioned implant difficult. The dentist should plan on augmenting alveolar processes that have receded to enable adequate position, form, and function of the implant and final crown to prevent failure.

Imaging of success
The CT radiographic imaging of dental implants postplacement is often challenging because of the presence of metal artifact surrounding the implants (**Fig. 13**), and often two-dimensional intraoral imaging is more useful in detecting bony defects. The alveolar bone should surround the implant with about 1- to 2-mm thickness of bone all around and no visible peri-implant bone loss. The implant should not violate any of the adjacent anatomy, including the teeth and adjacent implants if present. Imaging should be supplemented by clinical examination and probing to detect peri-implant loss of attachment. When planning the implants' angulation and insertion, special consideration is made for the final function and esthetics of the final tooth prosthesis (crown).

Imaging of complications
An implant that fails to osseointegrate loses radiographic bone attachment (peri-implant bone loss) (**Fig. 14**).[5,6] An implant that violates anatomy should also be evaluated clinically to correlate the symptoms to this violation of anatomy.[7] Graft material that is used to augment the bone for

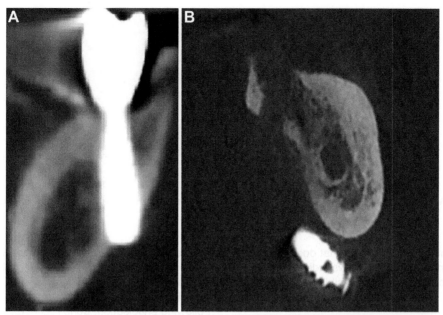

Fig. 12. (A, B) Coronal CBCT shows varying degrees of submandibular fossa violation.

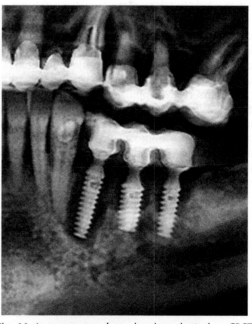

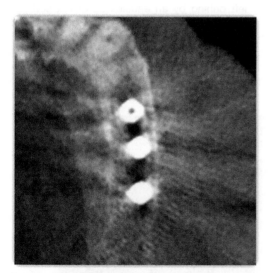

Fig. 13. Axial CBCT demonstrates the metal artifact typical in the presence of implants, particularly of multiple implants adjacent to one another. The artifact resembles bone loss even though the bone may be intact.

Fig. 14. In some cases, bone loss is evaluated on CBCT through changing the windowing and leveling and changing the slice thickness. Creation of a custom cross-section in the axial plane passing through the centers of the implants helps to generate a sagittal oblique section that may show the bone loss. In most cases, the bone loss is best evaluated through clinical evaluation and plain film vertical bitewing radiography.

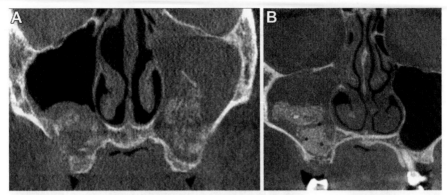

Fig. 15. (*A, B*) Coronal CBCT shows fragmentation and infection of particulate grafts placed in the maxillary sinuses.

placement of the implant but that does not resorb into the underlying bone shows radiographic signs of detachment and possible fragmentation (**Fig. 15**).

IMAGING OF SURGICAL MANAGEMENT OF BENIGN LESIONS
Enucleation and Marsupialization

Indications
When a benign lesion of the jaws (odontogenic or nonodontogenic) is present, it often requires surgical removal. The surgical management of the lesion depends on the size, extent, and location of the lesion, which dictates the surgical technique used. Smaller, less aggressive lesions require a more conservative approach, such as enucleation and excisional biopsy, whereas large cysts that inhabit a large portion of the jaws may require a marsupialization approach, which involves creation of a small opening and placing a drain in the cyst wall to relieve the hydraulic pressure of the growing cyst and evacuation of the fluid, allowing

for the deposition of bone on the inner surfaces of the cyst cavity, reducing the size of the defect before the removal of the cyst lining to prevent a pathologic fracture from occurring (**Fig. 16**).[8,9] Following enucleation, bone regeneration is more rapid than after marsupialization. However, marsupialization minimizes the danger of damage to adjacent structure and pathologic fracture.

Other large benign lesions may require marginal or complete mandibulectomy or maxillectomy. The more aggressive the lesion and the higher the risk for recurrence, the more aggressive the approach and the wider the excision margin should be.

Imaging of success
The remineralization of the inner portion of the cavity left behind by an enucleated or excised cyst should start to appear radiographically at around 6 to 8 weeks and the cavity should fill in with bone at 6 to 9 months if it is not grafted (**Fig. 17**), depending on the size of the lesion removed (longer if larger). The lumen of the cavity shrinks

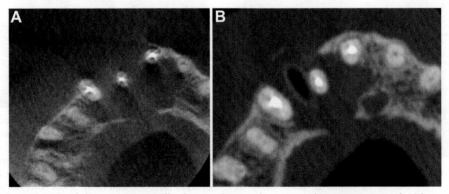

Fig. 16. (*A*) Axial CBCT of the anterior maxilla shows a large odontogenic keratocyst treated with marsupialization that has reduced in size over the course of 4 months. The drain is seen in *B*. (*Courtesy of* M Noujeim, DDS MS, San Antonio, TX.)

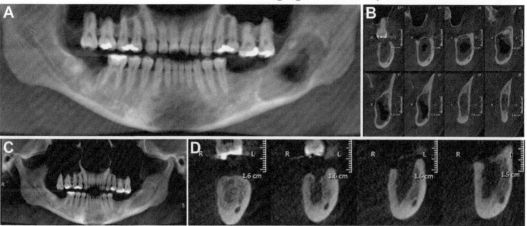

Fig. 17. CBCT panoramic and coronal cross-sections show the normal healing pattern of a benign cyst that has been enucleated. (*A, B*) shows the defect immediately postoperatively. (*C, D*) Eight months postoperatively, there is deposition of bone on the internal surface of the cyst margins. This may fill in completely with bone, or may retain some fibrous scar tissue in the center, which should be differentiated from recurrence. (*Courtesy of* M Noujeim, DDS MS, San Antonio, TX.)

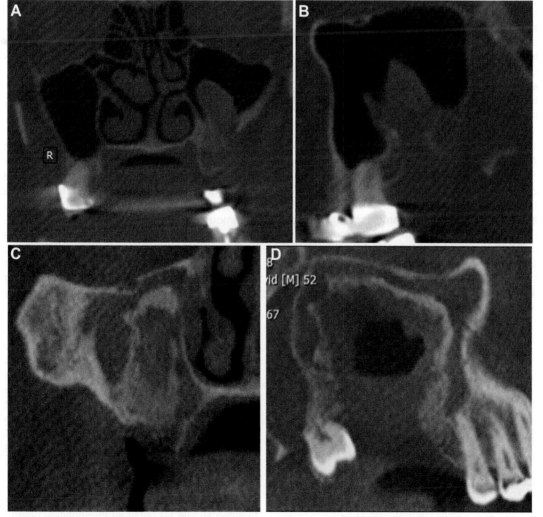

Fig. 18. Coronal and sagittal CBCTs of two separate patients (*A, B*) and (*C, D*) show the healing pattern of odontogenic cysts that have been either drained or enucleated through the oral cavity. The walls of the cyst collapse toward the center of the lumen leaving behind a sclerotic, irregular, and thickened cortex. This appearance is called a "collapsed" or "involuted" cyst. (*Courtesy of* M Noujeim, DDS MS, San Antonio, TX.)

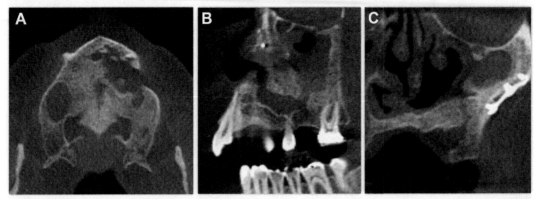

Fig. 19. Axial (*A*), sagittal (*B*), and coronal (*C*) CBCT shows fibrous healing of an odontogenic keratocyst. The bony margins are irregular, but well-defined and corticated. The underlying bone is often sclerotic. (*Courtesy of* M Noujeim, DDS MS, San Antonio, TX.)

concentrically from the outside in mandibular lesions. In maxillary lesions that extend into the maxillary sinus, the shrinking cystic walls in a marsupialized or self-draining cyst leave behind an irregular high-density structure called an involuted or collapsed cyst (**Fig. 18**). Sometimes, the defect exhibits fibrous healing, which shows soft tissue between the well-defined corticated but irregular margins of the often sclerotic bone (**Fig. 19**).

Imaging of complications
An inflammatory cyst that is not completely removed can persist as a residual cyst, which is often a perfectly circular unilocular low density in the area of the extracted tooth apex (**Fig. 20**), and an odontogenic keratocyst can recur (**Fig. 21**) because of incomplete removal of the cyst lining and the microscopic "daughter cysts" that are often associated with this lesion. There can also be secondary infection of the site, which shows irregular cortical boundaries of a previously well-defined cyst or neoplasia. Malignant

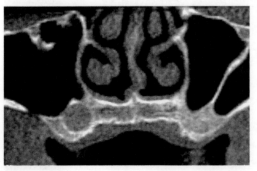

Fig. 20. Coronal view shows a residual cyst in the typical location where the tooth apex used to be. (*Courtesy of* M Noujeim, DDS MS, San Antonio, TX.)

transformation of a previously benign lesion should be ruled out in these cases.[10] Large cysts that were enucleated may leave behind a weakened mandible, so pathologic fracture should be ruled out especially with recent history of trauma to the area.

Excision and Marginal Mandibulectomy/ Maxillectomy

Indications
Benign tumors of the jaws require excision but, depending on the behavior of the lesion, the degree of aggressiveness, and rate of recurrence, the surgical approach may need to be more aggressive to decrease the rate of recurrence. Common benign lesions that have a high rate of recurrence are keratocysts and ameloblastomas. A wide margin of excision or removal of portions of the jaws are used for these lesions so the resulting defect does not retain the outlines of the original benign lesion, but rather has more angular or haphazard outlines radiographically.

Radiographic anatomic considerations
Identifying the anatomy that is in contact with the lesion before surgery helps in noting postprocedural changes. The IAN canal is often displaced by benign odontogenic lesions and may or may not return to a more normal alignment postexcision of the lesion (**Fig. 22**). Violation of the anatomy of the bony canals and decortication is important to note, because this may indicate either iatrogenic violation, or may indicate secondary infection or possible malignancy.

Imaging of success
Imaging should be obtained immediately postoperatively in the case of jaw resection to act as a baseline assessment to refer back to and compare

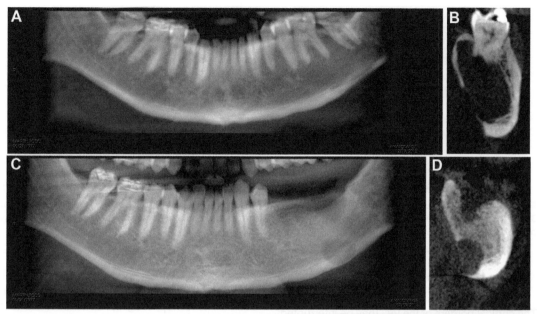

Fig. 21. CBCT panoramic and coronal view of an odontogenic keratocyst preoperatively (*A*, *B*) and 7 months post-enucleation (*C*, *D*) that largely show filling with bone and a recurrence in the lingual cortex of the mandible expanding into the submandibular gland fossa. (*Courtesy of* M Noujeim, DDS MS, San Antonio, TX.)

with on subsequent imaging. Small lesions that have been excised start to fill with bone that is radiographically visible at about 6 to 8 weeks post-operatively (**Fig. 23**). Large lesion defects may need to be reinforced to prevent fracture. This reinforcement is achieved through grafting (particulate, block, or rib/tibial grafts) or through fixation (**Fig. 24**). If the lesion is large enough to require removal of large sections of the mandible (partial or total mandibulectomy), the mandible may be replaced with a partial or total mandibular prosthesis metallic frame.

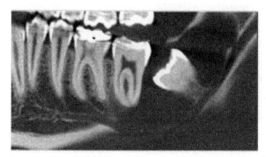

Fig. 22. CBCT custom reconstruction showing the course of an IAC that has been inferiorly displaced by a keratocyst. (*Courtesy of* D Hatcher, DDS, MS, Sacramento, California.)

Imaging of complications

- Recurrence of odontogenic keratocyst or ameloblastoma
- Graft rejection
- Fibrous union or nonunion (see **Fig. 19**)
- Loose screws or infection
- Inaccuracy of repositioning the segments

IMAGING OF SURGICAL MANAGEMENT OF MEDICATION-RELATED OSTEONECROSIS AND OSTEORADIONECROSIS
Indications

Sequestrectomy, bone debridement, bone curettage, marginal mandibulectomy, and segmental resection of the mandible are often used for the surgical management of medication-related osteonecrosis of the jaws (MRONJ), osteoradionecrosis, and osteomyelitis. Marginal mandibulectomy is used when the process leaves at least 10 mm of basal bone unaffected. Segmental resection of the mandible is used when the pathology involves the entire vertical height of the mandible or when a marginal resection would compromise the structural integrity of the mandible. The compromised portions of the mandible may be replaced by autogenous grafts, such as rib grafts, or may be replaced by a metal framework.[11]

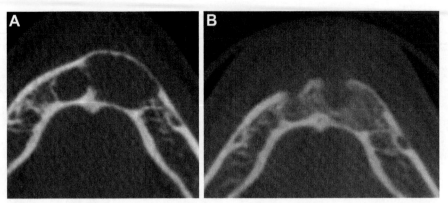

Fig. 23. (*A*, *B*) Axial CBCTs shows the healing pattern of a simple (traumatic) bone cavity over the course of 3 months. Note the deposition of new bone on the inner surface of the bone cavity from the outside in. (*Courtesy of* M Noujeim, DDS MS, San Antonio, TX.)

Radiographic Anatomy

Inferior alveolar canal
The cortical borders of the IAC may be interrupted in multiple areas when involved in osteonecrosis lesions.

Teeth
The teeth in contact with suspected areas of osteonecrosis most likely will be resected. When evaluating the postoperative imaging, any remaining teeth and bone should be evaluated for recurrence, especially in the case of MRONJ and particularly if the teeth show signs of infection (pulpal or periodontal), which may encourage the development of a separate MRONJ.

Imaging of Success

Imaging should be obtained immediately postoperatively to act as a baseline assessment to refer back to and compare with on subsequent imaging.

Marginal mandibulectomy
The margins should remain smooth and continuous on follow-up imaging. Bone sclerosis is a common finding postresection but should be monitored because stage 0 osteonecrosis can present with bone sclerosis (**Fig. 25**).[12]

Segmental mandibular resection
The resection margins should be smooth and may be sclerotic. All fixation screws should be intact and in place with no evidence of low-density bone surrounding them, which may indicate infection or recurrence. The metallic frame should be intact and not displaced or fractured. If graft material is used, it should be intact and assimilated into the adjacent bone.

Imaging of Complications

Irregular bony margins that were previously smooth and corticated should raise suspicion of recurrence or infection (**Fig. 26**). A challenge of

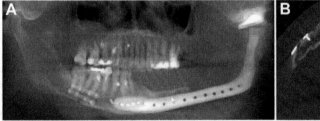
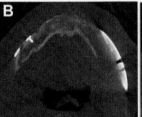
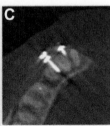

Fig. 24. (*A*) Panoramic and (*B*, *C*) axial CBCT views of a segmental mandibular resection following removal of a large benign tumor of the left mandible. A hollow tibial graft was initially used and had integrated into the anterior portion of the mandible. This was followed up with total joint replacement and replacement of the left ramus and body of the mandible with a metal frame. (*C*) Shows how the fixation screws are placed perfectly between the roots of the teeth without injury to the teeth. (*Courtesy of* A Serrano, DDS, Sao Paolo, Brazil and S Goncalves, MD, Sao Paolo, Brazil.)

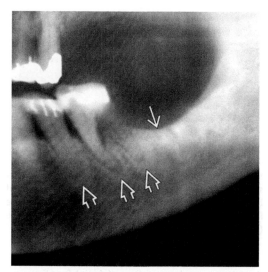

Fig. 25. Cropped panoramic radiograph shows the sclerosis of the alveolar crest (*thin arrow*) and lamina dura of the premolar and molar (*open arrows*) suggestive of stage 0 (nonspecific) bisphosphonate-related changes. (*Courtesy of* S Perschbacher, DDS, MSc; and *From* Koenig L, Tamimi D, Petrikowski G, Perschbacher S. Mandible-Maxilla Osteomyelitis. In: Koenig L, Tamimi D, Petrikowski G, Perschbacher S, editors. Diagnostic Imaging: Oral and Maxillofacial, 2nd Edition. USA: Elsevier; 2018. p. 387-390; with permission.)

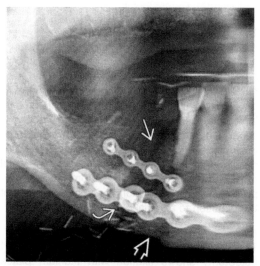

Fig. 26. Cropped panoramic radiograph shows osteoradionecrosis in a previous mandibulotomy site. Note the resorption along the surgical site (*arrow*) and destruction of the inferior cortex (*open arrow*). There is also fracture of the surgical plate (*curved arrow*). (*Courtesy of* S Perschbacher, DDS, MSc; and *From* Koenig L, Tamimi D, Petrikowski G, Perschbacher S. Mandible-Maxilla Osteomyelitis. In: Koenig L, Tamimi D, Petrikowski G, Perschbacher S, editors. Diagnostic Imaging: Oral and Maxillofacial, 2nd Edition. USA: Elsevier; 2018. p. 387-390; with permission.)

determining such a recurrence arises when the area surrounding the screws needs to be evaluated because metal artifact may obscure an area of low density or mimic one. A recurrence may be at the margins of the resection or may occur surrounding the adjacent teeth or bone segments, thus the remaining teeth and bone should be evaluated carefully. Injury of the adjacent teeth or the IAC by the fixation screws should be detected and noted. In the case of autogenous grafts, signs of fibrous union or graft rejection should be detected and noted. Single-photon emission CT can show areas of metabolic changes, but CT and CBCT can evaluate the fine anatomic and morphologic reactions more accurately.[13,14]

IMAGING OF ORTHOGNATHIC SURGICAL PROCEDURES
Introduction

There are several types of orthognathic procedures that aim to increase jaw volume, change the relationships of the jaws and teeth, improve esthetics and function, and to increase nasal cavity and oropharyngeal dimensions. These procedures are often used to correct significant developmental changes to the maxillofacial region that may have occurred because of a congenital malformation, to condylar height loss as a result of arthritis, idiopathic condylar resorption or condylar fractures, and to growth alteration from pathologic function.[7] The orthognathic surgery is usually performed with orthodontic treatment, but this is not always the case. The planning and execution of jaw surgery is complicated and requires complete diagnosis of the facial system, accurate three-dimensional planning, and detail-focused intraoperative and postoperative treatment.[15] Some of the most commonly used procedures are noted next.

Surgically Assisted Rapid Palatal Expansion

Indications
This procedure is used to increase the transverse dimension of the maxilla in adults or children whose midpalatine suture has fused and who are not candidates for the nonsurgical options of rapid palatal expansion or mini-screw-assisted rapid palatal expansion. The increase in transverse dimension is indicated in cases of maxillary or midface hypoplasia to increase nasal and oral cavity dimensions and create space for the tongue and to correct posterior crossbites of the dental occlusion.[16]

Radiographic anatomy

Surgically assisted rapid palatal expansion and its many similar but differently named procedures involve the presurgical placement of an intraoral expansion device on the palate. The surgery requires the separation of the midpalatine maxillary suture. It may also involve other cuts most often to one, two, or all of the maxillary buttresses: (1) piriform, (2) zygomaticomaxillary, and (3) pterygomaxillary midpalatine suture. After the surgery, the expansion device is activated daily, opening the midpalatal suture in the fashion on osseous distraction. Once adequate expansion has occurred, the device is retained until sufficient healing and bony union has occurred across the maxilla.

Imaging of success

Immediately after the procedure, there is a low-density zone of separation between the horizontal processes of the maxillae and palatine bones. This area then condenses and heals and becomes increasingly dense over time.

Imaging of complications

- Infection
- Inappropriate, asymmetric expansion (**Fig. 27**)
- Nonunion
- Tooth disruption (**Fig. 28**)

Le Fort I Osteotomy

Indications

The Le Fort I osteotomy is designed for the manipulation of the maxilla in three dimensions (anteroposterior, transverse, vertical and rotational) for the correction of the fit of the teeth, expansion of

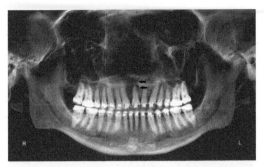

Fig. 28. CBCT reformatted Panorex postsurgically assisted rapid palatal expansion shows a failure of bone healing at the midline and disruption of the left maxillary central incisor's periodontal space (*arrows*).

the airway, and correction of facial function and esthetics. These movements address congenital defects, functional growth disturbances, dental malocclusions, and compromised airways. The maxilla is often operated in conjunction with the mandible: bilateral sagittal split osteotomies (BSSO), vertical ramus osteotomies, and/or genioplasty. When the Le Fort I and BSSO are performed together for airway expansion to treat patients with obstructive sleep apnea it is often referred to as maxillomandibular advancement.[17]

Radiographic anatomy

The Le Fort I osteotomy involves cuts axially from the piriform aperture to the pterygomaxillary junction. This cut goes through the lateral nasal walls and the walls of the maxillary sinuses. The axial cut is made above the dental root tips and below the infraorbital foramen and the zygomaticomaxillary buttresses. The pterygomaxillary junction is separated completely. The nasal septal foot plate is separated from the palate. Additional osteotomies may be performed vertically between dental roots and joined to palatal osteotomies to accomplish transverse expansion and vertical leveling of the dentition to an axial plane.

Imaging of success

The immediate successful result of a Le Fort osteotomy shows fixation with titanium plates and screws in the anterior and posterior along the piriform and zygomaticomaxillary buttresses. The midline of the anterior maxilla and maxillary central incisors aligns with the middle of the face and skull. The posterior segments align equidistant from the midsagittal plane of the face (no yaw). The canines and molar cusp tips lie level to the axial plane of the face. The nasal septum appears midline or appears in the same position as the septum preoperatively. The roots are intact

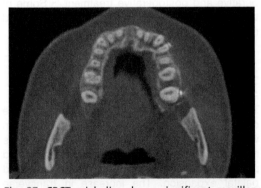

Fig. 27. CBCT axial slice shows significant maxillary arch form deformation and asymmetric encroachment of the left maxillary posterior arch and tuberosity toward the left mandibular ramus after surgically assisted rapid palatal expansion. Note the interval healing of the alveolar bone in the anterior midline.

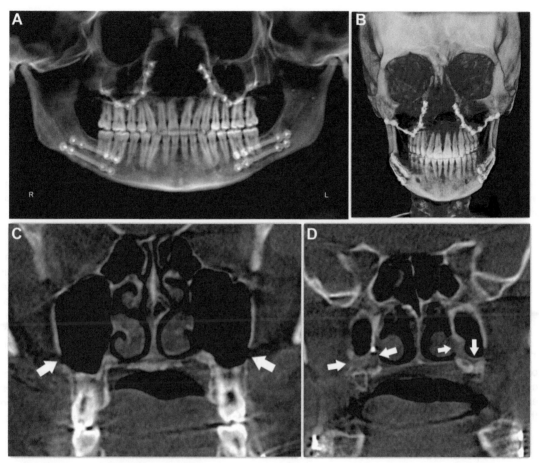

Fig. 29. (A) CBCT reformatted panoramic 9 months postmultisegment Le Fort I osteotomy and BSSO. Note symmetric overlap of dental structures, healing of the vertical osteotomies between the maxillary lateral incisors and canines, the centered mandibular condyles, and the bone healing at the piriform buttresses. (B) CBCT three-dimensional (3D) reformation. (C, D) Coronal views show the osteotomy margins (arrows).

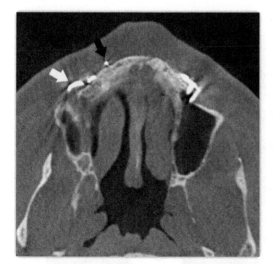

Fig. 30. CBCT axial oblique slice through the maxilla shows screws outside the bone (black arrow) and elevation of the plate from the cortical plate (white arrow) consistent with fixation failure.

without fracture or dislocation. The maxillary and mandibular teeth are aligned in an appropriate symmetric relationship. The TMJs fits into their fossae symmetrically in all three dimensions.

The long-term successful result shows intact fixation and the screws integrated in the bone. The three-dimensional position of the maxilla will have been maintained and the fit and alignment of the teeth. Bone healing is seen at the buttresses anterior and posterior. The maxillary sinuses are clear and the mandibular condyles are without erosion or size loss (Fig. 29).

Imaging of complications

- Loose fixation (Fig. 30)
- Infection (Fig. 31)
- Septal deviation (Fig. 32)
- Nonunion (Fig. 33)
- Inaccuracy of jaw placement (Fig. 34)
- Malocclusion

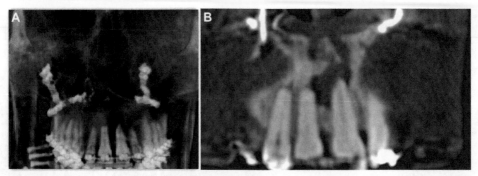

Fig. 31. CBCT 3D rendering (*A*) and Coronal slice though the anterior maxilla (*B*) in a patient several months post-multisegment Le Fort I osteotomy with a chronic infection in and around the anterior dentition. Note the resorption of the left maxillary central incisor root tip and the sequestration of bone under the septum of the nose.

- Injury of tooth roots (**Fig. 35**)
- Surgical Ciliated cyst (**Fig. 36**)
- Root resorption (**Fig. 37**)

Bilateral Sagittal Split Osteotomies

Indications
The purpose of BSSO is the same as the Le Fort I osteotomy but for the lower face. It provides correction of tooth fit, improvement of the esthetic and function of the face, and/or improvement in the size and shape of the airway.

Radiographic anatomy
BSSOs are performed with an axial cut through the medial cortex of the body of the mandible superior to the mandibular foramen and lingula. This cut is joined to a sagittal cut that is medial to the external oblique ridge and lateral to the mandibular molar roots. The sagittal cut is joined to a vertical cut through the lateral cortex of the body of the mandible. The final cut is in line with the vertical cut but through the cortex of the inferior border. The completion of the osteotomy is performed by "splitting" the medial cortex along the depression of the mylohyoid groove posteriorly and superiorly toward the lingula, joining the posterior aspect of the first axial cut. The design of the osteotomies minimizes encroachment on the dental and nerve structures, maximizes bone overlap for healing, and maintains TMJ function.

Imaging of success
The immediate successful result shows separation of the bones as described previously without

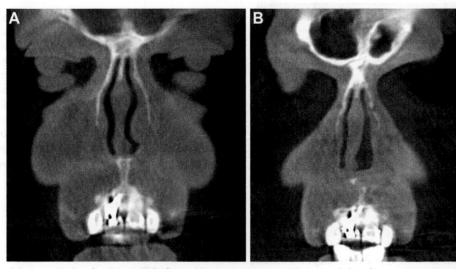

Fig. 32. (*A*) Coronal slice from a CBCT before Le Fort I osteotomy. (*B*) Coronal slice from a CBCT 9 weeks post Le Fort I osteotomy, which shows a significant right deviation of the bony septal foot plate with concomitant right deviation of the nasal septum.

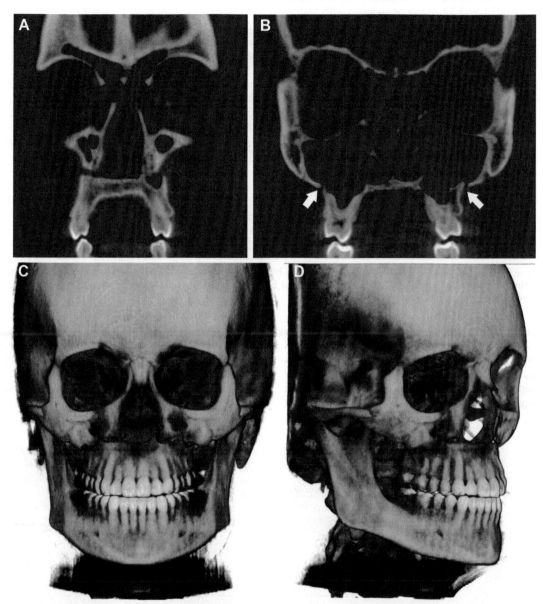

Fig. 33. (*A, B*) Coronal slices from a CBCT taken a few years after Le Fort I osteotomy (the fixation hardware was removed). (*A*) Failure of bony healing at the piriform buttresses bilaterally. (*B*) The posterior maxilla without bony union (*arrows*). (*C, D*) 3D reformation of the defect.

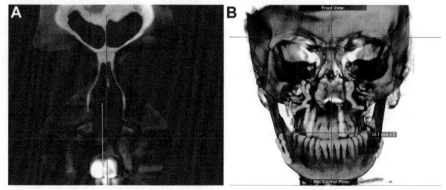

Fig. 34. (*A*) Coronal and (*B*) 3D CBCT reformats 3 years post Le Fort I osteotomy. The dental and maxillary midline is significantly to the right of the midsagittal plane.

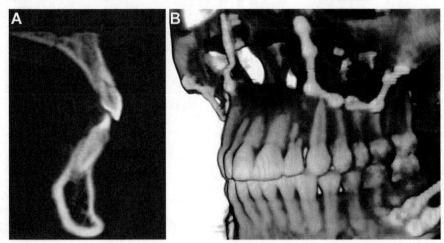

Fig. 35. CBCT (*A*) sagittal slice through the maxillary left lateral incisor and (*B*) lateral oblique 3D reformation postmultisegment Le Fort I osteotomy, which shows a horizontal root fracture from the vertical osteotomy between the canine and the lateral.

violation of the nerve canals by saw cuts, drill holes, or fixation screws. The mandibular condyles appear concentrically in their fossae in all three dimensions (Fig. 38). The chin, inferior borders, and angles are level to the axial plane of the face. The

anterior dental midlines appear on the midsagittal plane of the face and the posterior molars, angles and bodies are equidistant from the midsagittal plane (no yaw). The teeth appear to fit together and are in alignment with each other.

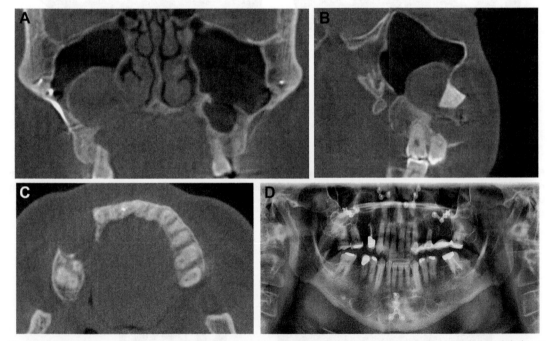

Fig. 36. Surgical ciliated cyst arising 12 years postmultisegment Le Fort I osteotomy. CBCT coronal view (*A*) shows a superiorly corticated expansile lesion with erosion through the alveolar and palatal bone, the sagittal slice (*B*) shows root blunting of the premolar and extension of the cyst between the roots of the teeth, and the axial slice (*C*) shows expansion laterally and palatally with significant bone loss throughout the alveolus. (*D*) Panoramic radiograph of a different patient with multiple surgical ciliated cysts. ([*D*] *Courtesy of* M. Nadim Islam, DDS, Gainsville, FL.)

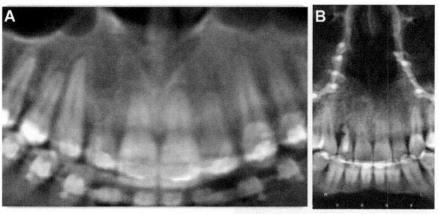

Fig. 37. (*A*) CBCT reformatted panoramic showing root blunting of the maxillary lateral and central incisors before Le Fort I osteotomy. (*B*) A year after Le Fort I osteotomy, the teeth show continued root resorption and complete resorption of the right lateral incisor with exposure of the root apex.

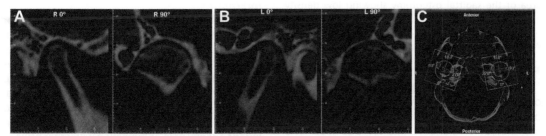

Fig. 38. (*A–C*) CBCT 2 weeks post-BSSO shows mandibular condyles centered in their fossae in all dimensions without eccentric displacement.

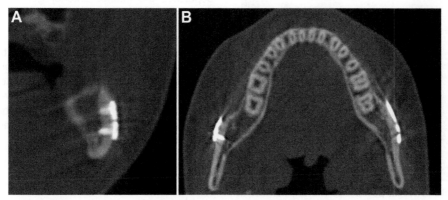

Fig. 39. (*A*) CBCT coronal view 9 months post-BSSO through the sagittal osteotomy site, which shows good cortical bone formation and medullary bone density. The screws are well integrated into the cortical bone with no signs of loosening. (*B*) Axial showing good bone density along the sagittal osteotomy gap areas.

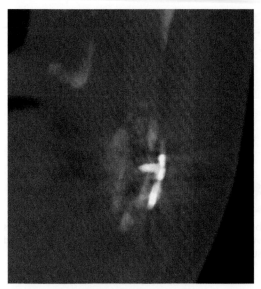

Fig. 40. Coronal CBCT 9 weeks post-BSSO through the area of the sagittal osteotomy showing low density around the screw and a lack of bone graft and bone healing at the sagittal gap. This indicates a nonunion with hardware failure.

The long-term successful result is as described previously without change from its immediate postoperative position. The mandibular condyles are without erosions or interval size loss. The

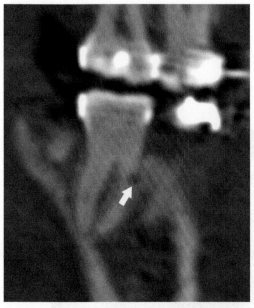

Fig. 41. CBCT 3 weeks post-BSSO. The sagittal slice at the right mandibular second molar shows the hypo-dense area in the mesial root (*arrow*) consistent with a drill-related injury.

fixation screws are well integrated into the bone. There is good healing between at the sagittal osteotomy between the distal and proximal segments (**Fig. 39**).[14]

Imaging of complications

- Nonunion (**Fig. 40**)
- Infection
- Injury to teeth (**Fig. 41**)
- Condylar displacement (**Fig. 42**)
- Condylar resorption (**Fig. 43**)
- Bad split (**Fig. 44**)
- Hardware failure
- Incorrect fixation hardware placement (**Fig. 45**)
- Violation of the mental foramen or IAN canal
- Asymmetric result (**Fig. 46**)

Genioplasty

Indications
The genioplasty is performed to increase or reduce the anteroposterior projection of the chin, decrease or increase the vertical dimension of the lower third of the face, and/or correct asymmetries in the anterior mandible. Genioplasties are made for esthetic reasons but also for functional reasons, such as decreasing lip incompetence to promote nasal breathing. Genioplasties are done independently or in combination with other orthognathic surgeries.

Radiographic anatomy
The genioplasty osteotomy is made from an intraoral incision. The cut is axial and starts more superiorly in the anterior and descends inferiorly as it goes posterior. The anterior cut is well below the roots of the mandibular teeth. The posterior cut is well below the mental foramen and the anterior descending loop of the IAN canal. The osteotomy separates the inferior anterior genial projection from the rest of the mandible superiorly.

Imaging of success
Fixation is in place with the middle of the genial segment centered to the midsagittal plane. The genial segment is without eccentric posterior rotation (yaw) and the inferior borders are level to each other and the axial plane of the face. The osteotomy is away from the IAN canals and mental foramen.

Imaging of complications

- Fixation failure (**Fig. 47**)
- Asymmetry
- Encroachment of the osteotomy on the mental foramen or IAN canal (**Fig. 48**)

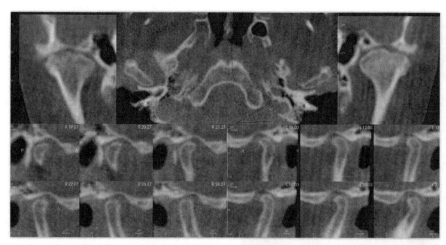

Fig. 42. CBCT TMJ cross-sections 4 weeks post-BSSO, which shows severe medial rotation of the right condyle with the lateral pole forward and the medial pole posterior to the fossa. The left condyle is posterior in the fossa.

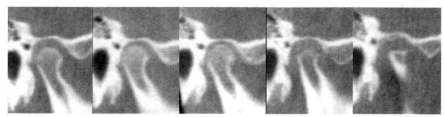

Fig. 43. Multiple CBCTs with sagittal slices through the right condyle. Time points left to right are preoperative, 12 days, 9 weeks, 6 months, and 1 year. The radiographs show progressive hypodensity of the condyles cortex leading to global bone loss and ending with hypercortication secondary to repair.

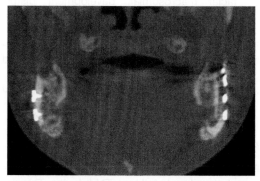

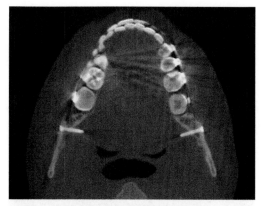

Fig. 44. Coronal CBCT 2 weeks post-BSSO shows a left buccal cortical plate fracture with separation from the inferior border of the proximal segment. Compare with the right side where the buccal plate is intact.

Fig. 45. Axial CBCT 2 years post-BSSO. The 2-mm-thick axial slice shows bicortical screw fixation with the screw tips almost 8 mm beyond the lingual cortex bilaterally. The position of the screws could violate the lingual nerve and this correlates with the patient's clinical complaint of lingual nerve paraesthesia.

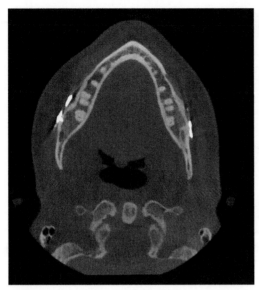

Fig. 46. CBCT axial view several years post-BSSO shows mandibular asymmetry in shape and alignment. The shape of the right ramus is more laterally projected than the left, the whole mandible is rotated (anterior left, posterior right) with the genial midline to the left, and asymmetry of the airway can also be seen.

IMAGING OF TEMPOROMANDIBULAR SURGICAL PROCEDURES
Definitions

TMJ surgery is varied and ranges from diagnostic and exploratory (eg, diagnostic arthroscopy) to disk replacement to total joint replacement (TJR). This section discusses the imaging success and failure of some disk replacement procedures and

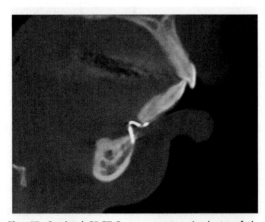

Fig. 47. Sagittal CBCT 2 years postgenioplasty of the anterior mandible shows posterior displacement of the fixation completely underneath the superior osteotomy and a total lack of bony union between the genial segment and the mandible above it.

TJR. Most TMJ treatments are palliative or aim to offer a biologic or chemical solution to TMJ dysfunction. TJR is a biomechanical answer rather than a biologic solution to management of severe and debilitating end-stage joint disease. It is often used as a last resort when all other treatments have failed or when the destruction of the condyle is so extensive that it cannot perform its functions. The parts replaced can be the condyle, the condyle and ramus, or both condyles and the entire mandible (in cases where the entire mandible needs to be replaced because of rampant disease). In many cases, the fossa is also replaced or lined by a titanium mesh backing and ultrahigh-molecular-weight polyethylene-bearing surface. Disk replacement is autogenous (eg, a muscle or fat flap placed between the osseous surfaces) or alloplastic. In the past, Teflon-Proplast grafts were used, but have been discontinued because of the severe and locally destructive foreign body reaction that tended to occur. These tend to surface from time to time in the radiologist's practice so familiarity with this is important.[18–20]

Indications

- End-stage degenerative joint disease that cannot be managed otherwise.
- End-stage inflammatory arthritides with excessive condyle volume loss that cannot be managed otherwise, such as rheumatoid arthritis and juvenile idiopathic arthritis.
- Ankylosis (fibrous or bony), where the bone is sectioned to create two separate segments and the TJR creates a new articulation.
- Failed autogenous tissue grafts, such as rib, auricular cartilage, or others.
- Loss of vertical mandibular height and/or disturbance in dental occlusal relationship, such as in congenital abnormalities (eg, hemifacial macrosomia), development disturbances (eg, severe condylar hypoplasia or hyperplasia), or even early onset juvenile idiopathic arthritis or idiopathic condylar resorption, both of which can affect the growth and development of the mandible (**Fig. 49**).
- Neoplasia (primary or secondary TMJ involvement).
- Trauma (intracapsular or extracapsular).

Radiographic Anatomy

For TJR, the condylar process of the mandible is resected and replaced by a TMJ device. This device may attach to the lateral aspect of the ramus through fixation screws. Determination of the position of the mandibular foramen and IAN canal is

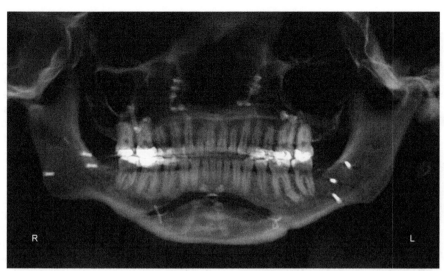

Fig. 48. CBCT reformatted panoramic shows the genioplasty osteotomy bisecting the left mental foramen and just inferior to the right mental foramen, likely through the right inferior alveolar nerve canal.

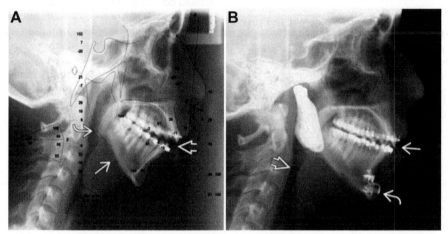

Fig. 49. (A) Pre-TMJ and (B) post-TMJ TJR lateral cephalometric analysis shows correction of a steep mandibular plane (*straight arrow*) and obtuse gonial angle. (A) Initial presentation with a long anterior face height, short posterior face height and anterior open bite (*open arrow*) that will be corrected through TJR. Note that on *B* the oropharyngeal dimensions have increased (*open arrow*) and the anterior open bite has closed (*straight arrow*) because of counterclockwise rotation of the mandible through the surgery. Genioplasty was also performed (*curved arrow*). (*Courtesy of* D. Kalant, DDS; and *From* Tamimi D, Hatcher D. Total Joint Replacement. In: Tamimi D, Hatcher D, editors. Specialty Imaging: Temporomandibular Joint. USA: Elsevier; 2017. p. 846-855; with permission.)

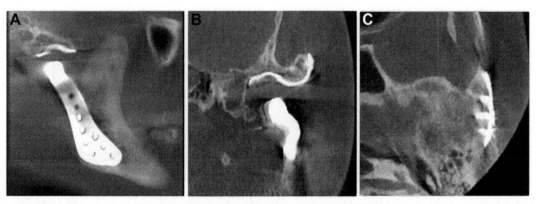

Fig. 50. The radiographic appearance of a successful TMJ TJR. Note the well-adapted fossa component to the outlines of the glenoid fossa with fixation screws in the lateral rim of the fossa (*A–C*). (*Courtesy of* L Mercuri, DDS; and From Tamimi D, Hatcher D. Total Joint Replacement. In: Tamimi D, Hatcher D, editors. Specialty Imaging: Temporomandibular Joint. USA: Elsevier; 2017. p. 846-855; with permission.)

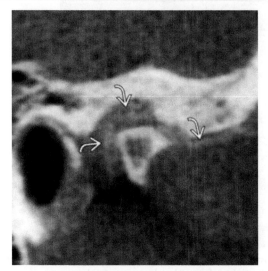

Fig. 51. Sagittal oblique CBCT of right TMJ shows the radiographic appearance of an alloplastic disk implant a slightly higher density membrane line structure separating the fossa and the condyle (*curved arrows*). Degenerative changes are seen in the condyle and the fossa, but these most likely preceded the implant placement. (*From* Tamimi D, Hatcher D. TMJ Disc Replacement. In: Tamimi D, Hatcher D, editors. Specialty Imaging: Temporomandibular Joint. USA: Elsevier; 2017. p. 856-857; with permission.)

For disk replacement surgery, the compromised temporomandibular disk is removed and replaced with either fat or the repositioning of a temporalis muscle flap into the joint space between the osseous components. The biologic and biomechanical properties of these tissues are not on par with those of the fibrocartilaginous disk, but have been used with varying success.

Imaging of Success

There should be proper adaptation of the ramus component of the device to the lateral aspect of the ramus and the fossa component to the lateral rim of the fossa and the zygomatic process of the temporal bone and posterior slope of the eminence. The fixation by the titanium alloy screws should be integrated with no radiographic signs of loosening. The screws should not violate any important anatomy. The condylar component should be in proper relationship with the fossa component when the teeth are in maximum intercuspation (**Fig. 50**). A disk replacement graft should be centered in the fossa and should surround the head of the condyle (**Fig. 51**). A ligation wire is often seen fixing the graft to the lateral rim of the fossa.

important to prevent perforation and injury to these structures. The fossa component is often fixed to the lateral rim of the fossa. Some types of TJR are CAD-CAM milled or three-dimensional printed to follow the exact contours of the fossa. Evaluation of the fossa for pneumatization by the mastoid air cells and integrity and thickness of the roof of the fossa should be performed to avoid perforation.

Imaging of Complications

- Infection
- Maladaptation or dislocation of the components (**Fig. 52**)
- Component or screw fracture (**Fig. 53**)
- Violation of the temporal fossa (**Fig. 54**)
- Heterogenous bone formation (**Fig. 55**)
- Foreign body reaction (seen in Proplast Teflon disk replacement)

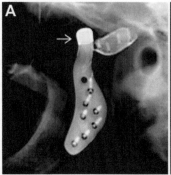
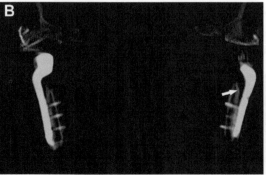

Fig. 52. (*A*) CBCT cropped panoramic reformation shows anterior dislocation of the ramus component (*arrow*) of a left TJR prosthesis. (*B*) Coronal CBCT shows a poorly adapted ramus portion of a TJR (*arrow*) with accompanying symptoms of discomfort. (*Courtesy of* M Ajami, DDS, Kirkland, WA.)

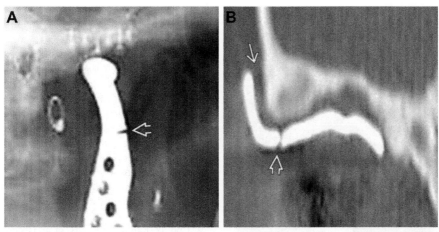

Fig. 53. Fractures of the components are noted here. (*A*) Panoramic radiograph shows the fracture (*arrow*) of the ramus component at the level of the condylar neck portion. (*B*) Coronal CT of an incompletely seated TMJ TJR fossa component where the metal mesh backing has fractured (*open arrow*) under functional loading because of poor adaptation (*thin arrow*). (*Courtesy of* L Mercuri, DDS; and *From* Tamimi D, Hatcher D. Total Joint Replacement. In: Tamimi D, Hatcher D, editors. Specialty Imaging: Temporomandibular Joint. USA: Elsevier; 2017. p. 846-855; with permission.)

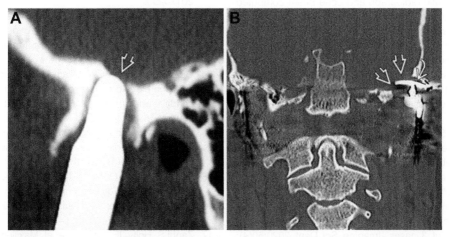

Fig. 54. Violation of the temporal fossa. (*A*) Sagittal view of a stock TMJ TJR without a fossa component that is migrating superiorly and eroding into the middle cranial fossa (*arrow*). (*B*) The stock fossa component of this TMJ TJR (*curved arrow*) has been driven into the middle cranial fossa (*open arrows*) by the trunnion of the ramus component because of failure of the polymethylmethacrylate condyle. (*Courtesy of* L Mercuri, DDS; and *From* Tamimi D, Hatcher D. Total Joint Replacement. In: Tamimi D, Hatcher D, editors. Specialty Imaging: Temporomandibular Joint. USA: Elsevier; 2017. p. 846-855; with permission.)

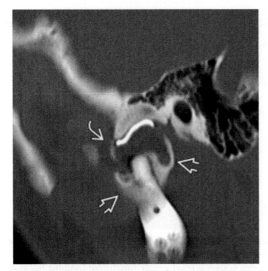

Fig. 55. Sagittal CT of the TMJ with a TJR shows heterotopic bone development around the ramus (*open arrows*) and fossa (*curved arrow*) components of the prosthesis (Courtesy, Louis Mercuri, DDS). (*Courtesy of* L Mercuri, DDS; and *From* Tamimi D, Hatcher D. Total Joint Replacement. In: Tamimi D, Hatcher D, editors. Specialty Imaging: Temporomandibular Joint. USA: Elsevier; 2017. p. 846-855; with permission)

DISCLOSURE

The authors have nothing to disclose.

REFERENCES

1. Patel PS, Shah JS, Dudhia BB, et al. Comparison of panoramic radiograph and cone beam computed tomography findings for impacted mandibular third molar root and inferior alveolar nerve canal relation. Indian J Dent Res 2020;31(1):91–102.

2. Menziletoglu D, Tassoker M, Kubilay-Isik B, et al. The assessment of relationship between the angulation of impacted mandibular third molar teeth and the thickness of lingual bone: a prospective clinical study. Med Oral Patol Oral Cir Bucal 2019;24(1): e130–5.

3. Blondeau F, Daniel NG. Extraction of impacted mandibular third molars: postoperative complications and their risk factors. J Can Dent Assoc 2007;73(4):325.

4. Shintaku WH, Ferreira CF, Venturin JS. Invasion of the canalis sinuosus by dental implants: a report of 3 cases. Imaging Sci Dent 2020;50(4): 353–7.

5. Clark D, Barbu H, Lorean A, et al. Incidental findings of implant complications on postimplantation CBCTs: a cross-sectional study. Clin Implant Dent Relat Res 2017;19(5):776–82.

6. Yepes JF, Al-Sabbagh M. Use of cone-beam computed tomography in early detection of implant failure. Dent Clin North Am 2015;59(1): 41–56.

7. Gaêta-Araujo H, Oliveira-Santos N, Mancini AXM, et al. Retrospective assessment of dental implant-related perforations of relevant anatomical structures and inadequate spacing between implants/teeth using cone-beam computed tomography. Clin Oral Investig 2020;24(9):3281–8.

8. Riachi F, Khairallah CM, Ghosn N, et al. Cyst volume changes measured with a 3D reconstruction after decompression of a mandibular dentigerous cyst with an impacted third molar. Clin Pract 2019;9(1): 1132.

9. Cho JY, Kim JW, Kim SB, et al. Decompression of large cyst invading the mandibular canal leading to reduced cyst volume and increased mandibular canal length. J Oral Maxillofac Surg 2020;78(10): 1770–9.

10. Gonçalves JM, Marola LHG, Modolo F, et al. Primary intraosseous carcinoma of the maxilla arising from an odontogenic keratocyst: a case report and review of the literature. Gen Dent 2019;67(6): 26–32.

11. Malina-Altzinger J, Klaeser B, Suter VGA, et al. Comparative evaluation of SPECT/CT and CBCT in patients with mandibular osteomyelitis and osteonecrosis. Clin Oral Investig 2019;23(12): 4213–22.

12. Shimamoto H, Grogan TR, Tsujimoto T, et al. Does CBCT alter the diagnostic thinking efficacy, management and prognosis of patients with suspected Stage 0 medication-related osteonecrosis of the jaws? Dentomaxillofac Radiol 2018;47(3): 20170290.

13. Silva LF, Curra C, Munerato MS, et al. Surgical management of bisphosphonate-related osteonecrosis of the jaws: literature review. Oral Maxillofac Surg 2016;20(1):9–17.

14. Gunson MJ, Arnet GW, Milam SB. Pathophysiology and pharmacologic control of osseous mandibular condylar resorption. J Oral Maxillofac Sure 2012; 70(8):1918–34.

15. Gunson MJ, Arnett GW. Orthognathic virtual treatment planning for functional esthetic results. Semin Orthod 2019;25(3):230–47.

16. Buck LM, Dalci O, Darendeliler MA, et al. Effect of surgically assisted rapid maxillary expansion of upper airway volume: a systematic review. J Oral Maxillofac Sure 2016;74(5):1025–43.

17. Zaghi S, Holty JE, Certal V, et al. Maxillomandibular advancement for treatment of obstructive sleep apnea: a meta-analysis. JAMA Otolaryngol Head Neck Surg 2016;142(1):58–66.

18. Gonzalez-Perez LM, Gonzalez-Perez-Somarriba B, Centeno G, et al. Prospective study of five-year

outcomes and postoperative complications after total temporomandibular joint replacement with two stock prosthetic systems. Br J Oral Maxillofac Surg 2020;58(1):69–74.

19. Mercuri LG. Avoiding and managing temporomandibular joint total joint replacement surgical site infections. J Oral Maxillofac Surg 2012;70(10): 2280–9.

20. Heffez L, Mafee MF, Rosenberg H, et al. CT evaluation of TMJ disc replacement with a Proplast-Teflon laminate. J Oral Maxillofac Surg 1987; 45(8):657–65.

Postoperative Computed Tomography for Facial Fractures

Elana B. Smith, MD[a], Lakir D. Patel, MD[b], David Dreizin, MD[c],*

KEYWORDS

- Facial trauma • Fracture fixation • Postoperative complications • Cinematic rendering

KEY POINTS

- Nasofrontal duct obstruction leads to suppurative complications, including mucopyocele development, osteomyelitis, and plate infection, which ultimately may result in intracranial and/or intraorbital spread. Patency is assessed best on sagittal images.
- Patients who have undergone obliteration or cranialization require periodic imaging surveillance to screen for developing mucopyocele.
- Small changes in the axis of rotation about the ZSS should be described on postoperative imaging. A small degree of rotation can lead to large changes in orbital volume and result in enophthalmos.
- Orbital floor implants should bridge the entire fracture defect. Any space that persists between fracture ledges may lead to postoperative entrapment and should be described objectively.
- Nonunion frequently accompanies osteomyelitis. In the mandible, this results from a combination of micromotion and the spread of infection from disrupted gingiva between incompletely mobilized tooth-bearing fragment surfaces.

INTRODUCTION

A recent analysis found that in 2017, more than 7.5 million new cases of facial fractures were diagnosed worldwide.[1] Fractures, such as isolated nasal pyramidal disruptions, small adult orbital floor blowouts, mildly displaced or angulated mandibular condyle fractures, and nondisplaced midface fractures, can be mechanically stable, have no cosmetically noticeable result, or have no long-term adverse effect on facial function and can be managed nonoperatively. Others may require open repair with titanium hardware to optimally restore premorbid function and aesthetics. Postoperative computed tomography (CT) scans commonly are performed and are useful in establishing a postoperative baseline and identifying complications that may require reoperation or revision.[2] In order for a radiologist to create reports that are meaningful to facial reconstructive surgeons, an understanding of the principles that guide surgical management and the hardware employed is imperative. This article is intended to promote efficient and salient reporting by illustrating surgeons' rationale for their approach. Hardware selection can be inferred and a defined set of potential complications anticipated when assessing the adequacy of surgical reconstruction on postoperative CT for midface, internal orbital, and mandible fractures.

[a] Trauma and Emergency Radiology, Department of Diagnostic Radiology and Nuclear Medicine, R Adams Cowley Shock Trauma Center, University of Maryland School of Medicine, 22 South Greene Street, Baltimore, MD 21201, USA; [b] Department of Diagnostic Radiology and Nuclear Medicine, University of Maryland School of Medicine, 22 South Greene Street, Baltimore, MD 21201, USA; [c] Trauma and Emergency Radiology, Department of Diagnostic Radiology and Nuclear Medicine, R Adams Cowley Shock Trauma Center, University of Maryland School of Medicine, 655 W Baltimore Street, Baltimore, MD 21201, USA
* Corresponding author.
E-mail address: daviddreizin@gmail.com

Neuroimag Clin N Am 32 (2022) 231–254
https://doi.org/10.1016/j.nic.2021.08.004

NASO-ORBITO-ETHMOIDAL FRACTURES
Surgically Relevant Anatomic Considerations

Naso-orbito-ethmoidal (NOE) fractures are characterized by a single or comminuted central fragment resulting from fractures along at least 4 of the following 5 cardinal tracts: the lateral nose and piriform aperture, the nasomaxillary buttress (NMB), the inferior orbital rim and floor, the medial orbital wall, and the frontomaxillary suture[3,4] (Fig. 1).

The central fragment serves as the insertion site of the anterior and posterior limbs of the medial canthal tendon (MCT), a support structure arising from the confluence of the upper and lower tarsal plates of the eyelids and orbicularis oculi.[5,6] Inadequate stabilization of the MCT can result in telecanthus (blunting of the medial palpebral fissure), hypertelorism (widening of the interpupillary and intercanthal distances), and enophthalmos.[6–9] The MCT may be functionally or truly avulsed secondary to lateral displacement of the central fragment or comminution at the MCT insertion sites on the lacrimal crest.[4]

Instability of the MCT (confirmed clinically through the application of pressure to the lower eyelid) largely determines the management.[4,6–8] Other considerations include the postreduction patency of the nasofrontal duct (NFD) and nasolacrimal duct (NLD), postreduction bone loss, posterior frontal sinus wall displacement, and depression of the frontal sinus wall—the last is important from a cosmetic standpoint.[8,10]

Surgical Goals and Approach

Surgical management goals of NOE fractures include restoring preinjury canthal position, globe and anterior sinus wall position, nasal projection, and mucociliary clearance.[6]

The method of fixation is based on an initial assessment of Markowitz-Manson grade at CT and evaluation of the internal orbit.[4] Stepwise small plate fixation is applied through cosmetically favorable incisions until the MCT is immobilized intraoperatively.[11] Internal orbital disruptions are discussed later.

A fracture resulting in a single central fragment (Markowitz-Manson grade I injury) may be stable intraoperatively, requiring no fixation, such as with greenstick or hinged fractures about a single intact cardinal line.[3] A single plate can stabilize a mobile noncomminuted central fragment, which indirectly stabilizes an intact MCT. Using cosmetically favored incisions, a low-profile miniplate may be placed along the NMB or inferior orbital rim through the gingivobuccal sulcus or subconjunctival lower lid incisions, respectively (Fig. 2). Subconjunctival incisions can be complicated by lid lag or entropion; thus, an NMB plate may be preferred for single-plate fixation.[12] With persistent mobility on palpation, the fragment is plated at both locations, a technique often used with slightly comminuted grade II injuries.[4] Plating across the frontomaxillary suture may be required if the fracture through the central fragment results in the creation of an upper and lower fragment.

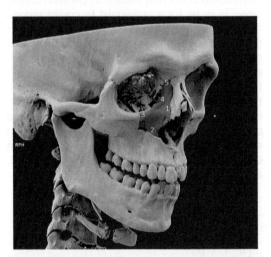

Fig. 1. NOE cardinal lines. Face CT cinematic 3-D rendering shows a type 1 right NOE fracture, with single central fragment isolated by fracture lines along the 5 cardinal tracts: the lateral nasal bone and piriform aperture (1), the NMB, (2), the inferior orbital rim and floor (3), the medial orbital wall (4), and the frontomaxillary suture (5).

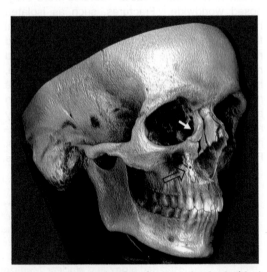

Fig. 2. Intraoral single-plate fixation via gingival incision. A 3-D volume-rendered maxillofacial CT of a patient status postfixation of a type 1 NOE fracture (solid arrow). Single-plate fixation of the NMB (open arrow) achieves adequate fixation.

Nasofrontal suture plating is used to restore anterior nasal projection.[2]

Severely comminuted high-energy grade III injuries result in a true or functional MCT avulsion, requiring transnasal canthopexy (**Fig. 3**). The reconstructive surgeon attaches a wire to the MCT and passes it through an intravenous cannula inserted via a posterior transnasal drillhole, typically made above and behind the posterior crest. The wire then is secured to a plate, screw, or mesh along the contralateral frontal bar.[4–6] Medial canthopexy is associated with a high failure rate, resulting in late telecanthus and globe malposition. Overtightening is performed in anticipation of expected lateral drift over time.[6,9,13]

If the nasal support is inadequate due to severe collapse or comminution of the nasal bone-cartilage framework, a dorsal nasal strut graft may be required. This often is fashioned out of the outer table of the calvarium and affixed to the glabella to restore anteroposterior nasal projection and reduce telecanthus.[7,8]

Severely comminuted fractures requiring canthopexy, reconstruction of the nasal pyramid, or repair of other subunits as part of a panfacial fracture pattern typically necessitate a coronal approach, which provides wider surgical access. In this approach, the facial soft tissues are reflected below the frontal bar following a cosmetically favorable behind-the-hairline incision.[6,8] The clinical rationale for the range of postoperative imaging findings after NOE fractures is summarized in **Table 1**.

Postoperative Assessment of Complications

Disruption and stenosis of the NLD and NFD, frontoethmoidal recess, and posterior walls of the frontal sinuses can lead to functional and septic complications. NFD patency is assessed intraoperatively by observing the passage of methylene blue dye from the frontal sinuses to the nares or pharynx, although passage may be obstructed due to mucosal swelling and nasal secretions.[10]

Postoperative CT assessment of the NFD is vital because obstruction eventually leads to development of mucopyocele with expansile bony remodeling, erosion, osteomyelitis, or plate infection. Orbital compartment syndrome or cellulitis may result from orbital spread, whereas intracranial extension results in meningitis, empyema, and brain abscess.[14–17] Postreduction NFD continuity is assessed best on sagittal imaging[18] (**Fig. 4**). Discontinuity also is strongly suggested by posterior intrusion of the nasal dorsum and collapse of the anterior and middle ethmoid air cells on axial images.[10] In ambiguous cases, serial CT over the first few weeks can be performed to assess for progressive aeration or filling of the frontal sinuses.[10,19]

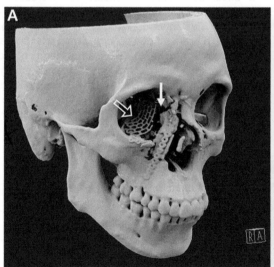
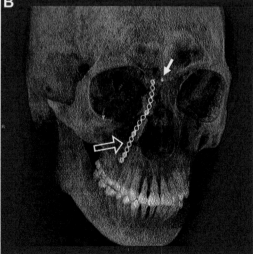

Fig. 3. Transnasal wire medial canthopexy. Face CT cinematic 3-D (*A*) and volume (*B*) renderings of a patient who sustained comminuted type III right NOE fractures. At surgery, the bony insertion of the MCT was fractured (*solid arrow [A]*) and mobile; the tendon also was detached. Transnasal wire canthopexy was performed. The wire is secured to a screw drilled into the frontal bone (*solid arrow [B]*). The titanium plate was prebent, mirrored from the normal left side using a patient-specific 3-D printed plastic model following virtual reconstruction during preplanning to restore the contour of the medial and inferior orbital defects (*open arrow [A]*). Fixation of the comminuted central fragment was achieved with an NMB plate (*open arrow [B]*).

Table 1
Summary of postoperative findings for naso-orbito-ethmoidal fractures

Postoperative Imaging Finding: Naso-orbito-ethmoidal Fractures	Clinical Rationale
Single-plate and screw fixation	Grade I fracture, unstable
Plate and screw fixation along the frontomaxillary suture and NMB	Unstable MCT insertion, with bone intact at the insertion site (grade II fracture)
Medial canthopexy	1. MCT avulsion OR 2. Severe comminution of the of the MCT-bearing fracture fragment (grade III) Canthopexy can be performed through existing incision or may require coronal incision.
Dorsal nasal strut graft	Severe collapse of the nasal bone-cartilage framework
Obliteration	1. Frontonasal duct obstruction OR 2. Noncomminuted fracture through the inner table of the frontal sinus with defect <25% total surface area posterior wall
Cranialization	Frontonasal duct obstruction AND 1. Severely comminuted or displaced fracture through the inner table of the frontal sinus (defect >25% posterior wall frontal sinus) OR 2. Traumatic brain injury requiring frontal craniotomy
Frontal sinus mesh	Anterior wall fracture with bone loss from the outer table of the frontal sinus

Elevated risk of septic complications corresponds with frontal sinus posterior wall defect size on postoperative imaging following reduction. In obliteration, the intracranial cavity is effectively separated from the external environment by filling the frontal sinus with free fat and plugging of the NFD with bone chips, fascia, and fibrin glue[14,16] (see **Fig. 4**). A defect less than 25% of the posterior wall surface area on postoperative CT is believed to have a lower risk of complications, and obliteration may be performed in lieu of more aggressive management with cranialization.[14,20] In such cases, associated dural defects are repaired or allowed to heal through fibrosis.[19] If defects from bone loss and displacement are large and comminuted, it becomes difficult to ensure all microscopic mucosal rests are removed, and cranialization is favored. This involves removal of the posterior wall and placement of a pericranial flap after frontal craniotomy[20,21] (**Fig. 5**). Because obliteration and cranialization involve mucoperiosteal stripping, even with meticulous removal, any remaining rests of mucosa during this process can serve as nidi for future mucopyocele.[16,20,21] Therefore, a relatively

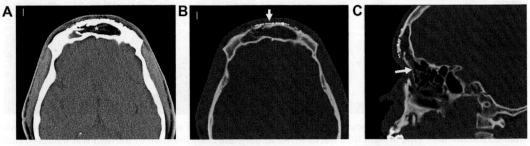

Fig. 4. Frontal sinus obliteration. Fractures of the anterior and posterior tables of the bilateral frontal sinuses status post-MVC. Axial CT images of the frontal sinuses in soft tissue (*A*) and bone windows (*B*) show frontal sinus obliteration with autologous abdominal fat (*asterisk* [*A*]) and the anterior table reconstructed with a mesh plate (*arrow* [*B*]). Sagittal CT image (*C*) shows the obstructed right frontal sinus outflow (*arrow*) as indication for sinus obliteration.

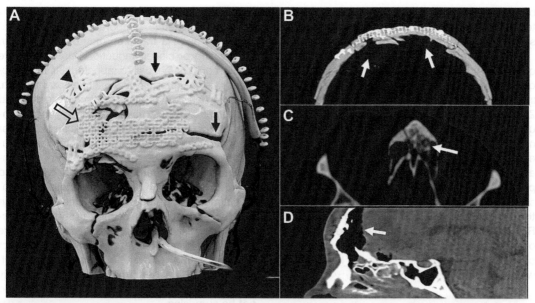

Fig. 5. Frontal sinus cranialization. Cinematic 3-D rendering (*A*) and axial (*B, C*) and sagittal (*D*) CT face images of a patient status postfrontal sinus cranialization for treatment of comminuted anterior and posterior table sinus fractures. Frontal craniotomy was performed to expose the frontal sinus (osteotomy planes [*solid arrows* (*A*)]). The posterior table and all sinus mucosa were removed (*arrows* [*B*]). Subsequently, the frontonasal ducts were obstructed using bone graft and chips (*arrow* [*C*]). Prior to closing the frontal skull, a pericranial flap was raised onto the frontal dura (*arrow* [*D*]). The craniotomy and fracture fragments were simplified using a variety of plates and screws (*open arrow and arrowhead* [*A*]).

conservative management approach frequently is employed.[14] Patients who have undergone obliteration and cranialization require some form of surveillance, such as yearly CT, to screen for developing mucopyocele.[16] Over time, the brain gradually expands until the frontal lobes come to rest against the anterior table after cranialization.[21]

Cosmetic management of the anterior frontal sinus wall
Depressed (and frequently comminuted) fractures of the anterior frontal sinus wall are elevated and plated for cosmetic reasons. These fractures commonly are reduced and fixed successfully with miniplates and 3-dimensional (3-D) matrix plates during surgical simplification[14,19] (see **Fig. 5**). Mesh is used in cases of severe bone loss either directly from injury, following gradual bone resorption after frontal craniotomy and cranioplasty or osteomyelitis.[22] Repair of panfacial fractures often is staged using a top-down or bottom-up approach, using either the frontal bar (glabella and superior orbital rims) or mandible and occlusion as a template for restoring premorbid dimensions of the midface.[23,24] If simplification of the upper face has not yet been performed on an initial postoperative CT in a patient requiring staged surgery, fragments depressed more than

1 table width should be described on postoperative imaging.[14,19]

The nasolacrimal duct
Postoperative CT assessment of the NLD does not have proved clinical value. The need for operative treatment of sequelae with dacryocystorhinostomy is based on persistence of symptoms (epiphora and recurrent dacryocystitis) beyond 6 months and confirmation with fluorescein dye or dacryocystogram.[6,25] If the NLD is reduced on postoperative CT, these sequelae may result from mucosal scarring and synechiae, which are not appreciable at CT.[25,26] This highlights the importance of recognizing both the strengths and limitations of postoperative imaging when communicating with facial reconstructive surgeons.

ZYGOMATICOMAXILLARY COMPLEX FRACTURES
Surgically Relevant Anatomic Considerations

The zygomaticomaxillary complex (ZMC) fracture fragment dissociates from the midface at 4 major points of failure: the zygomaticomaxillary buttress (ZMB), the zygomaticosphenoid suture (ZSS), frontozygomatic (FZ) suture, and zygomaticotemporal suture.[27,28] Because the lateral orbital floor almost always is involved, these fractures may be referred to orbitozygomatic fractures.[27] The terms, *malar fracture* and tetrapod *fracture*, also sometimes are used.[27,29]

The single most important feature of reduction quality on postoperative CT images is the status of the ZSS.[27,28,30,31] Telescoping or small changes in the axis of rotation of ZMC fractures about the ZSS lead to large increases in the bony orbital volume, potentially resulting in disfiguring enophthalmos.[27,32] Anatomic reduction of the ZSS along its entire oblique lateral orbital wall plane suggests anatomic reduction of the other aforementioned points of dissociation. The other involved sutures still should be assessed along with step-off at the orbital rim, particularly on coronal images.[30,33] Residual malar retrusion and offset about the ZMB on postoperative CT may result in poor aesthetic outcome, with asymmetric loss of lateral facial width and anterior projection.[31]

Surgical Goals and Approach

The primary goals of ZMC fracture management are to restore premorbid facial symmetry and orbital configuration.[28,30] Repairs of the orbital floor may be performed with preformed (kit) implants following ZMC repair or may be performed as a staged surgery for several reasons. First, orbital surgery requires globe retraction and excellent visibility of the posterior orbit, which is limited in the presence of posttraumatic edema.[32,34] A 7-day to-14-day delay may be warranted to ensure correct orbital implant placement, particularly along the far-posterior palatine ledge.[32,34] Second, patient-specific laser sintered titanium implants created through 3-D printing techniques from the mirrored intact contralateral side usually are made at an outside facility and require time for interactive surgical preplanning between surgeons and vendor, manufacturing, and shipping.[35]

Surgical approach is determined with the CT-based Zingg classification system and successive clinical assessment for fracture stability with each plate placement.[30,31,36]

Type A fractures involve a single limb of the zygoma (zygomatic arch—A1; lateral orbital wall—A2; and inferior orbital rim—A3).[28,30] Type A1 fractures typically exhibit a V-shaped depression of the zygomatic arch and are repaired for cosmetic and functional reasons because the arch can impinge on the mandibular coronoid process, limiting mouth opening and masticatory function.[28] Commonly, a surgical hook or elevator is introduced into the infratemporal space through a posterior buccal incision. The fragments then snap back into anatomic alignment with surgical instrument pressure.[28,30] Open repair is risky

because of the potential for facial nerve injury causing unilateral temporal hollowing.[28,30,37] Types A2 and A3 fractures may be treated with observation or closed reduction if fragments are stable and cosmetically inapparent. If instability and/or visible deformity is present on examination, reduction and small plate fixation are performed through cosmetically favorable subconjunctival incisions for inferior rim fragments and brow or blepharoplasty incisions for lateral rim/wall reduction along the FZ suture[28,30] (Fig. 6).

Zingg type B fractures are noncomminuted tetrapod fractures with a single liberated zygomatic fragment.[30] Observation or closed reduction may be appropriate, especially in the elderly for whom the risks of surgery and anesthesia are elevated and the relative desirability of a perfect cosmetic result is lower.[28] Follow-up CT in such patients may be performed to confirm stability following palpation; the lack of hardware should not be surprising.

When requiring internal fixation, 30% to 40% of type B fractures may be reduced and stabilized with a single plate.[28,30,31] Fixation along the ZMB and FZ sutures are most common, utilizing intraoral and upper blepharoplasty incisions, respectively.[27,28,30] ZMB plates are L-shaped and have a footplate for subapical fixation that avoids tooth roots.[28] There is no convincing evidence that one single-plate fixation approach is better than another for isolated ZMC fractures.[28,38] Fixation at the second site is used if instability persists during intraoperative palpation[28,31] (Fig. 7).

High-energy type C fractures with displacement and comminution are more likely to require fixation at a third site, in addition to orbital implant placement for concomitant large floor detects. Transconjunctival incisions have no external scar and are used for plating the inferior orbital rim in such cases.[12,28] The zygomatic arch rarely is plated except in the most unstable severely comminuted type C fractures that extend beyond the zygomaticotemporal buttress into the skull base.[28] If stability cannot be achieved without zygomatic arch plating, access is achieved through coronal incisions and temporal muscle dissection[27,28,30] (Fig. 8). A summary of postoperative findings for ZMC fractures is listed in Table 2.

Postoperative Assessment of Reduction Quality and Complications

Changes in the bony orbital volume associated with misalignment about the ZSS can result in visible (greater than 2-mm) enophthalmos, which worsens following resolution of posttraumatic and postsurgical orbital edema.[39] Revision often

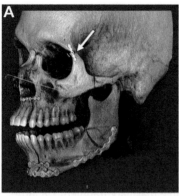
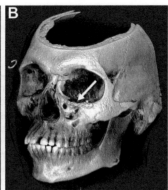
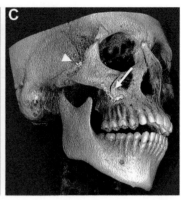

Fig. 6. Single-plate ORIF approaches to ZMC fractures; 3-D volume-rendered face CTs of 3 separate patients, each sustaining a different ZMC fracture type in the Zingg classification. Single-plate fixation of the left zygomatico-frontal suture (*arrow*) performed as the lateral orbital rim fracture was displaced and mobile at surgery in this Zingg B fracture (*A*). Additional fractures of the maxilla and mandible were fixed in staged fashion. Single-plate fixation at the inferior orbital rim (*arrow*) in a Zingg A3 fracture (*B*). Single L-shaped plate fixation at the ZMB (*arrow*) for a ballistic Zingg B fracture (*arrowhead* denotes bullet fragment) (*C*).

is necessary in such cases. If ZMC and internal orbital reconstruction are performed in stages, postoperative CT may reveal an orbital floor defect.[32,40,41] Unlike pure internal orbital disruptions, the process of ZMC fracture reduction often results in shifting of orbital floor fracture fragments, causing an increase or decrease in size of the orbital floor defect, depending in part on the reduction maneuver used.[32,40,41] Enophthalmos is the most common complication after both ZMC-related and pure orbital floor blowout fracture.[32] The contribution of floor defects to enophthalmos is described later. The postoperative CT

also should be examined for persistent internal rotation or malar retrusion that could result in postoperative malunion if uncorrected.[31,33] The soft tissues should be assessed for retrobulbar hematoma that could contribute to orbital compartment syndrome, evidenced by globe tenting from tension along the optic nerve.[32] Treatment involves

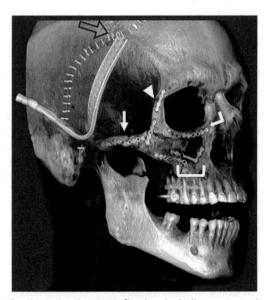

Fig. 8. A 4-point ZMC fixation including zygomatic arch. A 3-D volume-rendered maxillofacial CT shows ORIF of a right ZMC fracture via multiple approaches, achieving 4-point fixation across the zygomatic arch (*solid arrow*), zygomaticofrontal suture (*arrowhead*), inferior orbital rim (*angled arrow*), and ZMB (*bracket*). Penrose drain and skin staples over the temporalis region (*open arrow*) signify the hemicoronal approach required for arch fixation.

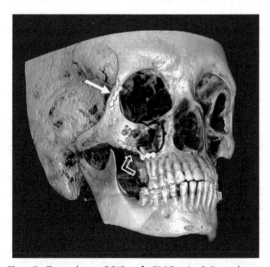

Fig. 7. Two-plate ORIF of ZMC. A 3-D volume-rendered face CT of a Zingg B ZMC fracture, with comminution at the maxilla. ORIF was performed with a zygomaticofrontal plate (*arrow*) and an L-shaped zygomaticomaxillary plate (*open arrow*).

Table 2
Summary of postoperative findings for zygomaticomaxillary complex fractures

Postoperative Imaging Findings: Zygomaticomaxillary Complex Fractures	Clinical Rationale
Single-point fixation	Zingg type B fracture, stable after 1 fixation point. Preferred when feasible due to improved cosmesis. ZMB L-shaped plates commonly are used (protect tooth roots); FZ suture can also be used. Plate choice is surgeon-dependent. Single-point fixation across the FZ suture 1. Zingg A2 (isolated lateral wall) OR 2. Zingg B fracture (single noncomminuted ZMC fragment), with unstable maxillary fragment OR large ZMB defect Single-point fixation across the inferior orbital rim Zingg A3 fracture (isolated inferior orbital wall)
Two-point fixation	Zingg type B fracture, stable after 2-point fixation (typically, both ZMB and FZ suture plates)
Three-point fixation	Zingg type B or type C fracture, stable after 3-point fixation Inferior orbital rim fixation is performed only as part of a 3-point fixation if fracture remains unstable after 2-point fixation (stability ultimately determined in operating room based on continued mobility after successive plate placement).
Four-point fixation	Fixation along the ZMB, FZ, inferior orbital rim, and zygomatic arch Rare but requires coronal incision and temporalis dissection for ZA plate placement. Can cause unilateral temporal hollowing but approach may be unavoidable for high-energy comminuted fractures

urgent lateral canthotomy at the bedside to relieve pressure.[32]

Suppurative complications, including dehiscence, plate migration, osteomyelitis, and nonunion, are rare in the highly vascularized and immobile midface. The low infection rate also is related to gravity drainage of secretions away from the nondependent maxillary gingivobuccal sulcus. When infection occurs, this usually involves fixation hardware along the ZMB placed using an intraoral approach.[42,43]

ORBITAL WALL FRACTURES
Surgically Relevant Anatomic Considerations

Although a detailed discussion of orbital anatomy is beyond the scope of this article, it is important to be aware of ledges and landmarks used as landing zones for orbital floor or combined floor and medial wall orbital implants. The junction of the lesser sphenoid wing with the orbital plate of the palatine bone forms a palatine ledge on which the implant rests posteriorly. The medial wall component of combined implants should ideally run in parallel and closely apposed to the intact portions of the lamina papyracea surrounding medial wall defects, coursing up toward the frontoethmoidal suture at the medial wall-roof junction (**Fig. 9**).

Surgical Goals and Approach

Orbital floor and medial orbital wall fractures
Due to the potential for postoperative lid complications, including entropion or lid lag, surgery is considered only when the benefits of preventing enophthalmos outweigh the risks.[12]

For every 1 mL of bony orbital volume change or tissue displacement beyond the orbital confines, 0.8 mm to 0.9 mm of enophthalmos results,[39,44] becoming noticeable when it exceeds 2 mm to 3 mm.[34] Effective volume changes sufficient to cause visible enophthalmos occur with floor or medial wall surface area blowout of greater than 2 cm^2,[45–47] equating to approximately 25% to 50% floor or medial wall involvement.[32] Collapse of the posterior junctional bulge can have a dramatic impact globe position, further magnifying

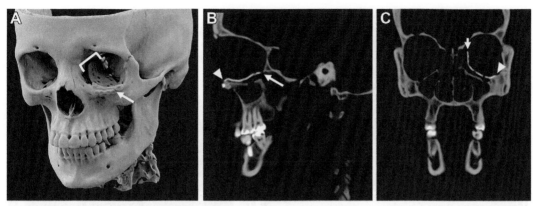

Fig. 9. ORIF for combined orbital medial wall and floor fractures. Cinematic 3-D volume-rendered face CT (*A*) and CT face images in the sagittal (*B*) and coronal (*C*) planes show plate fixation at the inferior orbital rim (*arrow* [*A*]) as well as placement of a patient-specific implant (*bracket* [*A*]) to cover orbital defects at the medial wall and floor. The implant adequately covers the fracture defects and adequately rests on the anterolateral rim (*arrowheads* [*B, C*]), posterior ledge (*arrow* [*B*]), and the upper border of the preserved medial wall (*arrow* [*C*]).

the risk of clinically significant enophthalmos.[34] CT guides decision making because the degree of enophthalmos is not evident clinically until edema has resolved and permanent soft-tissue architectural changes have begun to set in.[48]

Blowout fractures are not self-reducing in adults, unlike in children, and extraocular muscle (EOM) incarceration and infarction is rare in adult patients.[47] Entrapment of fibrofatty tissue within small (<3 mm) defects can cause EOM tethering in a small fraction of patients and may require orbital reconstruction if extraocular motility problems are confirmed with forced duction testing (the use of forceps to test for globe excursion following anesthetization of the sclera).[32,34,46,47]

If surgery is necessary, prefabricated implants or 3-D–printed patient-specific implants (PSIs) reconstitute the frequently collapsed upward-sloping posterior bulge. There is growing evidence that PSIs provide the best aesthetic result.[35]

Postoperative Assessment of Reduction Quality and Complications

Postoperative entrapment
Regardless of the type of implant used, ideally it should bridge the entire fracture defect and rest on all ledges on postoperative CT. Any space that persists between fracture ledges and the implant may result in herniation of EOMs or extraconal fibrofatty tissue, with potential for postoperative entrapment[32,34,48] (Fig. 10).

The extraconal fibrofatty tissue is composed of septa that are closely invested onto muscle. When herniated between fracture ledges and implants, tractional effects cause the adjacent EOM to have a hooked or kinked appearance with

displacement toward the defect.[46] The diagnosis of postoperative entrapment may be suspected based on CT, but clinicoradiologic discrepancies are frequent (eg, patients may have no ocular motility-related complaints despite presence of herniation).[32] Therefore, radiologists should describe gaps between implants and bony ledges, fibrofatty herniation, and EOM tractional changes objectively and refrain from subjective descriptors, such as "suboptimal reconstruction," in their reports. Entrapment ultimately is a clinical diagnosis confirmed with forced duction testing.[34] Additional uncommon postoperative complications include orbital cellulitis and orbital compartment syndrome.[49]

Orbital roof reconstruction and orbital apex decompression
Frontobasal skull fractures may involve the orbital roof. Fractures are characterized as nondisplaced, blowup, or blow-in. Blow-in fractures decrease the orbital volume and require prompt repair to avoid orbital compartment syndrome, whereas blow-up fractures initially increase the orbital volume. Orbital compression in the latter results from developing encephaloceles and retrobulbar hematomas. Surgical reconstruction typically involves mesh implants and dural repair using transfrontal techniques[50] (Fig. 11). Postoperative studies should be assessed for any gaps between implant and bone ledges, residual retrobulbar hematoma, and CT evidence of orbital compartment syndrome.

The International Optic Nerve Trauma Study[51] showed little benefit of surgical optic nerve decompression on outcomes in patients with traumatic optic neuropathy. Orbital apex syndromes

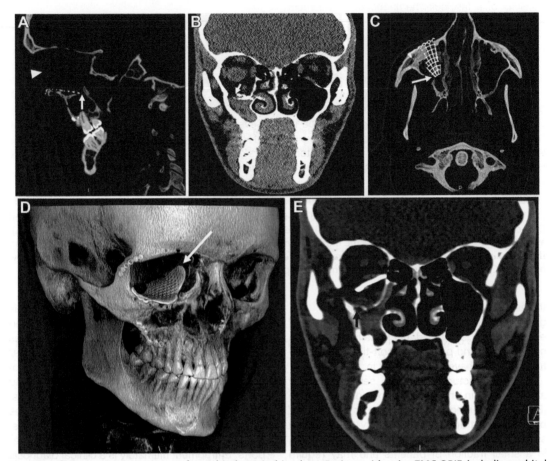

Fig. 10. Inferior rectus entrapment after orbital surgical implant. Patient with prior ZMC ORIF, including orbital floor implant presented with complaints of diplopia with upward and downward gaze. CT images in sagittal (A) coronal (B) and axial (C) planes show a malpositioned orbital implant, not seated on the posterior ledge (arrows [A, C]) with downward herniation of orbital fat and inferior rectus muscle (arrow [B]). These findings corresponded with clinical entrapment. Enophthalmos was also present (arrowhead [A]). After revision with a PSI (arrow [D]) herniated orbital contents are shown to be reduced (arrow [E]). Orbital volume also was restored with corrected enophthalmos (not shown).

include frequently transient ocular motor nerve palsies.[52] Decompressive surgery in this area is not without risk and rarely is performed in contemporary practice.[53] Evidence of orbital apex decompression includes drilling of the posterior lamina papyracea via transnasal endoscopic approaches or removal of the superior optic canal and portions of the sphenoid ridge via craniotomy[54–56] (Fig. 12).

Evaluation of the orbits with low-dose computed tomography technique

Postoperative imaging may be performed with low-dose technique to minimize radiation exposure.[57–61] A 2018 clinical pilot study demonstrated that low-dose CT technique using an exposure time product of 25 mAs led to an average 7-fold reduction in radiation dose compared with the standard institutional protocol without compromising diagnostic quality when using a soft tissue kernel, iterative reconstruction, and a contemporary dual source 128-section scanner[62] (Fig. 13).

MAXILLARY OCCLUSION-BEARING FRACTURES
Surgically Relevant Anatomic Considerations

In a series of complicated cadaver experiments, Le Fort described common lines of least resistance in facial fractures.[63] In the era preceding titanium hardware, the highest Le Fort level was used to determine stable points to affix wires.[64] Today it is recognized that Le Fort II and III fractures frequently represent combinations of ZMC, NOE, and maxillary occlusion-bearing fragments, the management of which is governed by specific principles unique to each midfacial subunit. The

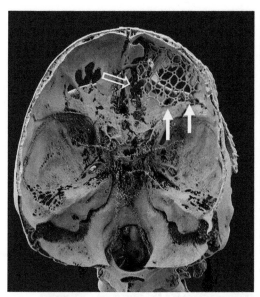

Fig. 11. Orbital roof mesh. Cinematic 3-D rendering of the skull base in a patient with frontobasal skull fractures status post–right anterior fossa and orbital roof mesh repair (*solid arrows*) via a right frontal craniotomy. The medial skull base was not sturdy enough to support screws to secure the medial edge of the mesh, resulting in persistent defect of the right ethmoid-cribiform complex (*open arrow*). There was no clinically evident meningocele.

lowest Le Fort level is of primary relevance from the standpoint of restoring the occlusion.[23]

Surgical Goals and Approach

Most occlusion-bearing fragments dissociate at the Le Fort I level. Le Fort I fractures propagate from the piriform aperture through the walls of the maxillary sinuses to the pterygomaxillary junction and pterygoid plates. When complete, these result in the classic floating palate.[65,66] The most difficult to treat Le Fort I fractures either are impacted or incomplete and require either forceps disimpaction or completion osteotomy before restoring the premorbid occlusion with mandibulomaxillary fixation (MMF).[67,68] Malocclusion greater than 2 mm to 3 mm cannot be corrected with dental resurfacing and requires revision surgery, whereas residual bone gaps of similar magnitude following restoration of facial symmetry and projection are masked by the soft tissue envelope.[67] Once the premorbid maxillary incline and occlusion are restored using either an intact or reduced and fixed mandible as a template, paramedian or lateral sagittal split fractures of the palate are fixed with miniplates along the buccal maxillary alveolar surface.[23] Direct plating of the hard palate leads to dehiscence and is

used less commonly.[69] Fixation may be supplemented with dental splints and side-to-side intermolar wiring to counteract buccal flaring of the hemi–Le Fort fragments.[69,70]

The restored occlusion is used along with an intact or reduced frontal bar as templates for top-down or bottom-up stepwise reconstruction of the NOE and ZMC regions using previously described subunit-specific reduction principles. Exact surgical sequencing largely is dependent on the surgeon. Finally, the reduced occlusion is reconnected to the reconstructed upper midface along the nasomaxillary and ZMBs[24] (**Fig. 14**).

Postoperative Assessment of Reduction Quality and Complications

The most common complication is malocclusion, which can lead to problems with mastication and speech. This is assessed best with a dental examination and impressions; however, gross malocclusions may be evident on volume-rendered CT images. Intraoperatively, difficult occlusion-bearing fragment disimpaction can result in insufficient anterior projection. This can be masked intraoperatively as the mandibular condyles are forced backwards to accommodate MMF but is not apparent as prognathism on postoperative 3-D CT images once the condyles return to their native position.[67,68]

Up to half of Le Fort fractures are associated with hard palate fractures.[70] Palatal collapse and buccal flaring in patients with palatal fractures may result in similarly obvious cross-bite malocclusions at postoperative CT. Tooth loss is common with associated comminuted dentoalveolar fractures, and bone loss of the hard palate in severely comminuted fractures can cause oronasal and oroantral fistulae.[70]

MANDIBLE

The mandible is a horseshoe-shaped structure divided into a horizontal strut containing the tooth-bearing symphyseal and parasymphyseal region, body, and angle, and the non–tooth-bearing vertical strut composed of the ramus, coronoid, and condyle.[71,72] Options for surgical management of mandibular fractures are determined by location and differ based on whether the tooth-bearing or non–tooth-bearing portions are involved, whether the fracture is bilateral or otherwise involves more than 1 region, the degree of comminution, and whether the patient is dentate or edentulous.[73]

The mandible is the only mobile bone of the face, and considerations for closed versus open reduction and hardware selection are based largely on

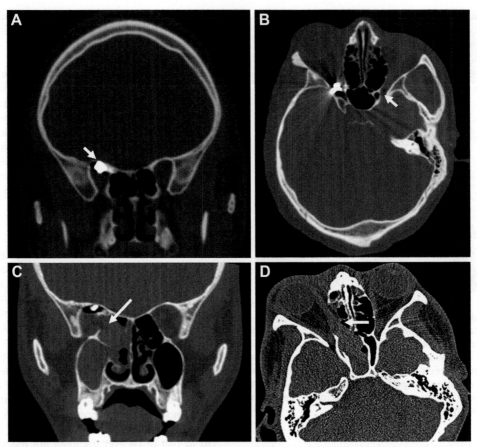

Fig. 12. Orbital apex decompression. Coronal (*A*) and axial (*B*) CT images through the orbits show a metallic pellet lodged at the right orbital apex (*arrow* [*A*]), narrowing the superior orbital fissure compared with the contralateral side (*arrow* [*B*]). Due to the patient's vision loss, endoscopic decompression of the medial orbital wall was performed. Postoperatively, there were adequate prolapse and decompression of orbital fat and medial rectus through the surgical medial wall defect (*arrows* [*C*, *D*]).

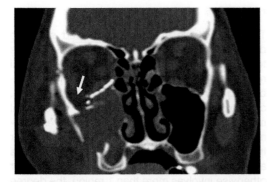

Fig. 13. Postoperative orbital low-dose CT technique. Coronal reformat CT image of the face in a patient status post–right orbital floor mesh repair. Low-dose technique (120 kV, 30 mAs) does not obscure soft tissue contrast between orbital contents (*arrow*) with use of iterative reconstruction and soft tissue kernel.

biomechanical principles. Most simple fractures of the tooth-bearing mandible are oriented perpendicular to the mandibular long axis, extending from the tooth row superiorly through the thick basal segment inferiorly. All fractures involving the tooth row are considered compound and contaminated.[72,74] Condylar fractures usually are closed and associated with disruption of the temporomandibular joint (TMJ) capsule, disc, and retrodiscal tissue.[75–77] The most common complications involving the tooth-bearing mandible are malocclusion, osteomyelitis, and nonunion.[78] The most common complications of the non–tooth-bearing mandible are malocclusion and TMJ ankylosis.[79]

Surgically Relevant Anatomic Considerations: Tooth-bearing Mandible

Nonunion frequently accompanies osteomyelitis and results from the combination of micromotion

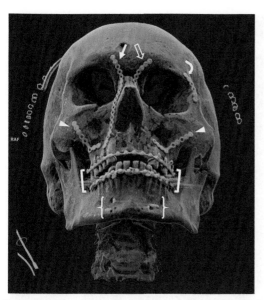

Fig. 14. Stepwise repair. Cinematic 3-D rendering of postoperative face CT for ORIF of bilateral Le Fort 1, Le Fort 2, and left ZMC fractures. A week prior, mandible symphyseal fractures were fixed using 2 lag screws (*braces*) and the patient was left in MMF (*brackets*) to serve as a template for occlusion. Subsequently, the upper Le Fort fractures were fixed; a long straight plate transfixes the right NOE fracture along the NMB (*arrow*). The left zygomaticofrontal suture was then fixed using a low-profile plate (*curved arrow*) and the left NOE fracture was fixed along the nasofrontal suture (*open arrow*). After ORIF of the upper midfacial subunits, the upper and lower midface were reconnected using L plates at the bilateral ZMBs (*arrowheads*).

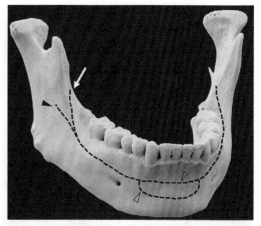

Fig. 15. Champy's lines of osteosynthesis. Cinematic rendering of the mandible from a face CT shows the ideal lines of osteosynthesis. Plates along these lines counteract distractive forces at the superior margin while promoting compression and bone contact inferiorly. At the angle, the plates can be placed along the external oblique ridge (*arrow*) or upper buccal cortex (*solid arrowhead*). In the parasymphyseal region, moments of torque can cause rotational splaying of the fracture segments; therefore, 2 plates are required in this region to neutralize the moments of torque (*open arrowheads*).

Surgical Goals and Approach: Tooth-Bearing Mandible

Load-sharing techniques: semirigid and rigid fixation

Semirigid (Champy) fixation provides functional stability to simple unilateral angle or body fractures using a single miniplate along the ideal fixation lines.[82] During occlusion, tensile stress is neutralized as the plate shares load with bone, and the basal fragments are brought into apposition.[83,84] Micromotion along the thick basal segment promotes callus formation and healing.[85] A meta-analysis of studies comparing semirigid (Champy) and rigid fixation at the mandibular angle shows that single-plate fixation is associated with fewer postoperative complications than 2-plate fixation.[86] The Champy technique is faster and requires less disruption of the soft tissue envelope. Miniplates are placed along the external oblique line or superior basal surface of the angle if the fracture is behind the tooth row[81,86] (Fig. 16). Monocortical screws are used along the ideal lines of fixation to prevent tooth root injury.[73] Semirigid techniques are not effective when bilateral mandibular fractures are present because these create moments of torque with in-plane bending of the miniplate and decreased bone contact.[87,88] At least 2 miniplates (placed superiorly and basally), an equivalent 3-D matrix plate, or a

and the spread of infection from disrupted gingiva between incompletely mobilized tooth-bearing fragment surfaces.[78,80] Micromotion results from opposing forces of mastication: anterior downward forces from the occlusion and suprahyoid mandibular depressors (the mylohyoid, geniohyoid, and digastric muscles) are opposed by posterior upward forces of the pterygomasseteric sling.[71] This results in a band of tensile forces along the upper mandible closer to the tooth row and compressive forces along the thick basal bone.[74,81] Champy and colleagues[82] determined ideal lines of fixation along which miniplates and screws are used to neutralize tensile stress while avoiding tooth roots and the inferior alveolar nerve canal (Fig. 15). In the parasymphyseal region, out-of-plane bending from rotational torque produced by contraction of the masseters necessitates rigid fixation with 2 plates.[82] Along the body and angle, several fixation methods are used.[74,81] These can be semirigid or rigid.

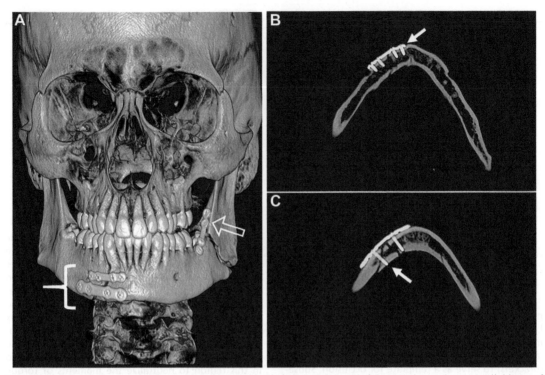

Fig. 16. Champy fixation. A 3-D volume-rendered maxillofacial CT (*A*) with fixation plates along parallel lines of osteosynthesis in the parasymphyseal mandible. Increased moments of torque in this region necessitate 2 plates (*brace*) to achieve adequate fixation. The patient also sustained a left mandibular angle fracture, fixated with a Champy plate along the external oblique ridge (*arrow* [*A*]). Axial CT images show the superior subapical miniplate (*arrow* [*B*]) uses monocortical screws. The larger inferior border plate is placed using bicortical screws, one of which has purchase in a basal triangle (*arrow* [*C*]) to achieve optimal fixation.

combination of a superior miniplate and stronger basal locking plate with bicortical screws are needed to convert at least 1 side to a rigid load-sharing fixation[71,81,89] (see **Fig. 16**; **Fig. 17**). For sagittally oriented midline symphyseal fractures, fixation may be performed using lag screws placed in a transverse orientation anterior to the mental foramina[74,83,90] (**Fig. 18**).

Arch bars typically are placed as the initial step in any reduction of the tooth bearing mandible to re-establish normal occlusion and may remain postoperatively to neutralize tensile forces, reinforce rigidity, and splint dentoalveolar fragments.[83,91,92] In patients expected to be noncompliant with a nonsolid diet, MMF is performed and involves wiring the jaw shut to promote proper healing. Self-drilling, self-tapping subapical intermaxillary fixation (IMF) screws can be placed quickly for occlusal reduction and inter-arch wiring provided that alveolar bone is noncomminuted and can be combined with or used as a faster alternative to arch bar MMF.[74,93–95]

Load-bearing fixation
Comminuted mandibular fractures are those with greater than 3 segments of bone in the same

anatomic region[96] and may be seen in 5% to 7% of mandibular fractures.[97] Mild comminution usually manifests with a fracture line perpendicular to the tooth row and either a triangular basal fragment (a basal triangle), a dentoalveolar fragment, or both[96] (see **Fig. 16**).

Whereas a combination of a subapical miniplate and a basal locking plate confers sufficient rigidity in cases of noncomminuted or mildly comminuted fracture, fully load-bearing heavy reconstruction plates are required to bridge areas of severe comminution. Load-bearing fixation prevents fragment telescoping, minimizes the risk of further periosteal stripping thereby preventing small fragment sequestration, and helps maintain the reduced buccal contour[97,98] (**Fig. 19**). Simplification with small plates and screws may be used to restore mandibular form and improve fragment contact prior to reconstruction plate fixation.[97] Severe comminution typically requires an extraoral surgical approach for adequate plate adaptation and monitoring of the reduction.[98]

Bone grafting and external fixation
Defect fractures with no contact between major bone fragments result most commonly from

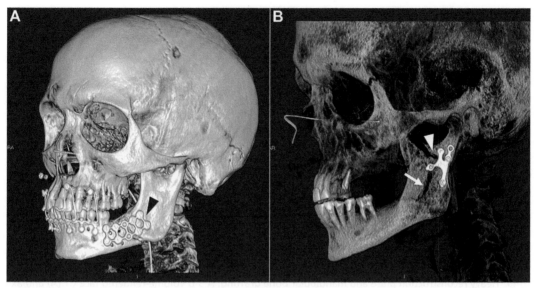

Fig. 17. Matrix plates for fracture fixation. Two 3-D volume-rendered CT examples of 3-D matrix plate fixation of a body fracture (*arrowhead* [*A*]) and subcondylar fracture (*arrowhead* [*B*]). At the subcondylar region, matrix plates are advantageous in that they can be applied from a variety of surgical approaches. The shape reduces the risk of inadvertent screw placement in the mandibular foramen (*arrow* [*B*]) .

cavitary gunshot wounds and less often from severe blunt trauma with comminution and bone loss.[91,97] Defects also may arise following resection of infected bone. If there is a healthy soft tissue cover, primary bone grafting is performed and bridged with a heavy reconstruction plate.[91] If there is gross infection or tissue loss, external fixation is used first to maintain facial form until flap reconstruction is performed[91,97] (**Fig. 20**). **Tables 3** and **4** summarize the commonly used hardware and types of fixation utilized for mandibular fractures.

Postoperative Assessment of Complications: Tooth-bearing Mandible

Nonunion and osteomyelitis
Nonunion and osteomyelitis are major complications requiring revision surgery with resection of bone ends, grafting, and load-bearing fixation.

Because the mandible is highly vascularized, nonunion is considered present after only 8 weeks of delayed healing[78,92] (**Fig. 21**). CT findings of mottled, resorbed, and irregular or rounded sclerotic bone; sequestered fragments; abscess; and persistent soft tissue edema are highly suggestive of osteomyelitis[99] (**Fig. 22**).

The primary predisposing factor to osteomyelitis is insufficiently stable fixation.[73,74,78,92] On postoperative CT, screws should be assessed for loosening and breakage. In split fractures, separating basal fragments into buccal and lingual components (so-called butterfly fragments) bicortical screws should be confirmed to engage both cortices. Screws inadvertently placed between fragments can have an adverse impact on stability and healing.[100] All major fragments should be fixed. Comminuted fragments missed preoperatively may be overlooked during open reduction and internal fixation (ORIF). For

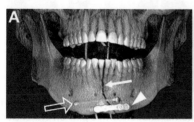
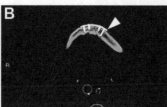
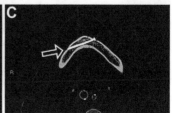

Fig. 18. Symphyseal lag screw. A 3-D volume rendering (*A*) and axial CT images (*B, C*) show fixation of a vertically oriented symphyseal fracture (*solid arrow* [*A*]) using a basal border plate (*arrowheads* [*A, B*]) and superior lag screw (*open arrows* [*A, C*]). There was no lingual gap.

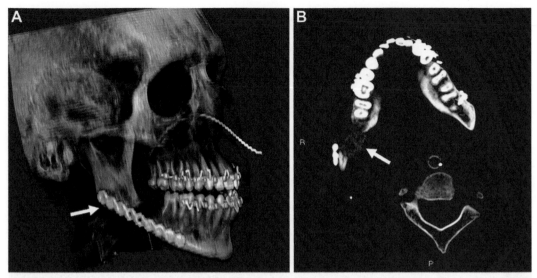

Fig. 19. Heavy reconstruction plate and mandibular bone grafting. A 3-D volume-rendered face CT (*A*) and axial CT image at the level of the mandible (*B*) show ORIF of the right mandibular body using a heavy reconstruction plate (*arrow* [*A*]), which was bent to contour the inferior buccal cortex. A segment of bone loss along the mandibular body resulted from nonunion secondary to osteomyelitis, which was filled with bone graft (*arrow* [*B*]).

example, semirigid Champy fixation is insufficient for an angle fracture with a missed basal triangle.[99] During staged reconstruction with external fixation, it is important to recognize pin loosening or displacement and telescoping of fracture segments.[101]

By definition, a major complication is one that requires revision surgery, such as grafting and placement of new hardware.[81] Hardware failure or soft tissue abscesses that develop following bone consolidation are considered minor complications, even if patient admission is required, because hardware can be removed safely, and

abscesses can be treated with drainage and intravenous antibiotics.[102,103]

Hematoma within tooth sockets is a rich culture medium that promotes infection, and the tooth socket acts as a potential portal of spread to bone. Teeth in the line of fracture, even when severely luxated, often are spared during reduction and can be treated with follow-up endodontic therapy provided they do not interfere with occlusion and there is no major periapical disease or caries. Severely comminuted dentoalveolar fragments can become devitalized and may be removed.[96]

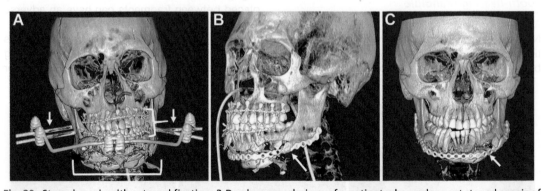

Fig. 20. Staged repair with external fixation; 3-D volume renderings of a patient who underwent staged repair of ballistic mandibular fractures (*bracket* [*A*]). Staged repair first involves external fixation with 2 pins on either side of the mandible attached to a U rod (*arrows* [*A*]). Hybrid MMF was used (*brace*). Four days later (*B*), external fixation was removed and internal fixation performed with an inferior buccal reconstruction plate extending from angle to angle (*arrows* [*B, C*]). The patient remained in MMF for 6 weeks, after which MMF was removed (*C*).

Table 3
Commonly used hardware for treatment of mandibular fractures

Mandibular Hardware	Purpose
Monocortical screw	Fracture in close proximity to tooth root apices and/or the inferior alveolar canal and nerve Placed along external oblique line or upper buccal surface in semirigid load sharing fixation (ie, Champy fixation) Subapical and basal segment placement of 2 miniplates for rigid fixation
Bicortical screw	Provides stronger fixation and increased stability compared with rigid fixation with miniplates alone. Placed along the basal segment of the mandible
Arch bars, IMF screws	Used for MMF to achieve premorbid occlusion. Used to provide added stability followed by plate fixation Used to splint dentoalveolar fragments IMF screws are self-drilling and tapping and used alone following rigid fixation (ease of use, avoids sharps injury from wire ends to surgeon). Used as a complement to arch bars (hybrid technique) when an unstable midface or dentoalveolar fracture necessitates at least 1 arch bar as a splint
Reconstruction plate	(1) Severe comminution and bone loss OR; (2) edentulous, atrophic mandible
External fixator	(1) Staged repair for comminuted fracture with insufficient soft tissue coverage (especially after bone and soft tissue loss following gunshot wound) OR (2) Staged repair for revision of an infected, nonhealing fracture OR (3). Critically ill patient
Lag screw	Sagittally oriented fracture of the mandibular symphysis Rapid technique (no plate bending) that is anterior to and avoids the mental foramina

Malocclusion

Trifocal bicondylar and parasymphyseal mandibular fractures (sometimes referred to as flail mandible) are prone to cross-bite malocclusions, especially when comminuted.[72] Surgeons overbend reconstruction and locking plates to prevent this complication.[73,96] Postoperative CTs should be assessed for posteriorly divergent widening and persistent lingual gap in any patient with parasymphyseal fracture[104] (**Figs. 23** and **24**). Malocclusion following consolidation that cannot be corrected with dental resurfacing is considered a major complication requiring revision surgery.[98]

Surgically Relevant Anatomic Considerations: Non–Tooth-bearing Mandible

Condylar, subcondylar, ramus, and coronoid fractures involve the non–tooth-bearing mandible. The ramus is a strong strut of bone and the coronoid is protected by the zygomatic arch, making fractures of these structures uncommon.[105] The condyles are thin structures prone to indirect fracture from tensile stress following blows to the anterior mandible.[79] Because these fractures are closed, micromotion does not lead to infection. Condylar fractures can involve the subcondylar region (the base of the condyle below the sigmoid notch), the condylar neck, and the condylar head. The primary goal of treatment is prevention of malocclusion and ankylosis.[79] The risk of ankylosis is much greater for intra-articular condylar head fractures.[106]

Surgical Goals and Approach: Non–Tooth-bearing Mandible

Open surgery of condylar fractures is associated with a risk of facial nerve injury and devascularization of the condylar head. Because most patients develop functional adaptations that allow normal or near-normal mouth opening and biting into occlusion following malunion, they frequently are treated with closed therapy using arch bars and guiding elastics.[79,83]

Postoperative Assessment of Complications: Non–tooth-Bearing Mandible

Malocclusion

Superior telescoping of the ramus by more than 15 mm, angulation about the fracture apex greater than 35°, and bilateral condylar fractures increase

Table 4
Types of mandibular fixation

Type of Mandibular Fixation	Appearance	Purpose
Semirigid (Champy) fixation	1. Single miniplate along the mandibular angle *OR* 2. Two miniplates in the par-asymphyseal region	Simple unilateral fracture, without significant displacement or comminution Champy fixation is less disruptive to the soft tissue envelope. Allows for some micromotion at the mandibular angle inferior border, which promotes callus formation Considered semirigid because distraction from opposing forces of occlusion and masticatory muscles is neutralized
Rigid load-sharing fixation	1. Large locking plate along the inferior border and a miniplate along the zone of tension *OR* 2. Single locking plate along the inferior border with an arch bar *OR* 3. 3-D miniplates	1. Noncomminuted fracture *OR* 2. Basal triangle fragments
Load-bearing fixation	1. Placement of a reconstruction plate *OR* 2. Placement of multiple plates and screws (simplification), especially in combination with larger locking plates May be combined with bone graft for large defects, provided adequate soft tissue coverage	1. Atrophic edentulous fracture *OR* 2. Comminuted fracture
Biplanar fixation	Single plate along the lateral buccal margin or external oblique line and another along the inferior border of the mandible	Mandibular angle fractures not amenable to Champy fixation (eg, bone loss from third molar extraction or basal triangle).
Condylar plating	Single-plate or double-plate and screw fixation along the condyle or subcondylar region	1. Bilateral mandibular condyle fracture *OR* 2. Fractures as risk for resulting in TMJ ankylosis (ramus telescoping, >35° angulation) *OR* 3. Moderate to severe unilaterally displaced fracture with dislocated/distracted condylar neck (implies damage to articular disk and retrodiscal tissue.

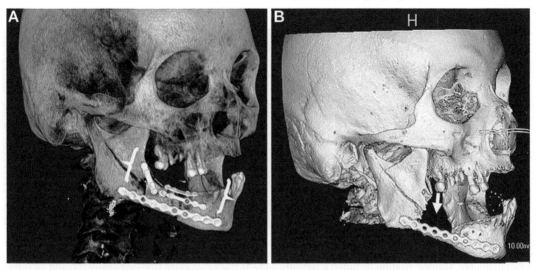

Fig. 21. Mandibular fracture nonunion requiring hardware revision; 3-D volume renderings of the face performed 2 months apart. Nonunion of the mandibular body fracture and infection of the fixation plates (*braces* [*A*]) required revision with removal of all plates except for the lower border plate. Osteotomy of the necrotic bone was performed (*arrow* [*B*]).

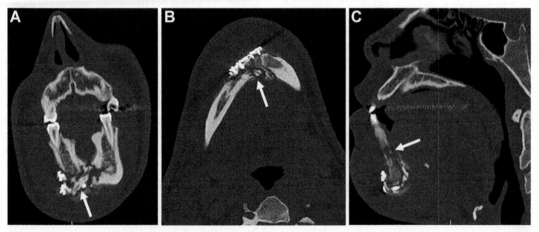

Fig. 22. Hardware failure with sequestrum. Multiplanar face CT images in the coronal (*A*) axial (*B*) and sagittal (*C*) planes in patient 7 weeks after trauma, shows nonunion manifested as bone erosion, sequestration (*arrows*), and prominent lucency around the existing fixation plate and monocortical screws. Devitalized bone was debrided, hardware removed, and the patient was placed in MMF with arch bars (not shown).

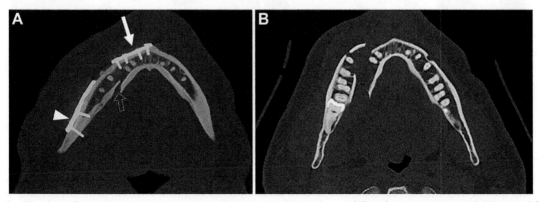

Fig. 23. Lingual gap. Postoperative maximum intensity projection image (*A*) and preoperative axial CT image (*B*) show reduction of lingual gap along the parasymphyseal mandible after ORIF, utilizing a parasymphyseal mini-plate with monocortical screws (*solid arrow* [*A*]) and a rigid reconstruction plate along the body (*arrowhead* [*A*]). Residual lingual gap measured 3 mm (*open arrow* [*A*]).

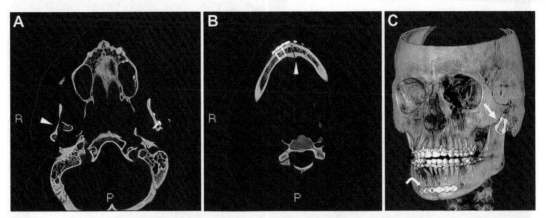

Fig. 24. Condylar plating for flail mandible. Axial CT (*A, B*) and 3-D volume rendering of the face (*C*). This patient sustained trifocal fractures, including bilateral condylar and symphyseal fractures (*arrowheads* [*A, B*]), resulting in a flail mandible. Surgical fixation included a left subcondylar trapezoid plate (*straight arrow* [*C*]) and an inferior border plate along the symphysis (*curved arrow* [*C*]). There is no lingual gap at the symphysis on the postoperative CT (*B*). The right intra-articular condylar head fracture was treated in a closed fashion with elastics.

the likelihood of a clinically significant malocclusion.[79,107,108] If any of these features is present on CT imaging following occlusal reduction with arch bars, ORIF with miniplate or 3-D matrix plate fixation may be favored. Hardware failure related to tensile stress is considerably higher following single-plate fixation than other plating schemes.[109]

Ankylosis

TMJ ankylosis results from a combination of increased bone contact and traumatic injury to the joint capsule, articular disc, and retrodiscal

tissue.[75,77] MRI is not performed routinely to assess TMJ dysfunction after condylar fractures due to high cost and limited scanner availability in the acute setting.[75] Several CT features are predictive of disc derangement and ankylosis. Fractures higher in the condyle, especially those with oblique fractures through the intra-articular condylar head and telescoping of the distal ramus segment, are at elevated risk of ankylosis because the ramus segment tends to abut the condylar eminence and root of the zygoma, increasing the surface area of contacting bone.[110] There is no widely accepted fixation

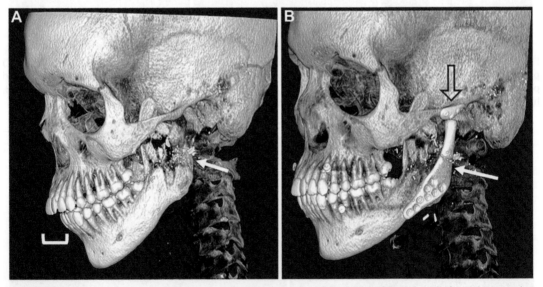

Fig. 25. TMJ arthroplasty after ballistic injury; 3-D volume-rendered face CTs before (*A*) and after (*B*) TMJ arthroplasty. Ballistic fragments surround the comminuted subcondylar fracture with extensive bone loss (*arrow* [*A*]). This resulted in malocclusion with anterior open bite (*bracket* [*A*]). A custom TMJ prosthesis was implanted, composed of a ramus component (*solid arrow* [*B*]) and glenoid fossa component (*open arrow* [*B*]). The occlusion is grossly normal at imaging after arthroplasty.

method for intracapsular condylar head fractures due to the risks associated with further capsular disruption. Total TMJ replacement may be necessary in the case of ankylosis or severe bone loss related to ballistic trauma[92] (**Fig. 25**).

SUMMARY

Concise clinically relevant reporting of postoperative CT imaging following facial fractures requires familiarity with commonly used surgical hardware, the anatomy-specific rationale for a given fixation method, and potential complications that may arise during the postoperative period.

CLINICS CARE POINTS

- NFD obstruction leads to suppurative complications, including mucopyocele development, osteomyelitis, and plate infection, which ultimately may result in intracranial and/or intraorbital spread. Patency is assessed best on sagittal images.

- Patients who have undergone obliteration or cranialization require periodic imaging surveillance to screen for developing mucopyocele.

- Small changes in the axis of rotation about the ZSS should be described on postoperative imaging. A small degree of rotation can lead to large changes in orbital volume and result in enophthalmos.

- Zygomaticomaxillary fracture fixation is determined using the CT-based Zingg classification system and intraoperative assessment for fracture stability with each plate placement.

- Orbital floor implants should bridge the entire fracture defect. Any space that persists between fracture ledges may lead to postoperative entrapment and should be described objectively.

- Nonunion frequently accompanies osteomyelitis. In the mandible, this frequently results from a combination of micromotion and the spread of infection from disrupted gingiva between incompletely mobilized tooth-bearing fragment surfaces.

- Basal triangle fragments should be included in mandibular fixation. Any residual lingual gaps should be described.

DISCLOSURE

The authors have nothing to disclose.

REFERENCES

1. Lalloo R, Lucchesi LR, Bisignano C, et al. Epidemiology of facial fractures: incidence, prevalence and years lived with disability estimates from the Global Burden of Disease 2017 study. Inj Prev 2020; 26(Supp 1):i27–35.
2. Reiter MJ, Schwope RB, Theler JM. Postoperative CT of the midfacial skeleton after trauma: review of normal appearances and common complications. AJR Am J Roentgenol 2017;209(4):W238–48.
3. Remmler D, Denny A, Gosain A, et al. Role of three-dimensional computed tomography in the assessment of nasoorbitoethmoidal fractures. Ann Plast Surg 2000;44(5):553–62 [discussion: 562–3].
4. Markowitz BL, Manson PN, Sargent L, et al. Management of the medial canthal tendon in nasoethmoid orbital fractures: the importance of the central fragment in classification and treatment. Plast Reconstr Surg 1991;87(5):843–53.
5. Kelly CP, Cohen AJ, Yavuzer R, et al. Medial canthopexy: a proven technique. Ophthal Plast Reconstr Surg 2004;20(5):337–41.
6. Baril SE, Yoon MK. Naso-orbito-ethmoidal (NOE) fractures: a review. Int Ophthalmol Clin 2013; 53(4):149–55.
7. Ellis E 3rd. Sequencing treatment for naso-orbito-ethmoid fractures. J Oral Maxillofac Surg 1993; 51(5):543–58.
8. Nguyen M, Koshy JC, Hollier LH Jr. Pearls of nasoorbitoethmoid trauma management. Semin Plast Surg 2010;24(4):383–8.
9. Kalavrezos ND, Graetz KW, Eyrich GK, et al. Late sequelae after high midface trauma. J R Coll Surg Edinb 2000;45(6):359–62.
10. Heller EM, Jacobs JB, Holliday RA. Evaluation of the frontonasal duct in frontal sinus fractures. Head Neck 1989;11(1):46–50.
11. Forrest CR, Hammer B, Manson PN, et al. Craniofacial Fractures. In: Prein J, editor. Manual of Internal Fixation in the Cranio-Facial Skeleton: Techniques Recommended by the AO/ASIF Maxillofacial Group. Berlin: Springer Berlin Heidelberg; 1998. p. 95–154.
12. Ridgway EB, Chen C, Colakoglu S, et al. The incidence of lower eyelid malposition after facial fracture repair: a retrospective study and meta-analysis comparing subtarsal, subciliary, and transconjunctival incisions. Plast Reconstr Surg 2009;124(5):1578–86.
13. Papadopoulos H, Salib NK. Management of naso-orbital-ethmoidal fractures. Oral Maxillofac Surg Clin North Am 2009;21(2):221–5, vi.
14. Bell RB, Dierks EJ, Brar P, et al. A protocol for the management of frontal sinus fractures emphasizing sinus preservation. J Oral Maxillofac Surg 2007; 65(5):825–39.
15. Sivori LA 2nd, de Leeuw R, Morgan I, et al. Complications of frontal sinus fractures with emphasis on

chronic craniofacial pain and its treatment: a review of 43 cases. J Oral Maxillofac Surg 2010; 68(9):2041–6.

16. Swinson BD, Jerjes W, Thompson G. Current practice in the management of frontal sinus fractures. J Laryngol Otol 2004;118(12):927–32.

17. Larrabee WF Jr, Travis LW, Tabb HG. Frontal sinus fractures–their suppurative complications and surgical management. Laryngoscope 1980;90(11 Pt 1):1810–3.

18. Jain SA, Manchio JV, Weinzweig J. Role of the sagittal view of computed tomography in evaluation of the nasofrontal ducts in frontal sinus fractures. J Craniofac Surg 2010;21(6):1670–3.

19. Rice DH. Management of frontal sinus fractures. Curr Opin Otolaryngol Head Neck Surg 2004; 12(1):46–8.

20. Donald PJ, Ettin M. The safety of frontal sinus fat obliteration when sinus walls are missing. Laryngoscope 1986;96(2):190–3.

21. Donald PJ. Frontal sinus ablation by cranialization. Report of 21 cases. Arch Otolaryngol 1982;108(3): 142–6.

22. Lakhani RS, Shibuya TY, Mathog RH, et al. Titanium mesh repair of the severely comminuted frontal sinus fracture. Arch Otolaryngol Head Neck Surg 2001;127(6):665–9.

23. Kelly KJ, Manson PN, Vander Kolk CA, et al. Sequencing LeFort fracture treatment (Organization of treatment for a panfacial fracture). J Craniofac Surg 1990;1(4):168–78.

24. Ali K, Lettieri SC. Management of Panfacial Fracture. Semin Plast Surg 2017;31(2):108–17.

25. Becelli R, Renzi G, Mannino G, et al. Posttraumatic obstruction of lacrimal pathways: a retrospective analysis of 58 consecutive naso-orbitoethmoid fractures. J Craniofac Surg 2004;15(1):29–33.

26. Gruss JS, Hurwitz JJ, Nik NA, et al. The pattern and incidence of nasolacrimal injury in naso-orbital-ethmoid fractures: the role of delayed assessment and dacryocystorhinostomy. Br J Plast Surg 1985; 38(1):116–21.

27. Lee EI, Mohan K, Koshy JC, et al. Optimizing the surgical management of zygomaticomaxillary complex fractures. Semin Plast Surg 2010;24(4):389–97.

28. Marinho RO, Freire-Maia B. Management of fractures of the zygomaticomaxillary complex. Oral Maxillofac Surg Clin North Am 2013;25(4):617–36.

29. Knight JS, North JF. The classification of malar fractures: an analysis of displacement as a guide to treatment. Br J Plast Surg 1961;13:325–39.

30. Zingg M, Laedrach K, Chen J, et al. Classification and treatment of zygomatic fractures: a review of 1,025 cases. J Oral Maxillofac Surg 1992;50(8):778–90.

31. Ellis E 3rd, Kittidumkerng W. Analysis of treatment for isolated zygomaticomaxillary complex fractures. J Oral Maxillofac Surg 1996;54(4):386–400 [discussion: 400–1].

32. Roth FS, Koshy JC, Goldberg JS, et al. Pearls of orbital trauma management. Semin Plast Surg 2010;24(4):398–410.

33. He D, Li Z, Shi W, et al. Orbitozygomatic fractures with enophthalmos: analysis of 64 cases treated late. J Oral Maxillofac Surg 2012;70(3):562–76.

34. Ellis E 3rd. Orbital trauma. Oral Maxillofac Surg Clin North Am 2012;24(4):629–48.

35. Gander T, Essig H, Metzler P, et al. Patient specific implants (PSI) in reconstruction of orbital floor and wall fractures. J Craniomaxillofac Surg 2015;43(1): 126–30.

36. Holmes KD, Matthews BL. Three-point alignment of zygoma fractures with miniplate fixation. Arch Otolaryngol Head Neck Surg 1989;115(8):961–3.

37. Kelley P, Hopper R, Gruss J. Evaluation and treatment of zygomatic fractures. Plast Reconstr Surg 2007;120(7 Suppl 2):5S–15S.

38. Davidson J, Nickerson D, Nickerson B. Zygomatic fractures: comparison of methods of internal fixation. Plast Reconstr Surg 1990;86(1):25–32.

39. Whitehouse RW, Batterbury M, Jackson A, et al. Prediction of enophthalmos by computed tomography after 'blow out' orbital fracture. Br J Ophthalmol 1994;78(8):618–20.

40. Czerwinski M, Izadpanah A, Ma S, et al. Quantitative analysis of the orbital floor defect after zygoma fracture repair. J Oral Maxillofac Surg 2008;66(9): 1869–74.

41. Tahernia A, Erdmann D, Follmar K, et al. Clinical implications of orbital volume change in the management of isolated and zygomaticomaxillary complex-associated orbital floor injuries. Plast Reconstr Surg 2009;123(3):968–75.

42. Francel TJ, Birely BC, Ringelman PR, et al. The fate of plates and screws after facial fracture reconstruction. Plast Reconstr Surg 1992;90(4):568–73.

43. Dreizin D, Nam AJ, Diaconu SC, et al. Multidetector CT of midfacial fractures: classification systems, principles of reduction, and common complications. Radiographics 2018;38(1):248–74.

44. Fan X, Li J, Zhu J, et al. Computer-assisted orbital volume measurement in the surgical correction of late enophthalmos caused by blowout fractures. Ophthal Plast Reconstr Surg 2003;19(3):207–11.

45. Manson PN, Grivas A, Rosenbaum A, et al. Studies on enophthalmos: II. The measurement of orbital injuries and their treatment by quantitative computed tomography. Plast Reconstr Surg 1986;77(2): 203–14.

46. Manson PN, Iliff N. Management of blow-out fractures of the orbital floor. II. Early repair for selected injuries. Surv Ophthalmol 1991;35(4):280–92.

47. Burm JS, Chung CH, Oh SJ. Pure orbital blowout fracture: new concepts and importance of medial orbital blowout fracture. Plast Reconstr Surg 1999;103(7):1839–49.

48. Ellis E 3rd, Tan Y. Assessment of internal orbital reconstructions for pure blowout fractures: cranial bone grafts versus titanium mesh. J Oral Maxillofac Surg 2003;61(4):442–53.

49. Simon GJB, Bush S, Selva D, et al. Orbital cellulitis: a rare complication after orbital blowout fracture. Ophthalmology 2005;112(11):2030–4.

50. Samii M, Tatagiba M. Skull base trauma: diagnosis and management. Neurol Res 2002;24(2):147–56.

51. Levin LA, Beck RW, Joseph MP, et al. The treatment of traumatic optic neuropathy: the International Optic Nerve Trauma Study. Ophthalmology 1999; 106(7):1268–77.

52. Jin H, Gong S, Han K, et al. Clinical management of traumatic superior orbital fissure and orbital apex syndromes. Clin Neurol Neurosurg 2018;165:50–4.

53. Dreizin D, Sakai O, Champ K, et al. CT of Skull Base Fractures: Classification systems. Complications, and Management. Radiographics; 2021. p. 200189.

54. Bell RB, Chen J. Frontobasilar fractures: contemporary management. Atlas Oral Maxillofac Surg Clin North Am 2010;18(2):181–96.

55. Archer JB, Sun H, Bonney PA, et al. Extensive traumatic anterior skull base fractures with cerebrospinal fluid leak: classification and repair techniques using combined vascularized tissue flaps. J Neurosurg 2016;124(3):647–56.

56. Raveh J, Laedrach K, Vuillemin T, et al. Management of combined frontonaso-orbital/skull base fractures and telecanthus in 355 cases. Arch Otolaryngol Head Neck Surg 1992;118(6):605–14.

57. Moritz JD, Hoffmann B, Sehr D, et al. Evaluation of ultra-low dose CT in the diagnosis of pediatric-like fractures using an experimental animal study. Korean J Radiol 2012;13(2):165–73.

58. Rozema R, Doff MH, van Ooijen PM, et al. Diagnostic reliability of low dose multidetector CT and cone beam CT in maxillofacial trauma-an experimental blinded and randomized study. Dentomaxillofac Radiol 2018;47(8):20170423.

59. Yi JW, Park HJ, Lee SY, et al. Radiation dose reduction in multidetector CT in fracture evaluation. Br J Radiol 2017;90(1077):20170240.

60. Bodelle B, Wichmann JL, Klotz N, et al. Seventy kilovolt ultra-low dose CT of the paranasal sinus: first clinical results. Clin Radiol 2015;70(7):711–5.

61. Widmann G, Dalla Torre D, Hoermann R, et al. Ultralow-dose computed tomography imaging for surgery of midfacial and orbital fractures using ASIR and MBIR. Int J Oral Maxillofac Surg 2015; 44(4):441–6.

62. Elegbede A, Diaconu S, Dreizin D, et al. Low-dose computed tomographic scans for postoperative evaluation of craniomaxillofacial fractures: a pilot clinical study. Plast Reconstr Surg 2020;146(2): 366–70.

63. Tessier P. The classic reprint. Experimental study of fractures of the upper jaw. I and II. Rene Le Fort, M.D. Plast Reconstr Surg 1972;50(5):497–506. contd.

64. Manson PN. Some thoughts on the classification and treatment of Le Fort fractures. Ann Plast Surg 1986;17(5):356–63.

65. Salvolini U. Traumatic injuries: imaging of facial injuries. Eur Radiol 2002;12(6):1253–61.

66. Daffner RH. Imaging of facial trauma. Curr Probl Diagn Radiol 1997;26(4):158–84.

67. Ellis E. Passive repositioning of maxillary fractures: an occasional impossibility without osteotomy. J Oral Maxillofac Surg 2004;62(12):1477–85.

68. Scolozzi P, Imholz B. Completion of nonreducible Le Fort fractures by Le Fort I osteotomy: sometimes an inevitable choice to avoid postoperative malocclusion. J Craniofac Surg 2015;26(1):e59–61.

69. Moss WJ, Kedarisetty S, Jafari A, et al. A Review of Hard Palate Fracture Repair Techniques. J Oral Maxillofac Surg 2016;74(2):328–36.

70. Chen CH, Wang TY, Tsay PK, et al. A 162-case review of palatal fracture: management strategy from a 10-year experience. Plast Reconstr Surg 2008; 121(6):2065–73.

71. Morrow BT, Samson TD, Schubert W, et al. Evidence-based medicine: Mandible fractures. Plast Reconstr Surg 2014;134(6):1381–90.

72. Mehta N, Butala P, Bernstein MP. The imaging of maxillofacial trauma and its pertinence to surgical intervention. Radiol Clin North Am 2012;50(1): 43–57.

73. Schilli W, Stoll P, Bähr W, et al. Mandibular Fractures. In: Prein J, editor. Manual of Internal Fixation in the Cranio-Facial Skeleton: Techniques Recommended by the AO/ASIF Maxillofacial Group. Berlin: Springer Berlin Heidelberg; 1998. p. 57–93.

74. Goodday RH. Management of fractures of the mandibular body and symphysis. Oral Maxillofac Surg Clin North Am 2013;25(4):601–16.

75. Dwivedi AN, Tripathi R, Gupta PK, et al. Magnetic resonance imaging evaluation of temporomandibular joint and associated soft tissue changes following acute condylar injury. J Oral Maxillofac Surg 2012;70(12):2829–34.

76. Sullivan SM, Banghart PR, Anderson Q. Magnetic resonance imaging assessment of acute soft tissue injuries to the temporomandibular joint. J Oral Maxillofac Surg 1995;53(7):763–6 [discussion: 766–7].

77. Takaku S, Yoshida M, Sano T, et al. Magnetic resonance images in patients with acute traumatic injury of the temporomandibular joint: a preliminary report. J Craniomaxillofac Surg 1996;24(3):173–7.

78. Mathog RH, Toma V, Clayman L, et al. Nonunion of the mandible: an analysis of contributing factors. J Oral Maxillofac Surg 2000;58(7):746–52 [discussion: 752–3].

79. Kisnisci R. Management of fractures of the condyle, condylar neck, and coronoid process. Oral Maxillofac Surg Clin North Am 2013;25(4):573–90.

80. Mendonca D, Kenkere D. Avoiding occlusal derangement in facial fractures: An evidence based approach. Indian J Plast Surg 2013;46(2):215–20.

81. Braasch DC, Abubaker AO. Management of mandibular angle fracture. Oral Maxillofac Surg Clin North Am 2013;25(4):591–600.

82. Champy M, Lodde JP, Schmitt R, et al. Mandibular osteosynthesis by miniature screwed plates via a buccal approach. J Maxillofac Surg 1978;6(1):14–21.

83. Ellis E 3rd, Miles BA. Fractures of the mandible: a technical perspective. Plast Reconstr Surg 2007; 120(7 Suppl 2):76S–89S.

84. Ellis E 3rd. An algorithm for the treatment of non-condylar mandibular fractures. J Oral Maxillofac Surg 2014;72(5):939–49.

85. Mehra P, Murad H. Internal fixation of mandibular angle fractures: a comparison of 2 techniques. J Oral Maxillofac Surg 2008;66(11):2254–60.

86. Al-Moraissi EA, Ellis E 3rd. What method for management of unilateral mandibular angle fractures has the lowest rate of postoperative complications? A systematic review and meta-analysis. J Oral Maxillofac Surg 2014;72(11):2197–211.

87. Susarla SM, Swanson EW, Peacock ZS. Bilateral mandibular fractures. Eplasty 2014;14:ic38.

88. Ellis E 3rd. Open reduction and internal fixation of combined angle and body/symphysis fractures of the mandible: how much fixation is enough? J Oral Maxillofac Surg 2013;71(4):726–33.

89. Singh V, Puri P, Arya S, et al. Conventional versus 3-dimensional miniplate in management of mandibular fracture: a prospective randomized study. Otolaryngol Head Neck Surg 2012;147(3):450–5.

90. Agnihotri A, Prabhu S, Thomas S. A comparative analysis of the efficacy of cortical screws as lag screws and miniplates for internal fixation of mandibular symphyseal region fractures: a randomized prospective study. Int J Oral Maxillofac Surg 2014;43(1):22–8.

91. Chrcanovic BR. Open versus closed reduction: comminuted mandibular fractures. Oral Maxillofac Surg 2013;17(2):95–104.

92. Vega LG. Reoperative mandibular trauma: management of posttraumatic mandibular deformities. Oral Maxillofac Surg Clin North Am 2011;23(1):47–61. v-vi.

93. Rai A, Datarkar A, Borle RM. Are maxillomandibular fixation screws a better option than Erich arch bars in achieving maxillomandibular fixation? A randomized clinical study. J Oral Maxillofac Surg 2011; 69(12):3015–8.

94. Ansari K, Hamlar D, Ho V, et al. A comparison of anterior vs posterior isolated mandible fractures treated with intermaxillary fixation screws. Arch Facial Plast Surg 2011;13(4):266–70.

95. Arosarena O, Ducic Y, Tollefson TT. Mandible fractures: discussion and debate. Facial Plast Surg Clin North Am 2012;20(3):347–63.

96. Ellis E 3rd, Muniz O, Anand K. Treatment considerations for comminuted mandibular fractures. J Oral Maxillofac Surg 2003;61(8):861–70.

97. Alpert B, Tiwana PS, Kushner GM. Management of comminuted fractures of the mandible. Oral Maxillofac Surg Clin North Am 2009;21(2):185–92, v.

98. Futran ND. Management of comminuted mandible fractures. Oper Tech Otolaryngol Head Neck Surg 2008;19(2):113–6.

99. Dreizin D, Nam AJ, Tirada N, et al. Multidetector CT of mandibular fractures, reductions, and complications: a clinically relevant primer for the radiologist. Radiographics 2016;36(5):1539–64.

100. Prein J, Kellman RM. Rigid internal fixation of mandibular fractures–basics of AO technique. Otolaryngol Clin North Am 1987;20(3):441–56.

101. Braidy HF, Ziccardi VB. External fixation for mandible fractures. Atlas Oral Maxillofac Surg Clin North Am 2009;17(1):45–53.

102. Kumar S, Prabhakar V, Rao K, et al. A comparative review of treatment of 80 mandibular angle fracture fixation with miniplates using three different techniques. Indian J Otolaryngol Head Neck Surg 2011;63(2):190–2.

103. Ellis E 3rd. A study of 2 bone plating methods for fractures of the mandibular symphysis/body. J Oral Maxillofac Surg 2011;69(7):1978–87.

104. Gerbino G, Boffano P, Bosco GF. Symphyseal mandibular fractures associated with bicondylar fractures: a retrospective analysis. J Oral Maxillofac Surg 2009;67(8):1656–60.

105. Boffano P, Kommers SC, Roccia F, et al. Fractures of the mandibular coronoid process: a two centres study. J Craniomaxillofac Surg 2014;42(7):1352–5.

106. Xiang GL, Long X, Deng MH, et al. A retrospective study of temporomandibular joint ankylosis secondary to surgical treatment of mandibular condylar fractures. Br J Oral Maxillofac Surg 2014;52(3):270–4.

107. Bhagol A, Singh V, Kumar I, et al. Prospective evaluation of a new classification system for the management of mandibular subcondylar fractures. J Oral Maxillofac Surg 2011;69(4):1159–65.

108. Forouzanfar T, Lobbezoo F, Overgaauw M, et al. Long-term results and complications after treatment of bilateral fractures of the mandibular condyle. Br J Oral Maxillofac Surg 2013;51(7):634–8.

109. Bischoff EL, Carmichael R, Reddy LV. Plating options for fixation of condylar neck and base fractures. Atlas Oral Maxillofac Surg Clin North Am 2017;25(1):69–73.

110. He D, Yang C, Chen M, et al. Intracapsular condylar fracture of the mandible: our classification and open treatment experience. J Oral Maxillofac Surg 2009;67(8):1672–9.

Imaging of Facial Reconstruction and Face Transplantation

Gopi K. Nayak, MD[a],*, Zoe P. Berman, MD[b],
Eduardo D. Rodriguez, MD, DDS[b], Mari Hagiwara, MD[a]

KEYWORDS

- Facial reconstruction • Orthognathic surgery • Facial feminization • Face transplantation

KEY POINTS

- Three commonly used orthognathic procedures include the Le Fort type I osteotomy, bilateral sagittal split osteotomy (BSSO), and osseous genioplasty. These procedures are used to correct deformities of the midface, lower face, and chin, respectively.
- Reference to the surgeon's operative note, or direct communication with the surgical team is extremely helpful and highly recommended to avoid language in the imaging report which may be incorrect, misleading, or results in unnecessary patient concern or confusion.
- Commonly addressed areas in facial feminization surgery (FFS) include the frontal and periorbital region, the nose, chin, and jawline, as these areas have been shown to play an important role in gender discrimination.
- Interdisciplinary preparation for the face transplant recipient and donor imaging is of paramount importance for operative planning.
- At our institution, preoperative imaging for both the donor and recipient consists of a high-resolution craniofacial CT, arterial, and venous phase CT angiogram of the head and neck, and 6-vessel digital subtraction angiography (DSA).

INTRODUCTION

Pre- and postoperative imaging is increasingly used in plastic and reconstructive surgery for evaluation of bony and soft tissue anatomy. Imaging plays an important role in preoperative planning and can also be used for computerized surgical planning and 3D modeling. In the postoperative setting, imaging is used for the assessment of surgical positioning, bone healing and fusion, and early or delayed surgical complications. This article will focus on imaging performed for surgical reconstruction of the face, including orthognathic surgery, facial feminization procedures for gender dysphoria, and face transplantation.

Orthognathic surgery

Orthognathic surgery involves repositioning of the maxilla and mandible to correct facial deformities that may be genetic, posttraumatic or otherwise cosmetically or functionally impairing. The maxilla and mandible, or components of each, can be deficient or excessive in any of the 3 orthogonal planes resulting in facial deformity of various types, and often dental malocclusion. Multiple surgical options are available for correcting dentofacial deformities; however, 3 commonly used procedures include the Le Fort type I osteotomy, the bilateral sagittal split osteotomy (BSSO), and osseous genioplasty. The Le Fort type I osteotomy

[a] Department of Radiology, NYU Langone Health, 222 East 41st Street, 5th Floor Radiology, New York, NY 10017, USA; [b] Hansjörg Wyss Department of Plastic Surgery, NYU Langone Health, 222 East 41st Street, 6th Floor, New York, NY 10017, USA
* Corresponding author.
E-mail address: Gopi.Nayak@nyulangone.org

neuroimaging.theclinics.com

is used to correct deformities of the midface, whereas the BSSO and osseous genioplasty involve the lower face and chin, respectively.

At our institution, a noncontrast craniofacial CT [Box 1] is often performed preoperatively, particularly for patients with complex syndromic conditions such as Treacher Collins, Crouzon, or Apert syndrome. CT imaging is also frequently performed in the immediate postoperative period to assess overall osseous alignment and hardware positioning, or performed in the delayed setting if there is a concern infection, nonunion, or hardware fracture.

Le Fort type I osteotomy

The Le Fort type I osteotomy allows the manipulation of the position of the upper lip and nose without affecting the orbit and zygomatic region. The surgeon may use Le Fort type II or III procedure to alter the nasomaxillary region, or the orbits and zygoma, respectively.[1] A typical Le Fort type I osteotomy is a horizontally oriented maxillary osteotomy, approximately 5 mm above the tooth root apices, involving the inferior aspect of the nasal septum, the lateral nasal walls, and the anterior and posterolateral maxillary sinus walls to the junction of the pterygoid plates and maxillary tuberosity.[1,2] As opposed to the classic Le Fort fracture patterns, the Le Fort type osteotomies typically do not include the pterygoid plates, though unintentional fractures through the pterygoid plates do occur and may be encountered on postoperative imaging.[3,4] Positioning of the anterior nasal spine affects the nasolabial angle and may or may not be included in the osteotomized segment.[1] The maxilla can be advanced, vertically distracted, or segmented and laterally distracted to correct maxillary hypoplasia. Similarly, impaction or bone removal can be used to decrease dental protrusion and correct vertical maxillary excess or a long inferior face; rotation

or asymmetric positioning can be used to correct a slanted bite or asymmetric face.[5,6] (**Figs. 1–4**). During surgery, impacted third molar teeth may be removed, or large inferior turbinates may require reduction.[1]

At our institution, imaging is often performed in the immediate postoperative period (usually postoperative day 1). Prominent, extensive soft tissue edema and infiltration, and high-density fluid levels in the sinuses are expected findings. However, larger hematomas or hemorrhages can occur and may be venous or arterial, involving the pterygoid plexus, the internal maxillary artery, or palatine branches arising from the facial, ascending pharyngeal, or maxillary arteries.[1,7,8] Arteriovenous fistulas and pseudoaneurysm related to orthognathic surgery have been described and may not be obvious at the time of the surgery due to the deep location of the vessels, or may occur in the delayed postoperative setting[8] (**Fig. 5**). Recurrent epistaxis should raise suspicion for a vascular injury and CT or conventional angiography should be considered with attention to appropriate regional vessels.

Asymmetric osteotomies, step-off, or gaps between bone segments are frequently intentional and should be noted, but not reported as abnormal findings. Reference to the surgeon's operative note or direct communication with the surgical team is extremely helpful and is highly recommended to avoid language in the imaging report which may be incorrect, misleading, or results in unnecessary patient concern or confusion. Knowledge of expected osteotomy patterns is helpful to avoid mislabeling osteotomies as fractures. Mild comminution at the level of the osteotomies, particularly involving the thinner maxillary sinus walls or nasal septum, is also frequently encountered. However, both unplanned fractures and fracture fragment displacement do occur and should be described, particularly if extending to the skull base, vascular canals, or orbit, as this may require a return to the operating room (**Fig. 6**). Separation of the pterygomaxillary junction is technically challenging and may result in uncontrolled fractures through the maxillary tuberosity or pterygoid plates, which may contribute to operative complications.[3]

Other described complications that may present in the later postoperative period include oronasal fistulas following palatal expansion with sagittal segmental maxillary osteotomies, or alveolar/periodontal bone loss or dental devitalization due to vascular compromise.[9,10]

Box 1
Craniofacial CT

- Helical scan from vertex to below mandible, include entire face and calvarium in anteroposterior dimension

- Slice thickness 0.75 mm. Axial, coronal, sagittal reconstruction in soft tissue and bone windows

- Voltage ~120kVp, Reference mAs ~300

- 3D volumetric images created on a separate workstation and sent to PACS

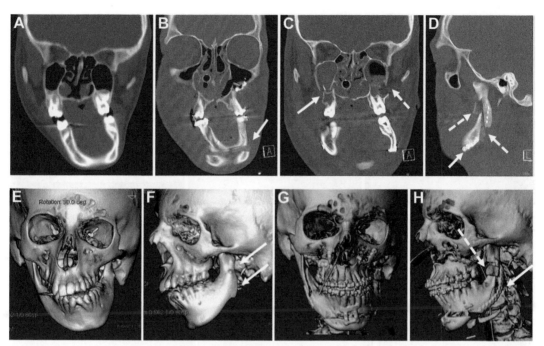

Fig. 1. Pre- and postoperative CT images in a patient who underwent Le Fort Type I osteotomy, BSSO, and advancement genioplasty for congenital left hemifacial microsomia. Preoperative coronal image (*A*) demonstrates hypoplasia of the left maxilla and mandible resulting in facial asymmetry and malocclusion. Postoperative coronal image of the anterior face (*B*) demonstrates asymmetric distraction of the left aspect of genioplasty osteotomy with the placement of bone graft material (*solid arrow*). Postoperative coronal CT image more posteriorly (*C*) demonstrates Le Fort type I osteotomies through the inferior maxillary sinus, lateral nasal cavity walls, and nasal septum with intentional asymmetric mild impaction on the right (*solid arrow*) and distraction of osteotomies on the left (*dashed arrow*). Postoperative sagittal CT image (*D*) demonstrates the reconstruction of the foreshortened, dysplastic left mandibular ramus and condyle using a curved plate and screw construct (*solid arrow*) and bone graft material (*dashed arrow*). Preoperative volume-rendered images (*E, F*) demonstrate hypoplasia of the left maxilla and mandible with a foreshortened, dysplastic left mandibular ramus and condyle (*solid arrow in F*), resulting in facial asymmetry and malocclusion. Postoperative volume-rendered images (*G, H*) demonstrate improved facial symmetry and occlusion. Note the mandibular reconstruction using a curved plate and screw construct (*solid arrow* in *H*) and bone graft material (*dashed arrow* in *H*).

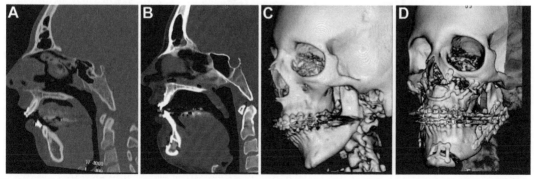

Fig. 2. Pre- and postoperative CT imaging in a patient who underwent Le Fort type I osteotomy, osseous genioplasty, and BSSO for left hemifacial macrosomia. Preoperative sagittal (*A*) and volume-rendered (*C*) images demonstrate mandibular retrognathia with a small chin. Postoperative sagittal (*B*) and volume-rendered (*D*) images demonstrate improved mandibular positioning, facial symmetry, and occlusion.

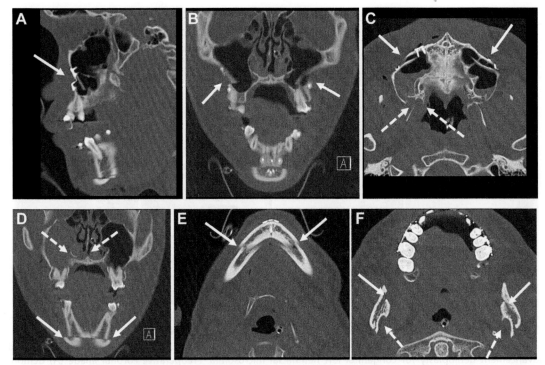

Fig. 3. Postoperative CT following Le Fort Type I osteotomy, osseous genioplasty, and bilateral sagittal split osteotomies for Class III malocclusion ("underbite"). Sagittal (*A*), coronal (*B*), and axial (*C*) images demonstrate maxillary advancement with an expected step off at the Le Fort osteotomy site and fixation with malleable "L" plates (*solid arrows*). Fractures through the right pterygoid plates are frequently encountered on imaging (*dashed arrows* in *C*). Coronal (*D*) and axial (*E*) images demonstrate the expected step off at the genioplasty site (*solid arrows*). Osteotomies through the lateral nasal walls and nasal septum are also noted (*dashed arrows* in *D*). Axial image through the mandible (*F*) demonstrates bilateral sagittal split osteotomies (*solid arrows*) coursing lateral to the mandibular foramen (*dashed arrows*).

Bilateral sagittal split osteotomy

The BSSO originally described by Obwegeser in 1955 is used to correct mandibular retrognathism or prognathism by advancement or setback, respectively, of the mobilized mandibular arch. The procedure involves horizontal osteotomies through the medial half of the mandibular rami, and sagittally oriented osteotomies through the ramus and posterior mandibular body, anteriorly exiting the buccal cortex and posteriorly involving

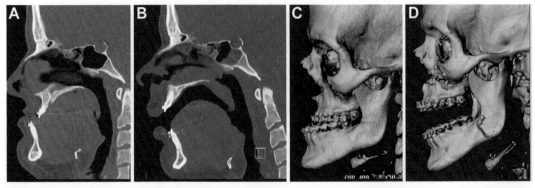

Fig. 4. Pre- and postoperative CT images of a Le Fort type I osteotomy and BSSO for class III malocclusion in a patient with mandibular prognathism. Preoperative sagittal (*A*) and volume-rendered (*C*) images demonstrate anterior positioning of the mandible relative to the maxilla. Postoperative sagittal (*B*) and volume-rendered (*D*) images demonstrate markedly improved maxillary-mandibular alignment.

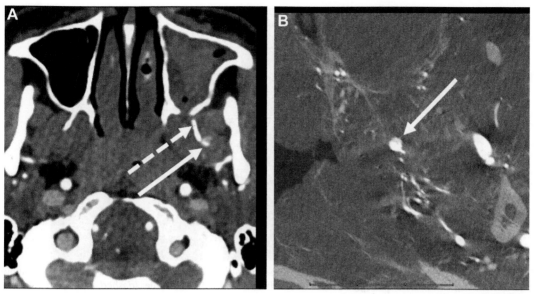

Fig. 5. Postoperative pseudoaneurysm. Axial CT angiogram image (*A*) and cone-beam CT image during catheter angiogram (*B*) demonstrate a pseudoaneurysm (*solid arrows*) secondary to the unanticipated fracture of the left lateral pterygoid plate (*dashed arrow*).

the lingual cortex, separating the tooth-bearing portion of the mandible from the bilateral lateral ramus segments. The horizontal osteotomy is performed superior and posterior to the mandibular foramen. The sagittal osteotomy should be lateral to the course of the inferior alveolar nerve to avoid injury (see **Figs. 1–4; Fig. 7**).

Unanticipated fractures during a BSSO may involve the condylar neck, the buccal plate, or lingual plate. The inferior alveolar nerve is at high risk during a BSSO, and violation of the mandibular foramen or nerve canal by the osteotomy, fixation hardware, or unintentional fractures may occur and should be communicated to the surgeon

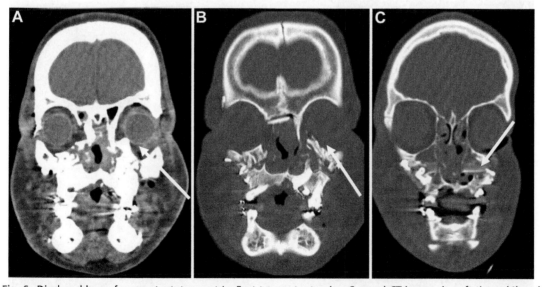

Fig. 6. Displaced bone fragments status post Le Fort type osteotomies. Coronal CT images in soft tissue (*A*) and bone (*B*) windows demonstrate a displaced fracture fragment abutting the left globe. Coronal CT image in a different patient (*C*) status post Le Fort type 1 osteotomy demonstrates planned mild leftward shift and distraction of the left maxillary segment; note however the bone graft material extending into the left nasal cavity (*arrow*), which required removal and graft repositioning.

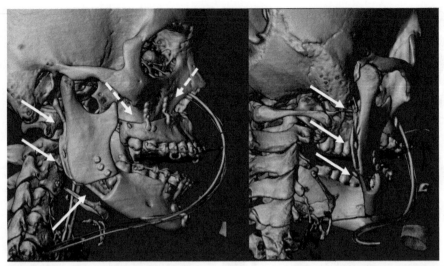

Fig. 7. BSSO. Volume-rendered images demonstrate the sagittal osteotomy (*solid arrows*) of the mandible, allowing repositioning of the mandibular arch, seen here with Le Fort type I osteotomies (*dashed arrows*) for improved dental occlusion.

(Fig. 8). Arteries at risk during the procedure include the inferior alveolar artery, facial, lingual, and internal maxillary arteries.[10]

Condylar resorption has been described by several authors following orthognathic surgery including the BSSO and Le Fort type I osteotomy and is a risk factor for relapse of maloccusion.[11]

Condylar resorption can occur from 6 months postoperatively to well beyond the first postoperative year.[12] Findings on CT include unilateral, bilateral, or asymmetric flattening and erosion of the condyle in anteroposterior, transverse, or craniocaudal dimensions.[13]

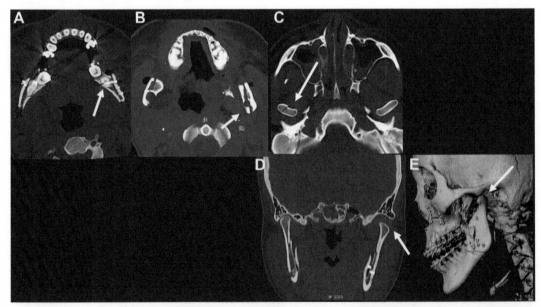

Fig. 8. Unintentional outcomes. (A) Unfavorable screw placement through the left mandibular molar tooth. (B) Unintentional osteotomy extension through left inferior alveolar nerve canal. (C) Unfavorable fracture through right mandibular condyle. Coronal (D) and volume-rendered (E) CT images demonstrate anterior subluxation of the left mandibular condyle.

Osseous genioplasty

The osseous genioplasty involves a horizontal osteotomy through the anterior inferior mandibular body 5 to 6 mm below the tooth root apices and mental foramen. The separated segment can be advanced or distracted to correct a small chin in the anteroposterior or craniocaudal dimensions, set back for an overly prominent chin, or tilted in the horizontal plane to correct an asymmetry. Parallel osteotomies may be used for a stepwise advancement, or to remove bone to decrease vertical height of the chin.[14]

As described above, the mobilized osseous segments during orthognathic surgery can be variably set, rotated, or further segmented depending on the unique anatomy of the patient; therefore, the radiologist should be aware that gaps, asymmetry, or step-offs can all be expected postoperative findings and should not be referred to as malalignment. Similarly, depending on surgeon preference, bone graft, resorbable, or titanium plates, in variable bent or prefabricated shapes and configurations, may be used (see Figs. 1–3).

For any of the above procedures, additional pertinent postoperative imaging findings may include temporomandibular joint dislocation, particularly in the immediate setting, evidence of soft tissue infection, osseous nonunion, hardware loosening, infection, or fracture. Careful evaluation should also be conducted for areas of bone loss or erosion as this may reflect underlying osteomyelitis or avascular necrosis, and may result in delayed complications including relapse of the corrected facial deformity.

Facial feminization surgery

Gender-affirming surgery in the transgender population is being increasingly used in the United States.[15] At our institution, the transgender health program performs upwards of 550 gender-affirming surgeries per year, mirroring trends in the overall US population.[15,16] Facial reconstruction procedures are an important component of treatment options available for gender dysphoria and have been shown to improve psychosocial metrics in the transgender population.[17,18] Procedures for the male to female transition more commonly involve osseous reconstruction or remodeling, and therefore are more likely to use pre- and postoperative imaging than procedures for the female to male transition, which rely more heavily on soft tissue-based remodeling with injectable fillers and lipotransfer.

Facial feminization surgery (FFS), more inclusively referred to as facial gender confirmation surgery, includes a conglomerate of procedures aimed to address the phenotypically male characteristics of the craniofacial skeleton and soft tissues. Head and neck radiologists should be familiar with the types of procedures performed and pre- and postoperative considerations that may be relevant for the referring surgeon.

Imaging considerations and protocol

Care and considerations should be taken before, during, and after imaging to ensure a positive health care experience and to avoid transgender discrimination.[19] Front desk staff, technologists, nurses, and radiologists should be educated regarding the needs and experiences of the transgender population. All staff should seek out and use the preferred pronoun of the patient, which at our institution is indicated in the patient's electronic medical record. Similarly, the imaging facility must be appropriately equipped with gender-neutral bathrooms and changing areas to promote an inclusive environment.

A preoperative craniofacial CT is performed on all potential candidates for facial feminization procedures. The study is used to identify key features which may impact the type of procedures best suited for the individual needs and anatomy of the patient. Additionally, the craniofacial CT can be used with image-guided surgical navigation software for the construction of individualized surgical cutting guides, hardware, or implants, or used in a more qualitative fashion depending on the preference of the individual surgeon. The radiologist can highlight salient anatomic features which may be relevant to presurgical planning, and identify pathology which may need to be addressed before surgery, or may pose additional challenges during surgery. 3D volumetric images are also helpful for patients to visualize their own bony anatomy and understand planned surgical procedures.[20]

Surgical procedures and relevant imaging findings

The most common areas addressed in FFS include the frontal and periorbital region, the nose, chin, and jawline, as these areas have been shown to play an important role in gender discrimination.[21]

Upper face

The forehead and supraorbital region contribute strongly to gender identity.[22] A prominent supraorbital rim with frontal bossing and a more narrow nasofrontal angle have been shown to confer masculinity, whereas a smooth, gently curved forehead contour with a relatively wider nasofrontal angle is associated with female gender[22-26] (Fig. 9).

As described by Ousterhout, in addition to the degree of anterior supraorbital bone projection, the extent of frontal sinus pneumatization and the thickness of the outer table of the frontal sinus can dictate which operative procedure may be best suited for the patient.[25] Patients with extensive frontal sinus pneumatization and thin outer tables may require anterior wall osteotomies and setbacks with plate fixation to reduce the degree of frontal bossing. Underpneumatized frontal sinuses or thick anterior tables may be addressed with osseous burring and recontouring alone (Fig. 10). During forehead recontouring, the supraorbital neurovascular bundle may be freed from its foramen or notch,[20,25] and therefore, the location of the supraorbital foramen or any variations or asymmetry in positioning is relevant to avoid unanticipated injury. The degree of frontal sinus pneumatization, thickness of the outer table, and position of the supraorbital notch or foramen may be qualitatively described as at our institution, or measured and reported by the radiologist as described by Callen and colleagues.[27] Additionally, the presence of sinus disease, particularly involving the frontal sinuses should be mentioned, as this may need to be addressed preoperatively.

Nose

Rhinoplasty is a central component of FFS and involves unique considerations for the transgender population.[28,29] Surgical alterations may include an overall reduction in the size of the nose, dorsal hump reduction, nasal deprojection, and narrowing of the nose.[28-30] The radiologist plays an important role in identifying features that may be relevant to surgical planning or patient outcomes. These include traumatic fractures, prior rhinoplasty, or septal defects which may indicate prior septoplasty, cocaine use, or an underlying systemic condition, which sometimes may not be revealed during the patient history and may be unknown to the performing surgeon.[28] (Fig. 11).

Lower face

The lower face, predominantly the chin and jawline, demonstrates several anthropomorphic differences between men and women. The male jaw often demonstrates a more "square" appearance due to the overall larger size with greater soft tissue covering, a more acute, pronounced mandibular angle, as well as flaring of the lower mandible in the transverse plane.[31,32] In contrast, the female jaw demonstrates a narrower width with a broad mandibular angle and smaller, more softly contoured chin. The lower face may be addressed in FFS with mandibular angle osteotomies or contouring, with a reduction in overlying masseter and soft tissue bulk. CT provides information about the degree of osseous mandibular flare versus contributions from the masseter muscle and overlying soft tissues[33] (Fig. 12). The chin is also frequently addressed with an osseous genioplasty or bony contouring to narrow and soften the chin depending on the unique anatomy of the patient and relative proportions of the overall face.

Some surgical techniques use an intraoral approach and therefore odontogenic disease may need to be addressed preoperatively to

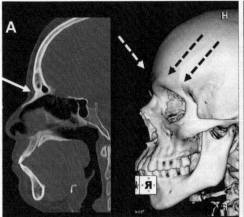
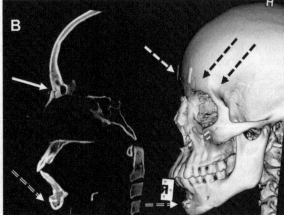

Fig. 9. Pre- and postoperative CT imaging for facial feminization. Preoperative sagittal and 3D volume-rendered images (*A*) demonstrate a relatively narrow nasofrontal angle (*solid white arrow*), frontal bossing (*dashed white arrow*), and supraorbital ridging (*dashed black arrows*). Postoperative sagittal and 3D volume-rendered images (*B*) status post frontal bone osteotomy with posterior setback and rhinoplasty demonstrate interval widening of the nasofrontal angle (*white arrow*), decreased frontal bossing (*white dashed arrow*), and decreased supraorbital ridging (*black dashed arrows*). Osseous genioplasty was also performed (*dashed double arrow*).

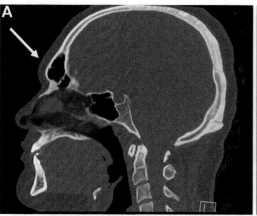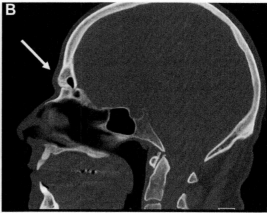

Fig. 10. Frontal sinus pneumatization. (*A*) Well-pneumatized frontal sinus with a thin outer table. (*B*) Underpneumatized frontal sinus with a thick outer table. Both images demonstrate frontal bossing and a relatively narrow nasofrontal angle.

reduce the risk of infection (**Fig. 13**). Impacted or unerupted molar teeth, odontogenic or other lesions of the mandible may be relevant to the surgical approach or technique. The inferior alveolar and mental nerves are in or near the operative site during mandibuloplasty. Mention of any variations or asymmetry in the position of the inferior alveolar nerve canal or mandibular and mental foramens may be useful for the performing surgeon and could impact the choice of procedure.[32]

It is known that transgender patients experience extremely high rates of discrimination, abuse, and violence.[34] Identification of prior facial trauma is of particular relevance to the plastic surgeon and may be encountered more frequently than in the general patient population. Evidence of prior subcutaneous injections, implants, or osseous reconstruction may be encountered and should be mentioned as they can produce scarring and fibrosis, and impact the health of the skin and subcutaneous soft tissues (**Figs. 14** and **15**). Prior trauma, injections, or surgery may present an additional challenge to the surgeon and impact healing, patient outcomes, and satisfaction. Preoperative identification of such pitfalls enables the surgeon to appropriately prepare, as well as preemptively manage patient expectations.

Face transplantation

Patients who suffer severe facial disfigurement now have the possibility of restoration of form and function with full facial allograft transplantation (**Fig. 16**). Full face transplant allograft includes soft tissue structures of the mid to lower face, eyelids, and variable portions of the forehead and scalp, as well as attached vascularized bone segments, sometimes including the components of the palate, jaw, teeth, and tongue, with successful graft healing in part dependent on the viability of the vascular anastomosis. Imaging plays a central role in preoperative planning, particularly for successful allograft harvesting and transplantation.

Interdisciplinary preparation for the transplant recipient and donor imaging is of paramount importance for operative planning. At our institution, multidisciplinary meetings are held with the transplant team, designated radiology faculty, and radiology administration well ahead of time to optimize recipient and donor arrival and imaging protocols, and to discuss relevant questions to be addressed by imaging. When potential recipient

Fig. 11. Rhinoplasty. Axial CT images demonstrate bilateral osteotomies through the frontal process of the maxilla (*arrows*) compatible with prior rhinoplasty. These findings may be difficult to differentiate from prior fractures.

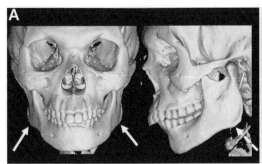
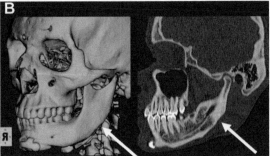

Fig. 12. Pre- and postoperative imaging for facial feminization. Preoperative volume-rendered images (*A*) demonstrate the characteristic appearance of a male jaw with lateral mandibular flare (*solid arrows*) and a "square" mandibular angle (*dashed arrow*). Postoperative volume-rendered and curved sagittal reformat CT images (*B*) in a different patient status post mandibuloplasty demonstrate a broadened mandibular angle (*arrows*). The patient also underwent masseter reduction for soft tissue contouring of jawline (not shown).

and donor patients are identified, the operative team can further refine patient-specific surgical planning and relevant imaging questions. Additionally, radiology technologists or information technology specialists must be prepared in advance to ensure prompt external imaging data transfer to the specified medical modeling company following scan acquisition as the time between donor identification and initiation of transplant surgery may be as short as 36 hours.

At our institution, preoperative imaging for both the donor and recipient consists of a high-resolution craniofacial CT, arterial and venous phase CT angiogram of the head and neck, and

6-vessel digital subtraction angiography (DSA), the protocols of which have been previously described.[35] Imaging for the recipient is often performed during the initial patient evaluation and may need to be repeated at the time of donor identification to ensure imaging information is current. Designated members of the radiology team should be notified and donor imaging should occur in house, as soon as an immunologically compatible donor is identified and arrives at the performing institution.

Craniofacial computed tomography

The craniofacial CT provides high resolution, detailed information about the patient's anatomy. Recipient patients may have extensive posttraumatic craniofacial bone loss and deformity and may also have undergone multiple prior reconstructive surgeries. During the initial workup of the potential recipient, the radiologist should describe the type and extent of bony defects, prior surgeries, and hardware (see **Fig. 16**). Even in recipient patients without significant osseous trauma and deformity, detailed imaging of osseous anatomy is necessary as full facial transplantation often includes vascularized bone segments to maintain the bony attachment sites of facial musculature, thereby optimizing soft tissue function.[36,37] Computerized surgical planning using craniofacial CT data is used to superimpose recipient and donor anatomy, allowing the surgeon to efficiently address the unique anatomic requirements of the recipient and donor, and thereby decrease operative time.[38]

The craniofacial CT data are concurrently sent to a medical modeling company for the creation of prefabricated, patient-specific operative cutting guides and reconstructive hardware. Various medical modeling companies are available for the production of cutting guides and hardware.

Fig. 13. Odontogenic disease. Curved sagittal CT reformat demonstrates mandibular odontogenic disease and osteitis, which may need to be addressed preoperatively and may impact the surgical approach.

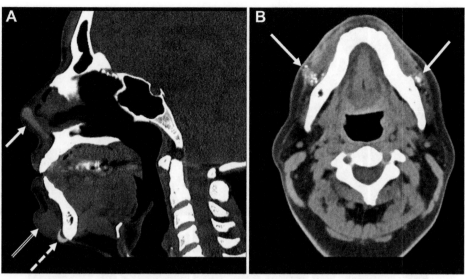

Fig. 14. Evidence of prior plastic surgery. Preoperative sagittal CT image (*A*) demonstrates nose (*solid arrow*) and chin (*dashed arrow*) implants with overlying fillers (*double arrow*). Axial CT (*B*) image demonstrates calcified injection granulomas in the premandibular soft tissues (*solid arrows*).

Company-specific imaging instructions such as scan parameters and reconstruction kernel algorithm guidelines should be sought well ahead of time and strictly adhered to avoid unnecessary delays.

Computed tomography angiogram and digital subtraction angiogram

Viability of the vascular anastomosis is of utmost importance to the success of transplant surgery and preoperative angiographic imaging plays an important role in determining adequate target donor and recipient vessels for anastomosis. Radiologists should be familiar with the transplant operation to provide appropriate and relevant vascular anatomic information to the surgical team. A CT angiogram and venogram and conventional DSA together provide a comprehensive road map of major arteries and veins and their functional status.

Patient-specific variability in normal anatomy combined with often extensive alterations or damage to native vasculature by prior injury and subsequent surgical procedures adds to the surgical complexity and case-by-case variability of each face transplant surgery. Therefore, detailed preoperative planning and evaluation are imperative to the success of the procedure. The CT angiogram allows the visualization of major vascular structures in relation to adjacent bony and soft tissue

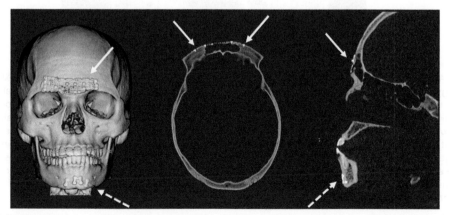

Fig. 15. Evidence of prior plastic surgery. Preoperative CT images demonstrate the evidence of prior facial feminization surgery including frontal osteotomy with mesh plate fixation (*solid arrows*) and prior osseous genioplasty (*dashed arrows*). The patient desired further contouring of the frontal bone, chin, and jawline.

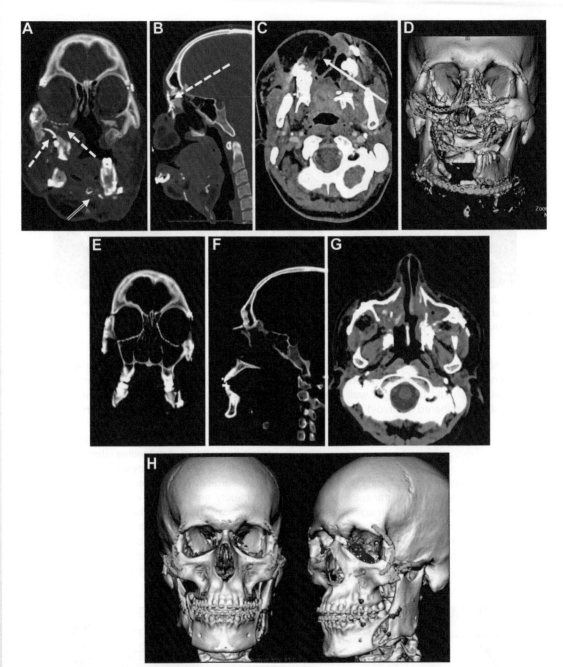

Figs. 16. (*A–D*): Pretransplant craniofacial CT with contrast of a face transplant recipient who had experienced high-energy ballistic injury to the face. Coronal (*A*) and sagittal (*B*) images in the bone window, axial image in soft tissue window (*C*), and volume-rendered image (*D*) demonstrate extensive soft tissue and osseous defects and evidence of multiple prior reconstructive surgeries with soft tissue flaps (*solid arrows*), retained ballistic fragments (*double arrow*), and surgical hardware (*dashed arrows*), with hardware highlighted in green in image D. (*E–H*): Posttransplant craniofacial CT of the same patient. Coronal (*E*) and sagittal (*F*) images in bone window, and axial images in soft tissue window (*G*) nearly 5 months postoperatively demonstrate restoration of osseous and soft tissue anatomy with marked functional improvement for the transplant recipient. Volume-rendered images (*H*) demonstrate dramatic restoration of normal osseous anatomy. Note as well the restoration of maxillary-mandibular occlusion.

landmarks, whereas DSA provides dynamic flow-related information including directionality of flow, collateral pathways of flow, and potential areas of arteriovenous shunting. The integration of these findings informs the surgeons' decisions for choosing sites of vascular anastomoses.

Prior transplants have been performed using unilateral or bilateral external carotid artery (ECA) or branch donor vessels, particularly the facial artery. Though controversial,[39] bilateral ECA anastomoses may be preferred if feasible.[37] Vessel caliber, course, and function all play a role in decisions regarding which parent and donor artery to be used for anastomosis. Important findings to be noted by the radiologist were previously described,[35] however, are resummarized here.

- The location of the donor and recipient carotid bifurcations with respect to the cervical spine and mandibular angle
- The caliber of donor and recipient ECA to determine the feasibility of end to end versus side to side anastomosis
- The branching pattern of the ECA including the distance between each vessel origin, and the proximal caliber of the branches, particularly the facial artery (Fig. 17)

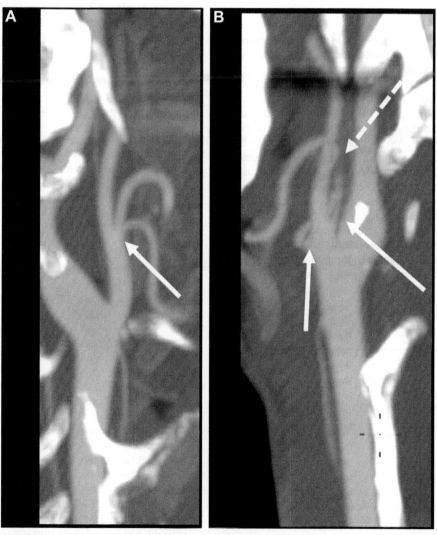

Fig. 17. ECA variations on pretransplant CT angiogram MIP images of a face transplant recipient. (*A*) The right external carotid artery demonstrates a 1 cm trunk proximal to the common origins of the facial and lingual branches (*arrow*). A variant origin of the occipital artery was noted approximately 4 cm beyond the carotid bifurcation (not shown). (*B*) The left external carotid artery demonstrates the origins of the lingual and occipital arteries (*arrows*) immediately beyond the carotid bifurcation with no significant ECA trunk. The left facial artery origin is approximately 1 cm above the bifurcation (*dashed arrow*).

- Any acquired or congenital variations in vascular anatomy, particularly variations which may predispose to complications (ie, prominent collateral networks from the native (recipient) ECA to internal carotid or vertebral artery territories which may become compromised following anastomosis to the donor ECA)
- Any vasculopathy such as atherosclerotic disease, dissection, luminal stenosis, or other alterations in flow dynamics.
- Venous phase imaging should describe the corresponding venous system including the facial vein and internal jugular veins

SUMMARY

Imaging plays an essential role in pre- and postoperative imaging in plastic and reconstructive surgeries including orthognathic surgery, facial feminization procedures for gender dysphoria, and face transplantation. Reporting of anatomic variations, prior facial trauma, surgery, and unexpected pathology provides important information to the surgeon for preoperative planning. In the postoperative setting, imaging allows the assessment of surgical positioning, bone healing and fusion, and early or delayed surgical complications. Ultimately, open communication between the radiology and surgical teams is necessary to distinguish expected and unintended postsurgical findings, optimize information included in reports, as well as establish appropriate protocols and workflow that ensure a positive, safe and efficient imaging experience for the patient.

CLINICS CARE POINTS

- Open communication between radiologists and surgical teams is of utmost importance for successful interpretation of perioperative imaging.

DISCLOSURE

No conflicts of interest to disclose.

REFERENCES

1. Patel PK, Novia MV. The surgical tools: the LeFort I, bilateral sagittal split osteotomy of the mandible, and the osseous genioplasty. Clin Plast Surg 2007; 34(3):447–75.
2. Buchanan EP, Hyman CH. LeFort I Osteotomy. Semin Plast Surg 2013;27(3):149–54.
3. Renick BM, Symington JM. Postoperative computed tomography study of pterygomaxillary separation during the Le Fort I osteotomy. J Oral Maxillofac Surg 1991;49(10):1061–5 [discussion: 1065–6].
4. Robinson PP, Hendy CW. Pterygoid plate fractures caused by the Le Fort I osteotomy. Br J Oral Maxillofac Surg 1986;24(3):198–202.
5. Obwegeser JA. Maxillary and midface deformities: characteristics and treatment strategies. Clin Plast Surg 2007;34(3):519–33.
6. Lim L, Heggie AA. Versatile facial osteotomies. Aust Dent J 2018;63(Suppl 1):S48–57.
7. Epker BN. Vascular considerations in orthognathic surgery. II. Maxillary osteotomies. Oral Surg Oral Med Oral Pathol 1984;57(5):473–8.
8. Lanigan DT, Hey JH, West RA. Major vascular complications of orthognathic surgery: false aneurysms and arteriovenous fistulas following orthognathic surgery. J Oral Maxillofac Surg 1991; 49(6):571–7.
9. Lanigan DT, Hey JH, West RA. Aseptic necrosis following maxillary osteotomies: report of 36 cases. J Oral Maxillofac Surg 1990;48(2):142–56.
10. Morris DE, Lo LJ, Margulis A. Pitfalls in orthognathic surgery: avoidance and management of complications. Clin Plast Surg 2007;34(3):e17–29.
11. Catherine Z, Breton P, Bouletreau P. Condylar resorption after orthognathic surgery: A systematic review. Rev Stomatol Chir Maxillofac Chir Orale 2016;117(1):3–10.
12. Hoppenreijs TJ, Freihofer HP, Stoelinga PJ, et al. Condylar remodelling and resorption after Le Fort I and bimaxillary osteotomies in patients with anterior open bite. A clinical and radiological study. Int J Oral Maxillofac Surg 1998;27(2):81–91.
13. He Y, Lin H, Lin Q, et al. Morphologic changes in idiopathic condylar resorption with different degrees of bone loss. Oral Surg Oral Med Oral Pathol Oral Radiol 2019;128(3):332–40.
14. Ward JL, Garri JI, Wolfe SA. The osseous genioplasty. Clin Plast Surg 2007;34(3):485–500.
15. Canner JK, Harfouch O, Kodadek LM, et al. Temporal Trends in Gender-Affirming Surgery Among Transgender Patients in the United States. JAMA Surg 2018;153(7):609–16.
16. Winter S, Diamond M, Green J, et al. Transgender people: health at the margins of society. Lancet 2016;388(10042):390–400.
17. Ainsworth TA, Spiegel JH. Quality of life of individuals with and without facial feminization surgery or gender reassignment surgery. Qual Life Res 2010; 19(7):1019–24.
18. Branstrom R, Pachankis JE. Reduction in Mental Health Treatment Utilization Among Transgender Individuals After Gender-Affirming Surgeries: A Total

Population Study. Am J Psychiatry 2020;177(8): 727–34.

19. Abeln B, Love R. Considerations for the Care of Transgender Individuals. Nurs Clin North Am 2019; 54(4):551–9.

20. Eisemann BS, Wilson SC, Ramly EP, et al. Technical Pearls in Frontal and Periorbital Bone Contouring in Gender-Affirmation Surgery. Plast Reconstr Surg 2020;146(3):326e–9e.

21. Brown E, Perrett DI. What gives a face its gender? Perception 1993;22(7):829–40.

22. Spiegel JH. Facial determinants of female gender and feminizing forehead cranioplasty. Laryngoscope 2011;121(2):250–61.

23. Hage JJ, Becking AG, de Graaf FH, et al. Gender-confirming facial surgery: considerations on the masculinity and femininity of faces. Plast Reconstr Surg 1997;99(7):1799–807.

24. Habal MB. Aesthetics of feminizing the male face by craniofacial contouring of the facial bones. Aesthet Plast Surg 1990;14(2):143–50.

25. Ousterhout DK. Feminization of the forehead: contour changing to improve female aesthetics. Plast Reconstr Surg 1987;79(5):701–13.

26. Farkas LG. Anthropometry of the head and face. 2nd edition. New York: Raven Press; 1994.

27. Callen AL, Badiee RK, Phelps A, et al. Facial Feminization Surgery: Key CT Findings for Preoperative Planning and Postoperative Evaluation. AJR Am J Roentgenol 2020. https://doi.org/10.2214/AJR.20.25528.

28. Spiegel JH. Considerations in Feminization Rhinoplasty. Facial Plast Surg 2020;36(1):53–6.

29. Berli JU, Loyo M. Gender-confirming Rhinoplasty. Facial Plast Surg Clin North Am 2019;27(2):251–60.

30. Bellinga RJ, Capitan L, Simon D, et al. Technical and Clinical Considerations for Facial Feminization Surgery With Rhinoplasty and Related Procedures. JAMA Facial Plast Surg 2017;19(3):175–81.

31. Morrison SD, Satterwhite T. Lower Jaw Recontouring in Facial Gender-Affirming Surgery. Facial Plast Surg Clin North Am 2019;27(2):233–42.

32. Mommaerts MY, Voisin C, Joshi Otero J, et al. Mandibular feminization osteotomy-preliminary results. Int J Oral Maxillofac Surg 2019;48(5):597–600.

33. Morris DE, Zhao L. Facial Gender Affirmation Surgery: Craniomaxillofacial Imaging. J Craniofac Surg 2019;30(5):1403–5.

34. Grant JML, Tanis J, Harrison J, et al. Injustice at every turn: a report of the national transgender discrimination survey. Washington, DC: National Centre for Transgender Equality and National Gay and Lesbian Task Force; 2011. p. 3.

35. Prabhu V, Plana NM, Hagiwara M, et al. Preoperative Imaging for Facial Transplant: A Guide for Radiologists. Radiographics 2019;39(4):1098–107.

36. Sosin M, Ceradini DJ, Levine JP, et al. Total Face, Eyelids, Ears, Scalp, and Skeletal Subunit Transplant: A Reconstructive Solution for the Full Face and Total Scalp Burn. Plast Reconstr Surg 2016; 138(1):205–19.

37. Rifkin WJ, David JA, Plana NM, et al. Achievements and Challenges in Facial Transplantation. Ann Surg 2018;268(2):260–70.

38. Dorafshar AH, Brazio PS, Mundinger GS, et al. Found in space: computer-assisted orthognathic alignment of a total face allograft in six degrees of freedom. J Oral Maxillofac Surg 2014;72(9): 1788–800.

39. Soga S, Pomahac B, Wake N, et al. CT angiography for surgical planning in face transplantation candidates. AJNR Am J Neuroradiol 2013;34(10): 1873–81.

Printed and bound by CPI Group (UK) Ltd, Croydon, CR0 4YY

03/10/2024

01040371-0006